Urological Cancer Management

Said Abdallah Al-Mamari
Salim Said Al-Busaidy
Editors

Urological Cancer Management

Springer

Editors
Said Abdallah Al-Mamari
Urology Department
The Royal Hospital
Muscat
Oman

Salim Said Al-Busaidy
Urology Department
The Royal Hospital
Muscat
Oman

ISBN 978-3-319-16300-0 ISBN 978-3-319-16301-7 (eBook)
DOI 10.1007/978-3-319-16301-7

Library of Congress Control Number: 2015938574

Springer Cham Heidelberg New York Dordrecht London

Printed on acid-free paper

Springer International Publishing AG Switzerland is part of Springer Science+Business Media
(www.springer.com)

Preface

This book endeavours to provide the reader with a brief and succinct text on common urological malignancies as opposed to comprehensive textbooks which are readily available describing all aspects of urology.

A handbook often implies a short text written for medical students, interns and paramedical trainees. We believe the information contained aptly matches the needs of urological residents as well and its depth may surprisingly challenge many consultants.

The chapters are written as informative guides on management with precise details on risk factors, clinical and investigative assessment, staging and treatment consistently supported by references. Emphasis has been placed on new concepts and advances reported in recent literature.

As a prominent feature of the book, we have included "Take home messages" summarizing the essential facts in all the chapters. These complement the principal aim of assisting the reader to assimilate the salient points through easy learning and memorizing.

A section on clinical scenarios has been added which in the editors' opinion is an excellent way to further stimulate and cement the learning process.

Abundant illustrations have been included which is rare for a book of this size.

It is my pleasure to acknowledge Dr. Said Al-Mamari for his initiative and inspiration in the writing of this practical book.

Muscat, Oman

Salim Said Al-Busaidy

Acknowledgement

1. The Editors and Authors are thankful to the following reviewers:
   - **Dr Pierre-Thierry PIECHAUD**, Chairman of Urological Courses in the IRCAD School, Strasbourg, Onco-Urologist, Laparoscopic and Robotic Surgeon in Saint-Augustin Clinic and Bergonié Oncological Institute, Bordeaux, France.
   - **Dr Jean-Luc HOEPFFNER**, Onco-Urologist, Laparoscopic and Robotic Surgeon in Saint-Augustin Clinic and Bergonié Oncological Institute, Bordeaux, France.
   - **Dr Hervé QUINTENS**, Onco-Urologist, Laparoscopic and Robotic Surgeon in Arnault Tzanck Institute, Saint-Laurent-du-Var, and University Hospital of Nice, Nice, France.
2. Our gratitude is also addressed to:
   - **Dr Sébastien NOVELLAS**, Radiologist, University Hospital of Nice, Nice, and Arnault-Tzanck Institute, Saint-Laurent-du-Var, France: for the relevant radiological images.
   - **Dr Anne DURLACH**, Pathologist, Pol Bouin Laboratory, University Hospital of Reims, France: for the beautiful pathological pictures.
   - **Dr Nicolas MOREL-JOURNEL**, Urologist, Penile Surgeon and Andrologist, University Hospital of Lyon, Lyon, France: for the nice pictures of penile cancer.
   - **Mrs Melissa MORTON**, Senior Editor, **Julia MEGGINSON**, Senior Editorial Assistant, and **Meena GOVINDAN**, Springer project manager, for their expert contribution in the final presentation and the publication of this book.

Contents

Contributors

Salim Said Al-Busaidy Urology Department, The Royal Hospital, Muscat, Oman

Qais Mohamed Al-Hooti Urology Department, The Royal Hospital, Muscat, Oman

Said Abdallah Al-Mamari Urology Department, The Royal Hospital, Muscat, Oman

Kurian George Urology Department, The Royal Hospital, Muscat, Oman

Santhosh Narayana Kurukkal Urology Department, The Royal Hospital, Muscat, Oman

Abbreviations

ACC Adrenocortical carcinoma
ADT Androgen deprivation therapy
AFP Alpha-fetoprotein
AJCC American Joint Committee on Cancer
AML Angiomyolipoma
AS Active surveillance
ASAP Atypical small acinar proliferation
BC Bladder cancer
BCG Bacillus Calmette-Guérin
BCR Biochemical relapse
BEP Bleomycin-etoposide-cisplatin
BHCG Beta-human chorionic gonadotrophin
BHD Birt-Hogg-Dubé syndrome
BMI Body mass index
BT Bladder tumour
BT Brachytherapy
CA Cryoablation
CAB Combined (or complete) androgen blockade
CC Choriocarcinoma
CCRCC Clear cell renal cell carcinoma
ChRCC Chromophobe renal cell carcinoma
CIS Carcinoma in situ
CN Cytoreductive nephrectomy
CRPC Castration resistant prostate cancer
cTNM Clinical TNM
DRE Digital rectal examination
EBRT External beam radiation therapy
EC Embryonal carcinoma
EDP Etoposide-doxorubicin-cisplatin
EGGCT Extragonadal germ cell tumour

EORTC	European Organization for Research and Treatment of Cancer
e-PLND	Extended pelvic lymph nodes dissection
EPO	Erythropoietin
F/T PSA	Free to total PSA ratio
G-C	Gemcitabine-cisplatin
G-CSF	Granulocyte colony-stimulating factor
GCT	Germ cell tumour
GS	Gleason score
HDIL-2	High-dose interleukin-2
HIF	Hypoxia-inducible factor
HIFU	High intensity focused ultrasound
HPR	Histopathological report
HPV	Human papilloma virus
HT	Hormonal therapy
i(12p)	Isochromosome of the short arm of chromosome 12
IIEF-5	International Index of Erectile Function (based on five items)
IL-2	Interleukin-2
ILND	Inguinal lymph nodes dissection
ITGCN	Intratubular germ cells neoplasia
LDH	Lactate dehydrogenase
LE	Life expectancy
LN	Lymph node(s)
LP	Laparoscopic radical prostatectomy
LPN	Laparoscopic partial nephrectomy
LRN	Laparoscopic radical nephrectomy
LUTS	Lower urinary tract infection
mCRPC	Metastatic castration resistant prostate cancer
MIBT	Muscle-invasive bladder tumour
MMC	Mitomycin C
MPC	Malignant phaeochromocytoma
mRCC	Metastatic renal cell carcinoma
MRI	Magnetic resonance imaging
MS	Metabolic syndrome
mTOR	Mammalian target of rapamycin (rapamycin = sirolimus)
MVAC	Methotrexate-vinblastine-Adriamycin-cisplatin (Adriamycin = doxorubicin)
NC	New cases
NEBT	Non-epithelial bladder tumour
NMIBT	Non-muscle-invasive bladder tumour
NSGCT	Non-seminomatous germ cell tumour
NSS	Nephron-sparing surgery
NVB	Neurovascular bundles
ONJ	Osteonecrosis of the jaw
OS	Overall survival
PC	Prostate cancer

PDGFR	Platelet-derived growth factor receptor
PFS	Progression-free survival
PIN	Prostatic intracytoplastic neoplasia
PLAP	Placental alkaline phosphatase
PLND	Pelvic lymph nodes dissection
PN	Partial nephrectomy
PNS	Paraneoplastic syndrome
PRCC	Papillary renal cell carcinoma
PSA	Prostate specific antigen
PSADT	PSA doubling time
PSM	Positive surgical margins
PTH-rP	Parathormone-related peptide
pTNM	Pathological TNM
QoL	Quality of life
RALP	Robotic assisted laparoscopic radical prostatectomy
RC	Radical cystectomy
RCC	Renal cell carcinoma
RFA	Radiofrequency ablation
RN	Radical nephrectomy
RNU	Radical nephroureterectomy
RP	Radical prostatectomy
RPLND	Retroperitoneal lymph nodes dissection
RT	Radiation therapy
SCC	Squamous cell carcinoma
SRM	Small renal mass
SRT	Salvage radiation therapy
SUVmax	Maximum standardized uptake value
SWOG	Southwest Oncology Group Study
TCC	Transitional cell carcinoma
TDM	Tomodensitometry
TKI	Tyrosine-kinase inhibitor
TNF- α	Tumour necrosis factor- α
TNM classification	Tumour lymph nodes and metastases-based classification
TRUS-biopsy	Transrectal ultrasound-guided prostatic biopsy
TURBT	Transurethral resection of bladder tumour
U/S	Ultrasound
UICC	Union Internationale Contre le Cancer (This French acronym which means International Union Against Cancer was later adapted in English language as Union for International Cancer Control)
UTI	Urinary tract infection
UTUC	Upper urinary tract urothelial cancer
VEGF	Vascular endothelial growth factor
VHL	Von Hippel-Lindau syndrome

Part I
Prostate Cancer

Said Abdallah Al-Mamari and Salim Said Al-Busaidy

Introduction

Prostatic specific antigen (*PSA*) screening has largely contributed to an increased incidence of *prostate cancer* (*PC*), particularly in the early stages of the disease. This has led to an increase in treatment options aimed at curing the disease. However the drawback to early detection is the increasing likelihood of diagnosing cancers with a low potential to progress during a patient's *life expectancy* (*LE*). This clinical scenario is psychologically stressful to both patients and their families and places the urologists in a dilemma in which he has to weigh the benefits of preventing the possibility of disease progression against the likelihood of unnecessary treatment. This may be detrimental to the patient's *quality of life* (*QoL*) and may lead to more serious consequences.

Several expert panels have proposed evidence-based guidelines. However, the guidelines are often too comprehensive and extensive for every urologist to digest. We have therefore endeavoured to provide a more concise and practical clinical aid without omitting essential information needed to tackle the various clinical problems.

In the present study, only adenocarcinoma has been considered under the terms prostate cancer, the other pathological entities such as sarcoma, primary lymphoma, neuroendocrine (small cell) carcinoma being extremely rare.

Chapter 1
Epidemiology, Aetiological Factors and Prevention

Said Abdallah Al-Mamari and Salim Said Al-Busaidy

1.1 Epidemiology

Prostate cancer (PC) is the most commonly diagnosed cancer in men. More than 1.1 million cases of PC were recorded worldwide in 2012 [1], and the estimated mortality of 307,481 showed a marked increase compared to the 258,000 deaths estimated in 2008 [2]. It is the second most common cause of cancer mortality in Western countries after lung cancer, and the incidence was estimated to be 417 new cases per 100,000 men in Europe in 2012 [3]. It is now fourth on the scale of the total economic cancer-related costs in Europe after lung, breast and colorectal diseases with an estimated cost of 8.43 billion euros in 2009 [4].

It has been estimated that 1 out of 7 men will be diagnosed with PC during his lifetime, but only one out of 37 will die from the disease [5]. *The risk of developing malignancy increases with age*, and an estimated 80 % of men who reach the age of 80 years will have PC. A study performing autopsies of deaths unrelated to prostatic diseases has revealed occult PC in 2, 29, 32, 55 and 64 % of men in their 3rd, 4th, 5th, 6th and 7th decades, respectively [6]. It is universally accepted that many patients will die *with* PC rather than *from* PC. Similarly patients undergoing radical cystoprostatectomy for bladder cancer were incidentally found to have an unsuspected PC, although the incidences varied significantly from 18 to 60 % in numerous studies [7–10]. Moreover, the stress related to the diagnosis of PC has been associated with an increased rate of cardiovascular deaths and suicide, especially in the early period following diagnosis [11].

S.A. Al-Mamari (✉)
Urology Department, The Royal Hospital, Muscat, Oman
e-mail: sabdal67@yahoo.com

S.S. Al-Busaidy
Senior Consultant and HOD, Urology Department, The Royal Hospital, Muscat, Oman
e-mail: salimalbusaidy@hotmail.com

S.A. Al-Mamari, S.S. Al-Busaidy (eds.), *Urological Cancer Management*,
DOI 10.1007/978-3-319-16301-7_1

1.2 Aetiological Factors

1.2.1 Age

The disease is very rare in men before the age of 40 years, and the incidence rises after 50. Approximately 60 % of cases are diagnosed in men over 65 years of age [5].

1.2.2 Race and Ethnicity

African-American population and Caribbean men of African origin seem to be at a higher risk than men of other races. *Martinique (a French West Indies territory in the Caribbean Sea) had the highest incidence of PC in the world with 227.2 new cases (NC) per 100,000* population reported in 2012, followed by Norway (129.7 NC/100,000) and Metropolitan France (127.3 NC/100,000) [3]. Moreover African-American men are also more likely to be diagnosed at advanced stages and die from the disease than white men [12].

1.2.3 Geography

North America, Western and Northern Europe, Australia and the Caribbean islands have a higher incidence than Asia, Africa and Latin America. Less intensive screening and under-reporting could partly explain the lower incidence in the latter group, but it has been shown that despite having a lower incidence than the white population, men of Asian origin living in the United States have an increased risk of developing PC compared to men with similar ethnic backgrounds living in Asia [13]. This fact suggests that life-style, food and environmental changes are possible contributing factors.

1.2.4 Family History

A Swedish Family-Cancer Database has suggested that approximately *9 % of prostate cancers are thought to be of true hereditary* origin which was defined as 3 or more affected individuals in the same family or 2 or more relatives having developed the disease at an age younger than 55 years [14]. Having a father with a history of PC doubles the risk of developing the disease. This is tripled by having a history of 2 affected generations, e.g. a grandfather and father, while the risk is multiplied by 17.7 when three brothers are affected. The risk is further increased

Table 1.1 Percentage of American men who develop prostate cancer over 10-, 20- and 30-year intervals according to their current age, 2008–2010

Current age	10 years	20 years	30 years
30	0.01	0.35	2.54
40	0.34	2.57	8.18
50	2.31	8.12	13.73
60	6.41	12.59	14.92
70	7.73	10.64	N/A

From Howlader et al. [5]

when the affected persons have got the disease at younger ages. The doubling or tripling risk has to be calculated from a baseline corresponding to the age (Table 1.1.) [5].

1.2.5 Genes

A preliminary result of the international IMPACT study has shown recently that inherited mutations of the BRCA1 or BRCA2 genes (already described in some families with breast and ovarian cancers) are associated with PC in a smaller number of cases, but have a higher proportion of aggressive disease [15]. There are ongoing research studies aiming at identifying genes associated with an increased risk of PC. These could be located on chromosome 17 and may also include HPC1, HPC2, HPCX and CAPB. Some gene overexpression (FUT8) was suggested in recent studies to be associated with the more aggressive PC [16] and with the progression to the androgen-independent state [17].

1.2.6 Foods

So far there is no evidence of their role. In a very large European Prospective Investigation into Cancer and Nutrition (EPIC) which included 150,000 men, it appeared that high intake of protein from dairy products had a link with the occurrence of PC [18]. Lycopene (tomatoes) could be protective, but the literature has provided inconsistent results [19, 20], while selenium and vitamin E did not show any protective effect in the large SELECT prospective clinical trial [21, 22].

1.2.7 Profession

Firefighters may be at risk due to their exposure to toxic combustion products [23, 24]. Exposure to heavy metals (cadmium) has also been incriminated [25], but the Strong Heart Mortality study did not show any significant association between cadmium and PC mortality [26].

1.2.8 Others

Studies have shown conflicting data and no evidence that link PC and sexually transmitted diseases, prostatitis, vasectomy, obesity or smoking. An epidemiologic study has linked the high incidence of PC in the French West Indies to chlordecone (Kepone®) use, an oestrogenic organophosphorate pesticide formerly extensively used in banana plantations in Martinique and Guadeloupe and now internationally banned [27]. However multivariate analysis showed that this association was stronger in subjects aged 60 years or older, in men with a family history of prostate cancer and in those who had previously lived in Western countries.

1.3 Prevention

Chemoprophylaxis with finasteride and dutasteride is not recommended due to their side effects and the lack of sufficient data relating to specific mortality [28, 29].

Take-Home Message: Aetiological Factors of PC
Apart from the age and the family history, there are no aetiological factors definitely linked to PC.
North American and Caribbean men with African ancestry are more at risk than white men.
About 9 % of PC is estimated to be hereditary, but genetic factors are still under study.
Alimentary factors are not yet proven.

References

1. Ferlay J, Soerjomataram I, Ervik M, Dikshit R, Eser S, Mathers C, Rebelo M, Parkin DM, Forman D, Bray F. GLOBOCAN 2012 v1.0, Cancer incidence and mortality worldwide: IARC CancerBase no. 11 [internet]. Lyon: International Agency for Research on Cancer; 2013.
2. Ferlay J, Shin HR, Bray F, et al. GLOBOCAN 2008 v1.2, Cancer incidence and mortality worldwide: IARC cCancerBase no. 10 [internet]. Lyon: International Agency for Research on Cancer; 2010.
3. Ferlay J, Steliarova-Foucher E, Lortet-Tieulent J, et al. Cancer incidence and mortality patterns in Europe: estimates for 40 countries in 2012. Eur J Cancer. 2013;49:1374–403.
4. Luengo-Fernandez R, Leal J, Gray A, Sullivan R. Economic burden of cancer across the European Union: a population-based cost analysis. Lancet Oncol. 2013;14(12):1165–74.
5. Howlader N, Noone AM, Krapcho M, Garshell J, Miller D, Altekruse SF, Kosary CL, Yu M, Ruhl J, Tatalovich Z, Mariotto A, Lewis DR, Chen HS, Feuer EJ, Cronin KA (eds). SEER Cancer Statistics Review, 1975–2011, National Cancer Institute. Bethesda, MD, http://seer.cancer.gov/csr/1975_2011/, based on November 2013 SEER data submission, posted to the SEER web site, April 2014.

6. Sakr WA, Grignon DJ, Crissman JD, Heilbrun LK, Cassin BJ, Pontes JJ, Haas GP. High grade prostatic intraepithelial neoplasia (HGPIN) and prostatic adenocarcinoma between the ages of 20–69: an autopsy study of 249 cases. In Vivo. 1994;8(3):439–43.
7. Alsinnawi M, Loftus B, Flynn R, McDermott T, Grainger R, Thornhill JA. The incidence and relevance of prostate cancer in radical cystoprostatectomy specimens. Int Urol Nephrol. 2012;44(6):1705–10.
8. Nevoux P, Ouzzane A, Ahmed HU, Emberton M, Montironi R, Presti Jr JC, Villers A. Quantitative tissue analyses of prostate cancer foci in an unselected cystoprostatectomy series. BJU Int. 2012;110(4):517–23.
9. Winkler MH, Livni N, Mannion EM, et al. Characteristics of incidental prostatic adenocarcinoma in contemporary radical cystoprostatectomy specimens. BJU Int. 2007;99:554–8.
10. Kouriefs C, Fazili T, Masood S, et al. Incidentally detected prostate cancer in cystoprostatectomy specimens. Urol Int. 2005;75:213–6.
11. Fang F, Keating NL, Mucci LA, Adami HO, Stampfer MJ, Valdimarsdóttir U, Fall K. Immediate risk of suicide and cardiovascular death after a prostate cancer diagnosis: cohort study in the United States. J Natl Cancer Inst. 2010;102(5):307–14.
12. Altekruse SF, Kosary CL, Krapcho M, et al. SEER cancer statistics review, 1975–2007. Bethesda: National Cancer Institute. http://seer.cancer.gov/csr/1975_2007/, based on November 2009 SEER data submission, posted to the SEER web site, 2010. Accessed 2 Apr 2011.
13. Kheirandish P, Chinegwundoh F. Ethnic differences in prostate cancer. Br J Cancer. 2011;105:481–5.
14. Hemminki K. Familial risk and familial survival in prostate cancer. World J Urol. 2012;30(2):143–8.
15. Bancroft EK, Page EC, Castro E, et al. Targeted prostate cancer screening in BRCA1 and BRCA2 mutation carriers: results from the initial screening round of the IMPACT study. Eur Urol. 2014;66(3):489–99.
16. Wang X, Chen J, Li QK, Peskoe SB, Zhang B, Choi C, Platz EA, Zhang H. Overexpression of alpha (1,6) fucosyltransferase associated with aggressive prostate cancer. Glycobiology. 2014;24(10):935–44.
17. Schinke EN, Bii V, Nalla A, Rae DT, Tedrick L, Meadows GG, Trobridge GD. A novel approach to identify driver genes involved in androgen-independent prostate cancer. Mol Cancer. 2014;13(1):120.
18. Key TJ. Nutrition, hormones and prostate cancer risk: results from the European prospective investigation into cancer and nutrition. Recent Results Cancer Res. 2014;202:39–46.
19. Wei MY, Giovannucci EL. Lycopene, tomato products, and prostate cancer incidence: a review and reassessment in the PSA screening era. J Oncol. 2012;2012:271063.
20. Ilic D, Misso M. Lycopene for the prevention and treatment of benign prostatic hyperplasia and prostate cancer: a systematic review. Maturitas. 2012;72(4):269–76.
21. Lippman SM, Klein EA, Goodman PJ, Lucia MS, Thompson IM, Ford LG, et al. Effect of selenium and vitamin E on risk of prostate cancer and other cancers: the Selenium and Vitamin E Cancer Prevention Trial (SELECT). JAMA. 2009;301:39–51.
22. Klein EA, Thompson IM, Tangen CM, Crowley JJ, Lucia MS, Goodman PJ, et al. Vitamin E and the risk of prostate cancer: the Selenium and Vitamin E Cancer Prevention Trial (SELECT). JAMA. 2009;306:1549–56.
23. Pukkala E, Martinsen JI, Weiderpass E, Kjaerheim K, Lynge E, Tryggvadottir L, Sparén P, Demers PA. Cancer incidence among firefighters: 45 years of follow-up in five Nordic countries. Occup Environ Med. 2014;71(6):398–404.
24. LeMasters GK, Genaidy AM, Succop P, Deddens J, Sobeih T, Barriera-Viruet H, Dunning K, Lockey JJ. Cancer risk among firefighters: a review and meta-analysis of 32 studies. Occup Environ Med. 2006;48(11):1189–202.
25. Julin B, Wolk A, Johansson JE, Andersson SO, Andrén O, Akesson A. Dietary cadmium exposure and prostate cancer incidence: a population-based prospective cohort study. Br J Cancer. 2012;107(5):895–900.

26. García-Esquinas E, Pollan M, Tellez-Plaza M, Francesconi KA, Goessler W, Guallar E, Umans JG, Yeh J, Best LG, Navas-Acien A. Cadmium exposure and cancer mortality in a prospective cohort: the strong heart study. Environ Health Perspect. 2014;122(4):363–70.
27. Multigner L, Rodrigue Ndong J, Giusti A, et al. Chlordecone exposure and risk of prostate cancer. J Clin Oncol. 2010;28(21):3457–62.
28. Thompson IM, Goodman PJ, Tangen CM, Lucia MS, Miller GJ, Ford LG, et al. The influence of Finasteride on the development of prostate cancer. N Engl J Med. 2003;349:215–24.
29. Andriole GL, Bostwick DG, Brawley OW, Gomella LG, Marberger M, Montorsi F, et al. Effect of dutasteride on the risk of prostate cancer. N Engl J Med. 2010;362:1192–202. Walsh PC. Chemoprevention of prostate cancer. N Engl J Med. 2010;362:1237–8.

Chapter 2
PSA Biology and PC Screening

Said Abdallah Al-Mamari and Salim Said Al-Busaidy

Prostate-specific antigen (PSA) is a serine protease of the tissue kallikrein family [1, 2].

The quantity of *PSA excreted* in the blood is increased in the presence of PC compared to a benign prostate. However, the *PSA concentration* in individual prostatic gland cells is higher in benign hyperplasia than in PC [3, 4]. Moreover, PSA has also been found at much lower levels in other tissues or organs (paraurethral glands, breast, thyroid, placenta, etc.), mainly in its free molecular form [5, 6]. Nonetheless, the PSA concentration in non-prostatic tissues is extremely low to be detectable by routine biochemical assays. Hence, in all practical purposes, *PSA is generally considered as an organ-specific and not a disease-specific marker since several physiological and pathological conditions may cause an increase in its level*:

- Ejaculation [7, 8]
- Urological manipulations (digital rectal examination, catheterization) or endourological procedures (especially transurethral resection of the prostate) [9, 10]
- Pathological conditions: acute urinary retention, urinary tract infections, chronic or acute prostatitis, prostatic infarction [11]
- Long-distance bicycle riding [12]

Hence the EAU expert panel recommends that *the first elevated PSA should not prompt an immediate biopsy* and advises a repeated test after a few weeks by the same assay, in the same laboratory and using the same method [13].

The PSA value is presently the cornerstone for early diagnosis of PC. However, *international guidelines do not recommend general PC screening in the population*

S.A. Al-Mamari (✉)
Urology Department, The Royal Hospital, Muscat, Oman
e-mail: sabdal67@yahoo.com

S.S. Al-Busaidy
Senior Consultant and HOD, Urology Department, The Royal Hospital, Muscat, Oman
e-mail: salimalbusaidy@hotmail.com

S.A. Al-Mamari, S.S. Al-Busaidy (eds.), *Urological Cancer Management*,
DOI 10.1007/978-3-319-16301-7_2

[14, 15], *but rather it should be tailored according to the individual's risk factors (men aged >50 years, or >45 years with family history of PC, Afro-American or Afro-Caribbean origin), all of whom should be individuals with good performance status (PS) and have at least a 10–15-year life expectancy (LE)* [16–18].

A large randomized European study showed that PSA-based screening for PC has reduced the disease-specific mortality rate by 20 % but was associated with a high risk of overdiagnosis and excessive treatment-related complications and mortality. This resulted in *a very modest absolute difference of 0.71 death per 1,000 men in favour of the screening group*, which means that *about 1,410 men would need to be screened to prevent 1 death* [19].

However, a Swedish study which included 21,000 men has shown that *PSA values ≥1 ng/ml at 45 years or ≥2 ng/ml at 60 years are associated with a significant increase in specific mortality risk and the risk of advanced or metastatic cancer later in life* [20]. This prompted the EAU experts[1] to propose the following protocol in 2013 [21]:

- First PSA value at 40–45 years for all men to initiate a risk-adapted follow-up.
- If PSA ≥ 1 ng/ml at 45–59 years, the test is to be repeated every 2–4 years.
- If PSA < 1 ng/ml at 45–59 years, the screening is to be repeated every 8 years.

Nonetheless, in the 2014 edition, the same expert panel seemed to attenuate this recommendation and *rather emphasized the early PSA testing of men with increased risks of developing PC who have the following criteria*: >50 years of age, >45 years with a family history of PC, African-American men, PSA >1 ng/ml at 40 years, and PSA >2 ng/ml at 60 years [22].

The French expert panel (CCAFU[2]) recommends a combination of PSA screening with DRE in healthy 50-year-old men and in high-risk men of 45 years [23].

The AUA[3] expert panel recommends that the decision to perform PSA measurement should be shared with men aged 55 to 69 years because the greatest benefit of screening is found in this age group. Screening may however be offered to high-risk men younger than 55 years but not below 40 [16].

The universal PSA cut-off for clinically suspicious PC is 4 ng/ml. There is a positive predictive value of 25–35 % when total PSA range is 4–10 ng/ml, with 70 % of diagnosed cancers being localized, and a positive predictive value of 50–80 % for values >10 mg/ml [24].

To enhance the specificity of the PSA interpretation, other parameters have been introduced:

- *The free to total PSA ratio (F/T PSA): It has been proposed as a second-line investigation after a first negative biopsy* [24]. In normal condition, about 70–90 % of PSA that enters the circulation is intact and becomes rapidly bound by the alpha 1-antichymotrypsin and other protease inhibitors. A portion of the PSA (10–30 %) is inactivated by internal cleavages which occur earlier in the seminal plasma and will not form complexes with protease inhibitors, remaining free in the peripheral blood.

[1] EAU: European Association of Urology.

[2] CCAFU: Comité de Cancérologie de l'Association Française d'Urologie.

[3] AUA: American Urology Association.

These cleavages are fewer in PC, leading to an increased fraction of the bound PSA and a lesser percentage of free PSA [1]. The consequence is *a lower F/T PSA ratio, with values ≤15 % being associated with an increased suspicion of cancer* [24]. Values of <10 % were associated with a diagnosis of cancer in 56 % of men, while values of>25 % were associated with a cancer diagnosis in only 8 % of men. *But this ratio is only useful when the total PSA is in the range of 4–10 ng/ml with a negative DRE. It has no role in total PSA values >10 or during follow-up of a known PC* [25].
- *The PSA kinetics:* Two parameters are used: *the PSA velocity* (defined as the absolute increase of serum PSA per year reported as ng/mL/year) and *the PSA doubling time (PSADT).* These are important prognostic factors often utilized during *active surveillance* or when monitoring early signs of biochemical relapse after curative intent treatments. *The higher the PSA velocity (>2 ng/ml/yr) or the shorter the PSADT (<6 months), the more aggressive the disease* [26–28].

Newer Biomarkers

- The Progensa urinary level of *PCA3 mRNA* (a gene specifically expressed in PC) is a promising test in patients suspected of having PC with an initial negative biopsy. It is done after prostatic massage. A ratio of >35 between this value and the urinary PSA is predictive of PC in subsequent biopsies [29].
- *ProPSA* is another biomarker now commercialized. This is a 244-amino-acid proenzyme which represents the early inactive form of the PSA when it is first secreted into prostatic ducts, before it becomes activated by cleavage of the seven N-terminal amino acids. Unfortunately, the high costs of these novel biomarkers limit their use [1, 30].
- The *cell cycle progression (CCP) test (Prolaris®)* is an ongoing prognostic assay that quantifies accurately the risk of developing prostate-cancer-specific disease progression and disease-specific mortality. It utilizes a gene-expression-based cell cycle progression score for clinically localized prostate cancers and aims at reducing overtreatment of patients with less aggressive disease [31, 32].
- A novel serum phospholipid panel was recently reported to have variable values in normal and prostate cancer sera and may serve as an early predictive marker for the presence of PC [33].

Take-Home Message: Screening of PC

PSA-based population screening for PC is not recommended by many authorities and should be limited to men with increased risks of developing the disease.

PSA is not a disease-specific marker for PC, and new parameters help to increase its specificity:

- The F/T PSA ratio used for early PC detection before prostatic biopsy or to justify a second biopsy after a negative result.
- The PSA kinetics (PSA velocity and PSADT) used in active surveillance and in follow-up of patients after curative treatment.

Promising newer biomarkers are under investigations, but the high costs may preclude their general use in the near future.

References

1. Balk SP, Ko YJ, Bubley GJ. Biology of prostate-specific antigen. J Clin Oncol. 2003;21(2):383–91.
2. Yousef GM, Diamandis EP. The new human tissue kallikrein gene family: structure, function, and association to disease. Endocr Rev. 2001;22:184–204.
3. Pretlow TG, Pretlow TP, Yang B, Kaetzel CS, Delmoro CM, Kamis SM, Bodner DR, Kursh E, Resnick MI, Bradley Jr EL. Tissue concentrations of prostate-specific antigen in prostatic carcinoma and benign prostatic hyperplasia. Int J Cancer. 1991;49(5):645–9.
4. Magklara A, Scorilas A, Stephan C, Kristiansen GO, Hauptmann S, Jung K, Diamandis EP. Decreased concentrations of prostate-specific antigen and human glandular kallikrein 2 in malignant versus nonmalignant prostatic tissue. Urology. 2000;56(3):527–32.
5. Diamandis EP, Yu H. Nonprostatic sources of prostate-specific antigen. Urol Clin North Am. 1997;24(2):275–82.
6. Howarth DJ, Aronson IB, Diamandis EP. Immunohistochemical localization of prostate-specific antigen in benign and malignant breast tissues. Br J Cancer. 1997;75(11):1646–51.
7. Tchetgen MB, Song JT, Strawderman M, Jacobsen SJ, Oesterling JE. Ejaculation increases the serum prostate-specific antigen concentration. Urology. 1996;47(4):511–6.
8. Herschman JD, Smith DS, Catalona WJ. Effect of ejaculation on serum total and free prostate-specific antigen concentrations. Urology. 1997;50(2):239–43.
9. Kravchick S, Bunkin I, Peled R, Yulish E, Ben-Dor D, Kravchenko Y, Cytron S. Patients with elevated serum PSA and indwelling catheter after acute urinary retention: prospective study of 63 patients with 7-year follow-up. J Endourol. 2007;21(10):1203–6.
10. Lin YH, Jiang YG, Li MC, Luo Y, Wang JS. Effects of prostate manipulation on serum total and free prostate specific antigen, and free-to-total prostate specific antigen ratio. Saudi Med J. 2010;31(9):999–1004.
11. Kiran PR. Markedly raised serum prostate specific antigen levels. Prostatic infarction rather than malignancy? Aust Fam Physician. 2001;30(5):458–60.
12. Mejak SL, Bayliss J, Hanks SD. Long distance bicycle riding causes prostate-specific antigen to increase in men aged 50 years and over. PLoS One. 2013;8(2):e56030. doi:10.1371/journal.pone.0056030.
13. Eastham JA, Riedel E, Scardino PT, Shike M, Fleisher M, Schatzkin A, Lanza E, Latkany L, Begg CB, Polyp Prevention Trial Study Group. Variation of serum prostate-specific antigen levels: an evaluation of year-to-year fluctuations. JAMA. 2003;289(20):2695–700.
14. Moyer VA. Screening for prostate cancer: US Preventive Services Task Force Recommendation Statement. Ann Intern Med. 2012;157:120–34.
15. Haute Autorité de Santé. Dépistage du cancer de la prostate chez les populations d'hommes présentant des facteurs de risque. Questions/Réponses 4 avril 2012. Available from www.has-sante.fr/portail/jcms/c_1238094/depistage- du- cancer- de- la- prostate- par- dosage- du- psa-interet- non- demontre- chez- les- hommes- presentant- des- facteurs- de- risque.
16. Carter HB, Albertsen PC, Barry MJ, Etzioni R, Freedland SJ, Greene KL, Holmberg L, Kantoff P, Konety BR, Murad MH, Penson DF, Zietman AL. Early detection of prostate cancer: AUA guideline. J Urol. 2013;190(2):419–26.
17. Salomon L, Azria D, Bastide C, Beuzeboc P, Cormier L, Cornu F, et al. Comité de Cancérologie de l'AFU. Recommandations en onco- urologie : cancer de la prostate. Prog Urol Association française d'urologie. Cancer de la prostate et dépistage. 12/04/12; from www.urofrance.org/À leadmin/medias/afu/communiques/2012-03-15_cancer- prostate.pdf.
18. Kamangar F, Dores GM, Anderson WF. Patterns of cancer incidence, mortality, and prevalence across five continents: defining priorities to reduce cancer disparities in different geographic regions of the world. J Clin Oncol. 2006;24(14):2137–50.
19. Schröder FH, Hugosson J, Roobol MJ, et al.; ERSPC Investigators. Screening and prostate-cancer mortality in a randomized European study. N Engl J Med. 2009; 360:1320–8.

20. Vickers AJ, Ulmert D, Sjoberg DD, Bennette CJ, Björk T, Gerdtsson A, Manjer J, Nilsson PM, Dahlin A, Bjartell A, Scardino PT, Lilja H. Strategy for detection of prostate cancer based on relation between prostate specific antigen at age 40–55 and long term risk of metastasis: case-control study. BMJ. 2013;346:f2023.
21. Heidenreich A, Abrahamsson PA, Artibani W, Catto J, Montorsi F, Van Poppel H, et al. Early detection of prostate cancer: European Association of Urology recommendation. Eur Urol. 2013;64:347–54.
22. Mottet N, Bastian PJ, Bellmunt J, et al. Guidelines on prostate cancer. The European Association of Urology. 2014, p. 17. Available from http://uroweb.org/wp-content/uploads/1607-Prostate-Cancer_LRV3.pdf#.
23. Salomon L, Bastide C, Beuzeboc P, et al. Les members du CCAFU. Recommandations en Onco-Urologie 2013 du CCAFU: Cancer de la Prostate. Prog Urol. 2013;23(Suppl 2): S69–101. p. 6.
24. Salomon L, Azria D, Bastide C, Beuzeboc P, Cormier L, Cornu F, et al. Comité de Cancérologie de l'AFU. Recommandations en onco- urologie : cancer de la prostate. Prog Urol. 2010;20:S217–51.
25. Catalona WJ, Partin AW, Slawin KM, Brawer MK, Flanigan RC, Patel A, Richie JP, deKernion JB, Walsh PC, Scardino PT, Lange PH, Subong EN, Parson RE, Gasior GH, Loveland KG, Southwick PC. Use of the percentage of free prostate-specific antigen to enhance differentiation of prostate cancer from benign prostatic disease, a prospective multicenter clinical trial. JAMA. 1998;279(19):1542–7.
26. Klotz LH. PSA recurrence: definitions, PSA kinetics, and identifying patients at risk. Can J Urol. 2006;13 Suppl 2:43–7.
27. Llorente C, de la Morena JM, Ardura MA. PSA doubling time as a new diagnostic and prognostic method for prostate cancer. Arch Esp Urol. 2006;59(10):1083–7.
28. Arlen PM, Bianco F, Dahut WL, D'Amico A, Figg WD, Freedland SJ, Gulley JL, Kantoff PW, Kattan MW, Lee A, Regan MM, Sartor O, Prostate Specific Antigen Working Group. Prostate Specific Antigen Working Group guidelines on prostate specific antigen doubling time. J Urol. 2008;179(6):2181–5; discussion 2185–6.
29. Crawford ED, Rove KO, Trabulsi EJ, Qian J, Drewnowska KP, Kaminetsky JC, et al. Diagnostic performance of PCA3 to detect prostate cancer in men with increased prostate specific antigen: a prospective study of 1,962 cases. J Urol. 2012;188:1726–31.
30. Sartori DA, Chan DW. Biomarkers in prostate cancer: what's new? Curr Opin Oncol. 2014;26(3):259–64.
31. Shore N, Concepcion R, Saltzstein D, Lucia MS, van Breda A, Welbourn W, Lewine N, Gustavsen G, Pothier K, Brawer MK. Clinical utility of a biopsy-based cell cycle gene expression assay in localized prostate cancer. Curr Med Res Opin. 2014;30(4):547–53.
32. Crawford ED, Scholz MC, Kar AJ, Fegan JE, Haregewoin A, Kaldate RR, Brawer MK. Cell cycle progression score and treatment decisions in prostate cancer: results from an ongoing registry. Curr Med Res Opin. 2014;30(6):1025–31.
33. Patel N, Vogel R, Chandra-Kuntal K, Glasgow W, Kelavkar U. A novel three serum phospholipid panel differentiates normal individuals from those with prostate cancer. PLoS One. 2014;6:9(3).

Chapter 3
Symptoms, Signs, Clinical Examination, Primary Diagnostic Methods and Disease Extension Investigations

Said Abdallah Al-Mamari and Salim Said Al-Busaidy

3.1 Symptoms and Signs

Localized PC is generally an asymptomatic disease. It may sometimes present with lower urinary tract symptoms (LUTS). Locally advanced disease may also be asymptomatic, but with time it will more likely present with urinary obstruction, urinary infections, haematuria, impotence, tenesmus, obstructive uropathy with uraemia, etc. Haematospermia is a rare symptom of PC, found in only 0.5 % of cases; but its presence should prompt screening for PC in selected patients since it has been associated with a PC diagnosis in 13.7 % of patients [1–3]. Metastatic disease generally present with complications. These may be *local* in keeping with locally advanced disease, *distant* (back pain, spontaneous fracture, paraplegia, obstructive jaundice caused by massive para-aortic and para-caval lymph nodes compressing the common bile duct) *or systemic* when the general health is affected by anorexia, loss of weight and anaemia.

3.2 Clinical Examination

The combination of DRE and the serum PSA level is the cornerstone in the initiation of a PC diagnosis before histopathological confirmation. Varying with teaching institutions and the practitioner's habits, the DRE techniques differ in the patient's positioning: the patient is placed in the supine, left lateral or genupectoral postures.

S.A. Al-Mamari (✉)
Urology Department, The Royal Hospital, Muscat, Oman
e-mail: sabdal67@yahoo.com

S.S. Al-Busaidy
Senior Consultant and HOD, Urology Department, The Royal Hospital, Muscat, Oman
e-mail: salimalbusaidy@hotmail.com

S.A. Al-Mamari, S.S. Al-Busaidy (eds.), *Urological Cancer Management*,
DOI 10.1007/978-3-319-16301-7_3

Correlating a raised PSA and the patient's age with the feeling of a "true nodule" on DRE is highly suggestive of PC. However there are several benign conditions which are associated with the feeling of a prostatic nodule: hyperplastic nodule, prostate stones, fibrosis in chronic prostatitis, granulomatous prostatitis and prominent ampulla of the vas deferens at the prostatic base [4, 5]. A large population-based screening study has revealed that the risk of cancer detection is only 5–30 % when there is *a suspicious DRE finding alone with a PSA level less than 4 ng/ml* [6], but a significant proportion of prostate cancers diagnosed in this scenario were associated with a clinically aggressive course [7].

Consequently any abnormal DRE is considered as sufficient to justify a transrectal ultrasound (TRUS)-guided biopsy of the prostate irrespective of the PSA value [8].

3.3 Imaging Techniques in Initial Diagnosis

The aim of these studies is to help the clinician to reach a positive diagnosis of PC.

1. *Ultrasonography (U/S)* is mostly commonly used for estimating the *prostate volume* and remains the standard imaging technique for *prostatic biopsy and focal therapy guidance*. However its sensitivity is poor in detecting PC (only 60 %). Its specificity remains also questionable since the finding of a *hypoechoic area in the prostatic outer gland* was proven to be benign prostatic hyperplasia in 9 % of patients after biopsy [5]. The combination of real-time elastography and microbubble contrast injection may significantly decrease false-positive results and improve the positive predictive value of the U/S examination [9].
2. Until a decade ago, *computerized tomography (CT)* was the standard imaging technique used for the detection of lymph nodes (LN) in intermediate- and high-risk patients. The following criteria were suggestive of positive results for malignant deposits: obturator LN ≥8 mm, aorto-lumbar LN ≥10 mm and oval-shaped LNs rather than the round-shaped.
3. *Magnetic resonance imaging (MRI)* performed for LN detection is no better, but *it has supplanted CT due to its better definition of early intraprostatic malignant changes* [10]. Its sensitivity and specificity for cancers >0.5 cc in volume are 86 and 94 %, respectively [11]. *Today CT is only indicated when MRI is contraindicated*, e.g. pacemaker, history of total hip replacement and claustrophobia. *Presently the use of MRI is mostly justified after an initial negative biopsy when there is clinical and biological suspicion of PC*. In this setting it will be helpful to define the suspicious areas more accurately and *provide guidance for the second biopsy, especially for anteriorly located tumours* [12, 13]. However MRI should be delayed after the initial negative biopsy to avoid artefacts and only be performed

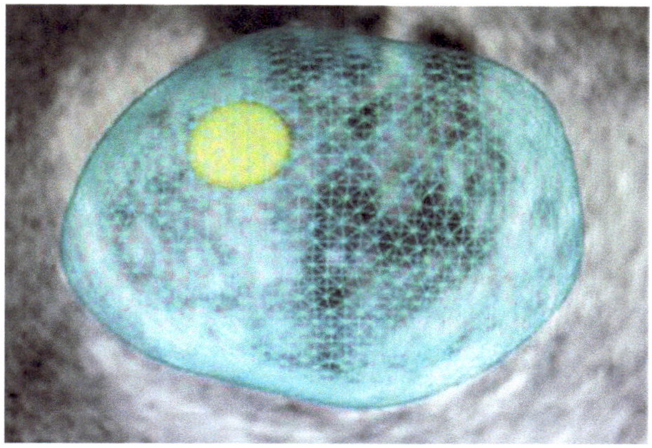

Fig. 3.1 Fusion of prerecorded MRI data with real-time U/S (Urostation®, Keolis): the *blue net* is an MRI 3-D reconstruction of U/S information collected before the procedure, delineating the whole prostatic gland. The *small yellow sphere* indicates the suspected lesion to be targeted during biopsy

after 8 weeks. Ongoing studies are evaluating the use of MRI *before the first biopsy* [12, 14]. The coupling of U/S and MRI images (Fig. 3.1) has also been shown to significantly improve PC detection rates in repeated biopsies, especially for clinically significant tumours [15–17]. In this technology prostate biopsy is performed using prerecorded MRI images fused with real-time ultrasound, optimizing therefore the accuracy in the targeting of the suspicious lesions.

Technically *a prostatic MRI should be multiparametric* providing morphological (T1- and T2-weighted) and functional information. *Morphological sequences* are consistent with axial[1] T1-weighted images and three-plane T2-weighted images including axial, coronal and sagittal. *Functional information* comprises of three phases (Fig. 3.2a–d):

- Perfusion phase: T1-weighted dynamic phase with gadolinium injection
- Diffusion phase
- Spectroscopy phase (spectro-MRI)

3.4 Primary Diagnosis

This is confirmed by the *histopathological examination of the prostate core specimens provided by a TRUS-guided biopsy*:

1. *Prior to the prostatic biopsy, a urine culture should always be performed to exclude urinary infection.* The recommended pre-procedural antibiotic prophylaxis continues to be second-generation fluoroquinolones, such as *Ciprofloxacin* (500 mg) which is more effective than ofloxacin (400 mg) [18]. The tablets are

[1] Axial plane is synonymous to transverse, horizontal or transaxial plane.

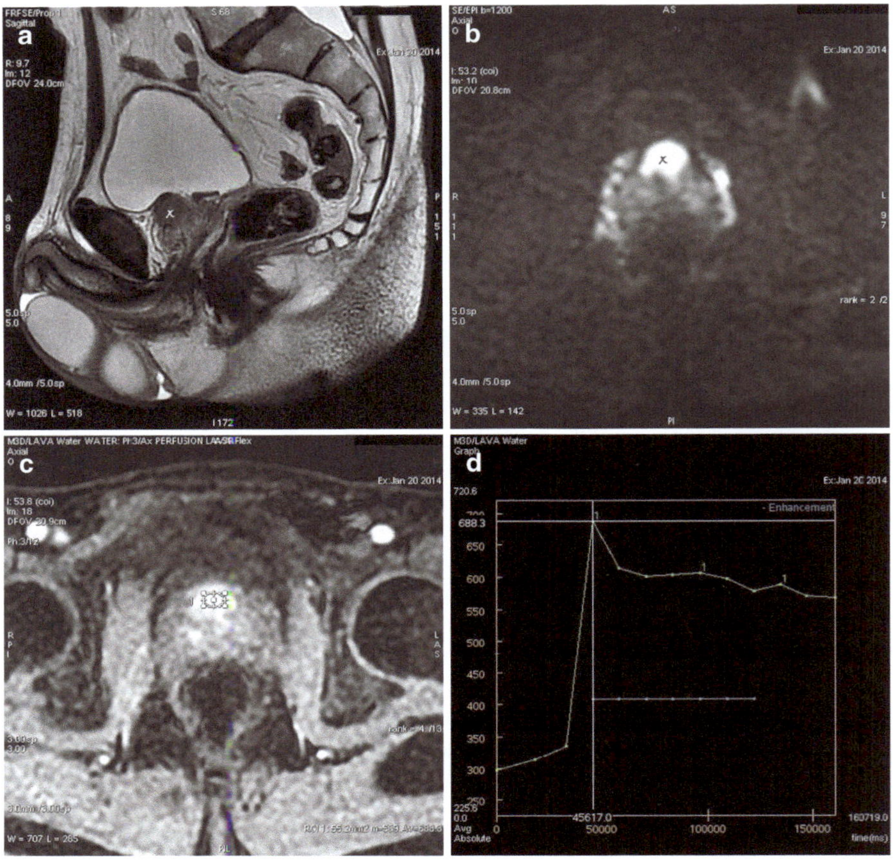

Fig. 3.2 (**a**–**d**) MRI prostate showing a cancer (x) developing from the anterior part of the prostate base (Courtesy of S. Novellas, Radiology, Arnault-Tzanck Institute, Saint-Laurent-du-Var and CHU Nice, Nice, France). (**a**) Is T2-weighted, (**b**) is a diffusion picture at b1000, (**c**) is a perfusion phase and (**d**) shows a type 3 enhancement according to PI-RADS classification. Contrary to adenoma, cancer has an early enhancement and a rapid washout

best taken 1–2 h before the procedure. Ceftriaxone is an alternative in cases of allergy to fluoroquinolones. There are reports of ciprofloxacin-resistant *Escherichia coli* in the faecal flora [19, 20] which may justify the combination with other antibiotics in some cases, e.g. ertapenem and amikacin [21–23].

Here again the patient's positioning varies according to teaching institutions, from the lithotomy position (doctor sitting between the legs like for a cystoscopy) to the left lateral position with flexed hips and knees (doctor sitting behind the patient). The former is the preferred position for high-risk patients undergoing the procedure under sedation and close monitoring in operating theatres.

TRUS-guided prostatic biopsy performed under *local anaesthesia through a periprostatic infiltration* has been proven superior to instillation of intrarectal anaesthetic creams such as 1 % lidocaine solution (Xylocaine® or lignocaine)

[24]. *Low-dose aspirin is no longer considered an absolute contraindication for prostatic biopsy* [8, 25]. Large studies have also suggested that discontinuation of warfarin is not necessary [26, 27] as long as the international normalized ratio (INR) is within the therapeutic range. However, if a history of coagulopathy is discovered, the patient should have his coagulation profile normalized prior to the prostatic biopsy. The recommended points of technique on performing the first biopsy are [28]:

- *12-core biopsy* if there are no clinical or imaging anomalies (i.e. a biopsy indicated only by an abnormal PSA level).
- *Additional biopsy at the suspected area* if there is an abnormality on clinical examination (nodule on DRE) or prostatic images.
- One-core biopsy in each lobe may be sufficient when there is clinical suspicion of locally advanced disease (≥T3b, see TNM classification later).

Complications: A retrospective review of nearly 6,000 TRUS-guided biopsies of the prostate performed over 10 years has revealed the following complications [29]:

- Minor: *haematospermia (36.3 %), haematuria (14.5 %)* and rectal bleeding persisting up to 2 days (2.3 %)
- Major: bacteraemia with fever requiring admission (0.8 %), persistent rectal bleeding for more than 2 days (0.6 %) and urinary retention (0.2 %)

Interestingly this study did not show increased morbidity when comparing three different protocols with 6, 10 and 15 core biopsies. Vasovagal reaction is also known to occur.

In a recent study the mortality rate within 120 days after prostate biopsy (0.1%) was not found to be higher than in a control group (0.18%), and the deaths were mainly associated with risk factors such as ischemic heart and respiratory diseases [30].

The transperineal prostate biopsy is an alternative to the transrectal route when the anal orifice is closed after previous rectal surgery. It is also a valuable approach for patients with initially negative TRUS-guided biopsies and persistently high PSA or MRI images showing suspicious *anteriorly located lesions* [31].

2. *The primary histopathological diagnosis* of PC should ideally be confirmed by two pathologists. After staining the prostate cores with *haematoxylin* and *eosin* (H&E stain), the pathologists will first study the *architectural patterns* (presence of small glands with haphazard distribution, cribriform, fused and poorly formed glands or solid sheets, cords or isolated cells), the *nuclear atypia* (increase nucleocytoplasmic ratio with prominent nucleoli) and the *prognostic factors* like invasive growth and presence of perineural infiltration [32] (Fig. 3.3a–c). Additional *immunohistochemical studies* are sometimes needed for small tumour foci to identify invasive adenocarcinoma which is characterized by a loss of basal cells and, consequently, *negative basal cell markers (34βE12 and p63).* Conversely there will be a positive study for *alpha-methylacyl-CoA racemase (AMACR,* also called *504 s)* which is upregulated in prostate carcinoma [32] (Fig. 3.4). Nonetheless *immunohistochemistry should be reserved only for equiv-*

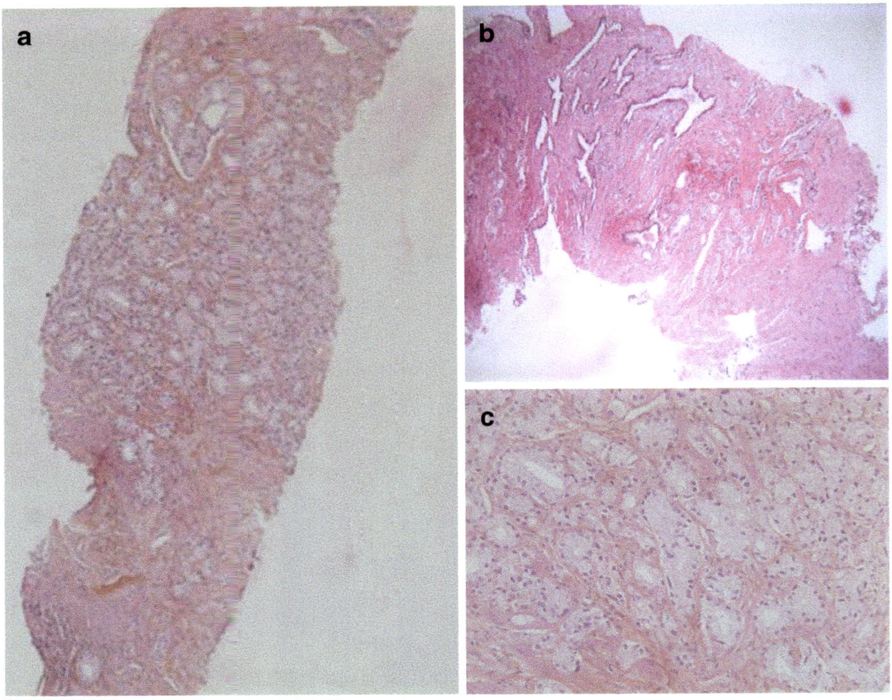

Fig. 3.3 (**a–c**) A prostatic core procured through TRUS-guided biopsy (H&E). This was a 3+3 (6) Gleason score, the most common pathological pattern (Courtesy of A. Durlach, Pol Bouin Laboratory, University Hospital of Reims, France)

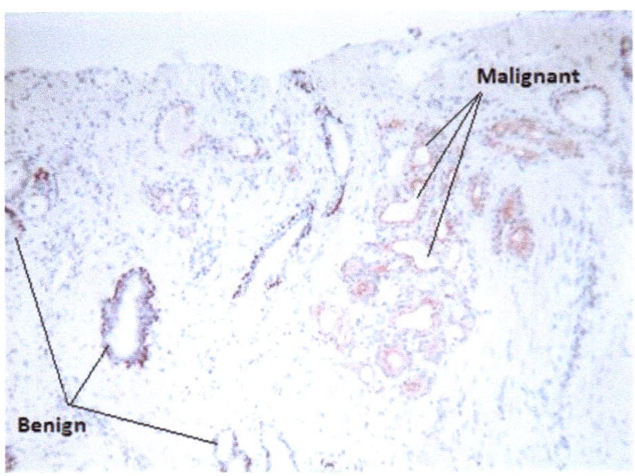

Fig. 3.4 Immuno-histochemistry using P63 and racemase: P63 stains the glands in brown and racemase in *red*. Being P63 negative and racemase positive, carcinomatous glands are stained in *red* (*right of the picture*), while the P63-positive and racemase-negative benign glands are stained in *brown* (*left of the picture*) (Courtesy of A. Durlach, Pol Bouin Laboratory, University Hospital of Reims, France)

Table 3.1 2005 ISUP modified Gleason system

Pattern 1	Circumscribed nodule of closely packed but separate, uniform, rounded to oval, medium-sized acini (larger glands than pattern 3)
Pattern 2	Like pattern 1, fairly circumscribed, yet at the edge of the tumour nodule, there may be minimal infiltration
	Glands are more loosely arranged and not quite as uniform as Gleason pattern 1
Pattern 3	Discrete glandular units
	Typically smaller glands than seen in Gleason pattern 1 or 2
	Infiltrates in and amongst nonneoplastic prostate acini
	Marked variation in size and shape
	Smoothly circumscribed small cribriform nodules of tumour
Pattern 4	Fused microacinar glands
	Ill-defined glands with poorly formed glandular lumina
	Large cribriform glands
	Cribriform glands with an irregular border
	Hypernephromatoid
Pattern 5	Essentially no glandular differentiation, composed of solid sheets, cords or single cells
	Comedocarcinoma with central necrosis surrounded by papillary, cribriform or solid masses

By Epstein et al. [35]. Reproduced with permission from Wolters Kluwer Health
Gleason scoring system: this is obtained by adding the two mostly represented patterns (i.e. the primary and the secondary grades), for example, 3+3, 3+4, 4+5, etc. The score is the sum of this addition. The secondary pattern has to be represented in not less than 5 %. Whenever present even in a very low percentage, grade 5 should be used as a tertiary pattern

ocal cases where conventional pathology is inconclusive [33]. PC histopathological grading was first reported by Gleason [34] and was modified later by the International Society of Urological Pathologists (ISUP) [35] (Table 3.1). The histopathological report must also include the localization and the number of positive cores out of the total number (generally 12), as well as the length of the malignant tissue in millimetres in every positive core. This is reported as a percentage of the total length of the positive cores. Several studies have demonstrated that the total tumour length in biopsy cores is an important prognostic factor. This was even suggested to have a stronger correlation with overall survival than the patient's age, serum PSA or Gleason score [36]. This factor is taken into account especially when considering a patient for active surveillance (see later).

3. *A repeat biopsy* is indicated within 3–6 months in the presence of *atypical small acinar proliferation (ASAP)* as this is associated with a subsequent PC diagnosis in 40 % of patients [37]. It is also performed when *extensive prostatic intraepithelial neoplasia (PIN) is seen on multiple sites (≥2 cores)* carrying a 20–30 % risk of cancer [38, 39], as well as when the *PSA is rising with the appearance of a prostate nodule* during regular follow-up. However *non-extensive (unifocal) high-grade PIN as an isolated finding is no longer considered an indication for*

repeat biopsy [40] unless there are new changes suggesting disease progression, i.e. PSA increase or appearance of a nodule on DRE during subsequent follow-up. Here it is recommended to perform *MRI in order to define the suspected zone. If MRI is not available, 4–6 biopsies should be taken at the apex and the transitional zone in addition to the standard 12 biopsies* [41]. *A saturation biopsy exceeding 20 cores* can also be recommended in highly suspicious cases with a previous negative biopsy. The incidence of PC detected in such circumstances is reported to be between 30 and 43 % [42].

3.5 Disease Extension Investigations

Once a positive diagnosis of PC is confirmed by histopathology, an image-based study is *sometimes* indicated to define *whether the disease is localized, locally advanced or metastatic*. After this study, the disease's *clinical* tumours-nodes-metastases (cTNM) staging can be documented as per the 2010 AJCC cancer staging which is identical to the UICC classification [43] (Table 3.2). The *pathological* (pTNM) *staging can only be established after radical prostatectomy*, when the pathologist will be provided with the complete prostate specimen including the seminal vesicles and sometimes the pelvic LN.

Therefore it is worthy of note to remember that by definition there is no pathological T1 stage. T1 staging is reached by fortuitously detecting malignant tissue in TURP specimens or positive prostatic biopsies following a high PSA, and none of the above criteria refer to a prostatectomy specimen. In order to minimize unnecessary exposure of patients to radiation and contrast media injection, and to improve cost-effectiveness, *investigations for disease extension are indicated only in clinically suspected intermediate- and high-risk groups* [44] (see D'Amico risk groups below).

MRI is the best imaging modality for local extension (T3a) as well as for regional or distant extension including regional LN detection and even bony metastases [45] (Fig. 3.5a–e).

The indications for a CT scan are confined to the contraindications of MRI (Fig. 3.6a–c). *Isotope bone scanning* is still extensively used to detect bony metastases. Apart from its *limited sensitivity* (46–70 %), the major drawback of isotope bone scanning remains its *low specificity* since hot zones can be due to benign conditions such as fracture, arthrosis, Paget's disease, etc. Conversely MRI has a higher sensitivity in T1 weighting [46].

- Low risk: cT1–cT2a, GS <7 and PSA ≤10 ng/ml.
- Intermediate risk: cT2b or GS = 7 or PSA >10 and ≤ 20 ng/ml.
- High risk: cT2c or GS >7 or PSA >20 ng/ml.

Table 3.2 The 2010 AJCC cancer staging for prostate cancer [43]

Primary tumour (T)	
TX	*Primary tumour cannot be assessed*
T0	*No evidence of primary tumour*
T1	*Clinically inapparent tumour neither palpable nor visible by imaging*
T1a	Tumour incidental histological finding in 5% or less of tissue resected
T1b	Tumour incidental histological finding in more than 5% of tissue resected
T1c	Tumour identified by needle biopsy (e.g. because of elevated PSA)
T2	*Tumour confined within the prostate* (tumour found in one or both lobes by needle biopsy, but not palpable or reliably visible by imaging, is classified as T1c)
T2a	Tumour involves one-half of one lobe or less
T2b	Tumour involves more than one-half of one lobe but not both lobes
T2c	Tumour involves both lobes
T3	*Tumour extends through the prostate capsule* (invasion into the prostatic apex or into, but not beyond, the prostatic capsule is classified not as T3 but as T2)
T3a	Extracapsular extension (unilateral or bilateral)
T3b	Tumour invades seminal vesicle(s)
T4	*Tumour is fixed or invades adjacent structures other than seminal vesicles such as the external sphincter, rectum, bladder, levator ani muscles and/or pelvic wall*
Pathologic (pT) (*There is no pathological T1 classification*)	
pT2	*Organ confined*
pT2a	Unilateral, involving one-half of one side or less
pT2b	Unilateral, involving more than one-half of one-half but not both lobes' sides
pT2c	Bilateral disease
pT3	*Extraprostatic extension*
pT3a	Extraprostatic extension or microscopic invasion of the bladder neck (*positive surgical margin should be indicated by an R1 descriptor: residual microscopic disease**)
pT3b	Seminal vesicle invasion
pT4	Invasion of the rectum, levator ani muscles and/or pelvic wall
Regional lymph nodes (N)	
Clinical	
NX	Regional lymph nodes were not assessed
N0	No regional lymph node metastasis
N1	Metastasis in regional lymph node(s)
Pathologic	
PNX	Regional nodes not sampled
pN0	No positive regional nodes
pN1	Metastases in regional node(s)
Distant metastasis (M) (*when more than one site of metastasis is present, the most advanced category is used. pM1c is most advanced*)	
M0	*No distant metastasis*
M1	*Distant metastasis*
M1a	Nonregional lymph node(s)
M1b	Bone(s)
M1c	Other site(s) with or without bone disease

Used with the permission of the American Joint Committee on Cancer (AJCC), Chicago, Illinois. The original source for this material is the *AJCC Cancer Staging Manual*, Seventh Edition (2010), published by Springer Science and Business Media LLC, www.springer.com

* In *R* classification for residual tumour, *R0* corresponds to complete resection with negative surgical margins, *R1* to microscopic residual tumour (or microscopic positive margins), *R2* to macroscopic residual tumour (or macroscopic positive margins)

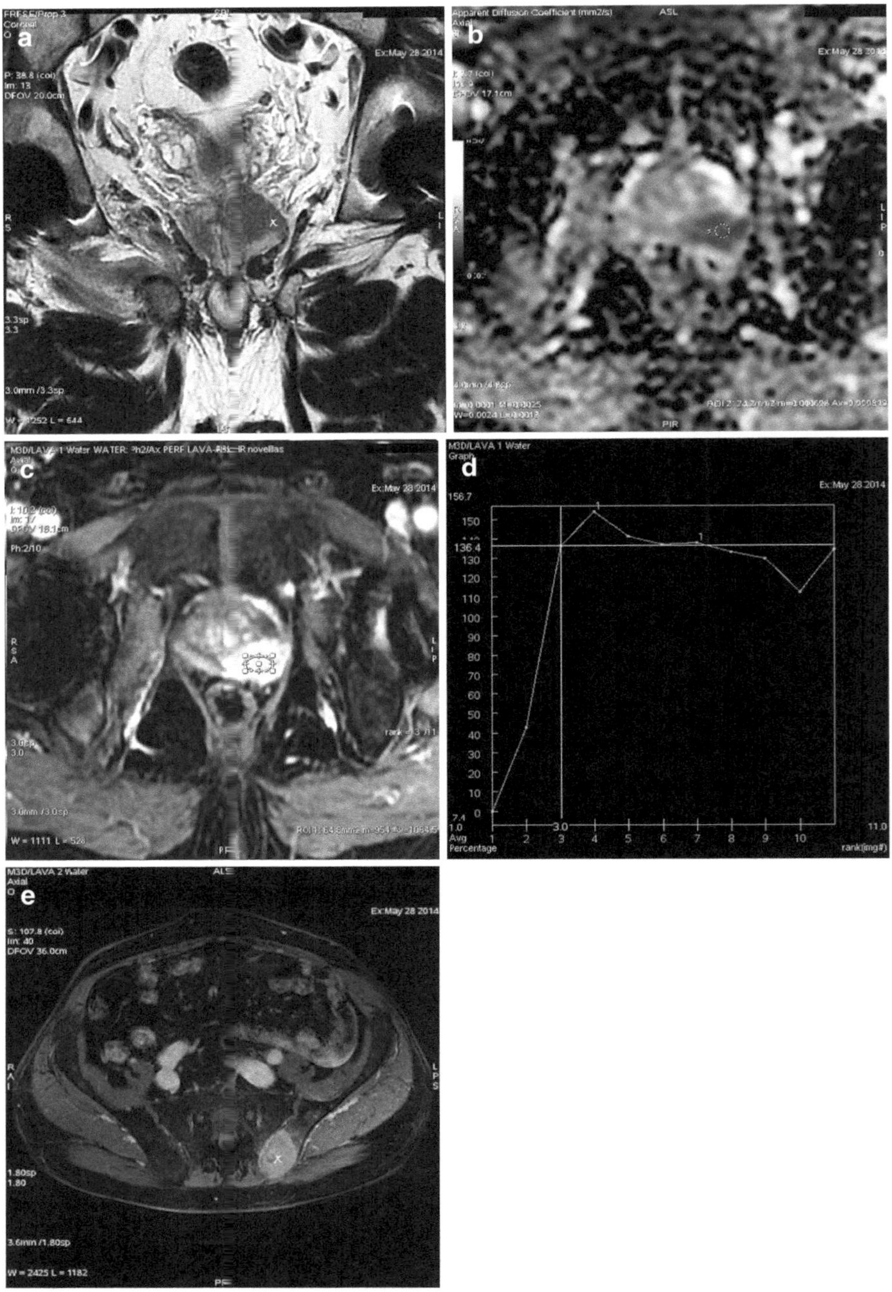

Fig. 3.5 (**a**–**e**) MRI showing a PC (x) invading the prostate capsule (**a**), ADC mapping (**b**), perfusion phase (**c**, **d**) as well as metastasis in the left iliac bone (**e**) (Courtesy of S. Novellas, Radiology, Arnault-Tzanck Institute, Saint-Laurent- du- Var and CHU Nice, Nice, France)

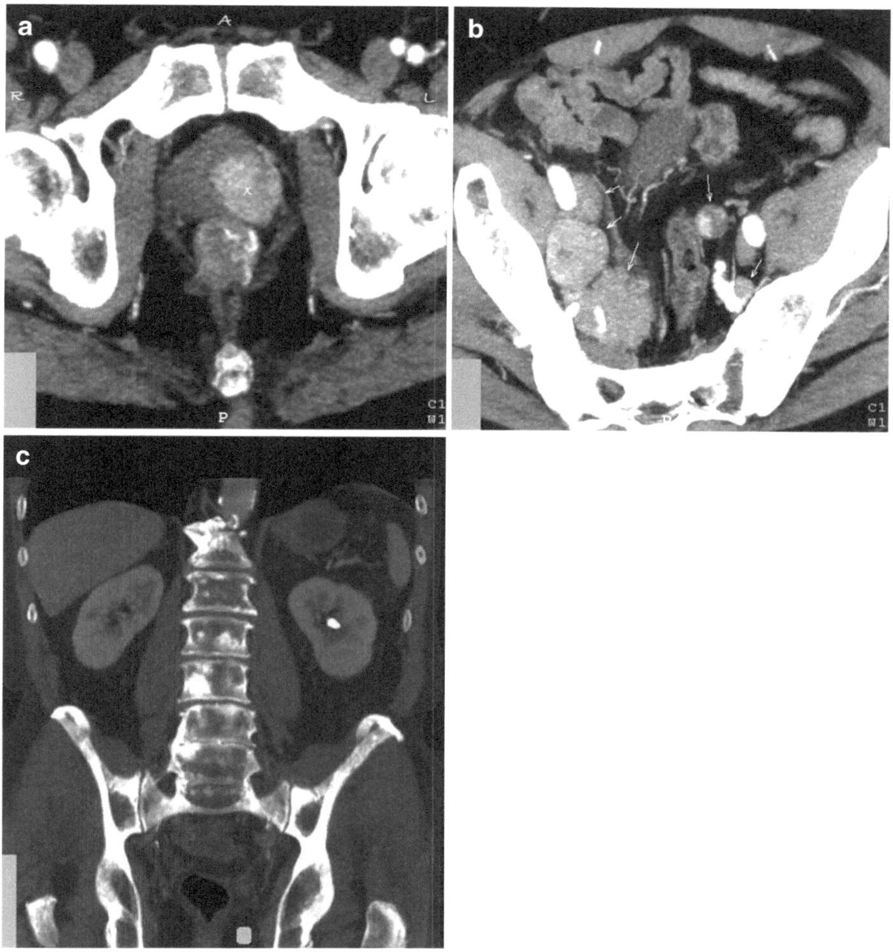

Fig. 3.6 (**a–c**) CT scan of the prostate showing a cancer involving the left lobe (**a**). There are also pelvic LN involvement (**b**) and bony metastases (**c**)

Knowing the serum PSA level, the cTNM staging and the Gleason score (GS), the clinician can categorize *the patients with localized disease* into one of the following three *D'Amico progression risk groups* [47]:

Note: Within the intermediate-risk group (GS 7), there is a prognosis difference between the Gleason grades 3 + 4 and 4 + 3, the latter being considered as a high-risk factor [46, 48].

Take-Home Message: Diagnosis of PC

- DRE and serum PSA measurements are the cornerstone for initiating the diagnosis of PC.
- An abnormal DRE is a sufficient finding to indicate a TRUS biopsy of the prostate irrespective of the PSA value.
- TRUS-guided prostatic biopsy is the standard way for core procurement. 12-core biopsy is recommended as first line. Local anaesthesia with periprostatic infiltration is the recommended technique to achieve adequate analgesia. Transperineal prostate biopsy may be helpful for anteriorly located lesions.
- The presence of ASAP or extensive (multifocal) PIN warrants a repeat prostate biopsy within 3–6 months; isolated high-grade (non-extensive) PIN is no longer considered an indication for a repeat biopsy.
- The modified Gleason score is the standard method for PC disease grading.
- MRI is the standard imaging modality for intraprostatic disease as well as for defining extraprostatic extension. It must be multiparametric.
- Localized PC is categorized into three progression risk groups based on PSA level, cTNM staging and GS (D'Amico risk groups).

References

1. Han M, Brannigan RE, Antenor JA, Roehl KA, Catalona WJ. Association of hemospermia with prostate cancer. J Urol. 2004;172(6 Pt 1):2189–92.
2. Ng YH, Seeley JP, Smith G. Haematospermia as a presenting symptom: outcomes of investigation in 300 men. Surgeon. 2013;11(1):35–8.
3. Stefanovic KB, Gregg PC, Soung M. Evaluation and treatment of hematospermia. Am Fam Physician. 2009;80(12):1421–7.
4. Liu X, Tang J, Yang JC, Zhang Y, Shi HY. An autopsy specimen study of benign hyperplastic nodules in the peripheral zone of the prostate. Zhonghua Nan Ke Xue. 2008;14(4):307–10.
5. Tang J, Li X, Wang N, Zhang S, Lin Q, Li J, Shi H. Correlation between hypoechoic nodules on ultrasonography and benign hyperplasia in the prostatic outer gland. J Ultrasound Med. 2005;24(4):483–8.
6. Carvalhal GF, Smith DS, Mager DE, Ramos C, Catalona WJ. Digital rectal examination for detecting prostate cancer at prostate specific antigen levels of 4 ng/ml or less. J Urol. 1999;161(3):835–9.
7. Okotie OT, Roehl KA, Han M, Loeb S, Gashti SN, Catalona WJ. Characteristics of prostate cancer detected by digital rectal examination only. Urology. 2007;70(6):1117–20.
8. Mottet N, Bastian PJ, Bellmunt J, et al. Guidelines on prostate cancer. The European Association of Urology. 2014. Available from http://uroweb.org/wp-content/uploads/1607-Prostate-Cancer_LRV3.pdf#.
9. Brock M, Eggert T, Palisaar RJ, Roghmann F, Braun K, Loppenberg B, et al. Multiparametric ultrasound of the prostate: adding contrast enhanced ultrasound to real- time elastography to detect histopathologically confirmed cancer. J Urol. 2012;189:93–8.
10. Hovels AM, Heesakkers RA, Adang EM, Jager GJ, Strum S, Hoogevee YL, et al. The diagnostic accuracy of CT and MRI in the staging of pelvic lymph nodes in patients with prostate cancer: a meta- analysis. Clin Radiol. 2008;63:387–95.
11. Puech P, Potiron E, Lemaitre L, Leroy X, Haber GP, Crouzet S, Kamoi K, Villers A. Dynamic contrast-enhanced-magnetic resonance imaging evaluation of intraprostatic prostate cancer: correlation with radical prostatectomy specimens. Urology. 2009;74(5):1094–9.

12. Puech P, Rouviere O, Renard-Penna R, Villers A, Devos P, Colombel M, et al. Prostate cancer diagnosis: multiparametric MR- targeted biopsy with cognitive and transrectal US- MR fusion guidance versus systematic biopsy: prospective multicenter study. Radiology. 2013;268: 461–9.
13. Singh AK, Kruecker J, Xu S, Glossop N, Neeman Z, Choyke P, et al. Initial clinical experience with real- time transrectal ultrasonography- magnetic resonance imaging fusion- guided prostate biopsy. BJU Int. 2008;101:841–5.
14. Turkbey B, Shah VP, Pang Y, Bernardo M, Xu S, Kruecker J, et al. Is apparent diffusion coefficient associated with clinical risk scores for prostate cancers that are visible on 3- T MR images? Radiology. 2010;258:488–95.
15. Maxeiner A, Fischer T, Stephan C, Cash H, Slowinski T, Kilic E, Durmus T. Real-time MRI/US Fusion-guided Biopsy Improves Detection Rates of Prostate Cancer in Pre-biopsied Patients. Aktuelle Urol. 2014;45(3):197–203. Mol Med Rep. 2014;9(5):1989–97.
16. Zhang J, Xiu J, Dong Y, Wang M, Han X, Qin Y, Huang Z, Cai S, Yuan X, Liu Q. Magnetic resonance imaging-directed biopsy improves the prediction of prostate cancer aggressiveness compared with a 12-core transrectal ultrasound-guided prostate biopsy. Mol Med Rep. 2014;9(5):1989–97.
17. Quentin M, Blondin D, Arsov C, Schimmöller L, Hiester A, Godehardt E, Albers P, Antoch G, Rabenalt R. Prospective evaluation of MRI-guided in-bore prostate biopsy versus systematic transrectal ultrasound (TRUS)-guided prostate biopsy in biopsy-naïve men with elevated prostate-specific antigen (PSA) levels. J Urol. 2014. doi:10.1016/j.juro.2014.05.090.
18. Aron M, Rajeev TP, Gupta NP. Antibiotic prophylaxis for transrectal needle biopsy of the prostate: a randomized controlled study. BJU Int. 2000;85(6):682–5.
19. Williamson DA, Roberts SA, Paterson DL, Sidjabat H, Silvey A, Masters J, Rice M, Freeman JT. Escherichia coli bloodstream infection after transrectal ultrasound-guided prostate biopsy: implications of fluoroquinolone-resistant sequence type 131 as a major causative pathogen. Clin Infect Dis. 2012;54(10):1406–12.
20. Taylor S, Margolick J, Abughosh Z, Goldenberg SL, Lange D, Bowie WR, Bell R, Roscoe D, Machan L, Black P. Ciprofloxacin resistance in the faecal carriage of patients undergoing transrectal ultrasound guided prostate biopsy. BJU Int. 2013;111(6):946–53.
21. Losco G, Studd R, Blackmore T. Ertapenem prophylaxis reduces sepsis after transrectal biopsy of the prostate. BJU Int. 2014;113 Suppl 2:69–72.
22. Gopal Rao G, Batura D. Emergency hospital admissions attributable to infective complications of prostate biopsy despite appropriate prophylaxis: need for additional infection prevention strategies? Int Urol Nephrol. 2014;46(2):309–15.
23. Kehinde EO, Al-Maghrebi M, Sheikh M, Anim JT. Combined ciprofloxacin and amikacin prophylaxis in the prevention of septicemia after transrectal Ultrasound guided biopsy of the prostate. J Urol. 2013;189(3):911–5.
24. Adamakis I, Mitropoulos D, Haritopoulos K, Alamanis C, Stravodimos K, Giannopoulos A. Pain during transrectal ultrasonography guided prostate biopsy: a randomized prospective trial comparing periprostatic infiltration with lidocaine with the intrarectal instillation of lidocaine-prilocain cream. World J Urol. 2004;22(4):281–4.
25. Giannarini G, Mogorovich A, Valent F, Morelli G, De Maria M, Manassero F, Barbone F, Selli C. Continuing or discontinuing low-dose aspirin before transrectal prostate biopsy: results of a prospective randomized trial. Urology. 2007;70(3):501–5.
26. Chowdhury R, Abbas A, Idriz S, Hoy A, Rutherford EE, Smart JM. Should warfarin or aspirin be stopped prior to prostate biopsy? An analysis of bleeding complications related to increasing sample number regimes. Clin Radiol. 2012;67(12):e64–70.
27. Ihezue CU, Smart J, Dewbury KC, Mehta R, Burgess L. Biopsy of the prostate guided by transrectal ultrasound: relation between warfarin use and incidence of bleeding complications. Clin Radiol. 2005;60(4):459–63; discussion 457–8.
28. Salomon L, Bastide C, Beuzeboc P, et al. Les members du CCAFU. Recommandations en Onco-Urologie 2013 du CCAFU: Cancer de la Prostate. Prog Urol. 2013;23(Suppl 2):S69–101. p. 6.

29. Berger AP, Gozzi C, Steiner H, Frauscher F, Varkarakis J, Rogatsch H, Bartsch G, Horninger W. Complication rate of transrectal ultrasound guided prostate biopsy: a comparison among 3 protocols with 6, 10 and 15 cores. J Urol. 2004;171(4):1478–80; discussion 1480–1.
30. Pinsky PF, Parnes HL, Andriole G. Mortality and complications after prostate biopsy in the Prostate, Lung, Colorectal and Ovarian Cancer Screening (PLCO) trial. BJU Int. 2014;113(2):254–9.
31. Dimmen M, Vlatkovic L, Hole KH, Nesland JM, Brennhovd B, Axcrona K. Transperineal prostate biopsy detects significant cancer in patients with elevated prostate-specific antigen (PSA) levels and previous negative transrectal biopsies. BJU Int. 2012;110(2 Pt 2):E69–75.
32. Humphrey PA. Diagnosis of adenocarcinoma in prostate needle biopsy tissue. J Clin Pathol. 2007;60(1):35–42.
33. Pavlakis K, Stravodimos K, Kapetanakis T, Gregorakis A, Athanassiadou S, Tzaida O, Constantinides C. Evaluation of routine application of P504S, 34betaE12 and p63 immunostaining on 250 prostate needle biopsy specimens. Int Urol Nephrol. 2010;42(2):325–30.
34. Gleason DF, Mellinger GT. Prediction of prognosis for prostatic adenocarcinoma by combined histological grading and clinical staging. J Urol. 1974;111(1):58–64.
35. Epstein JI, Allsbrook Jr WC, Amin MB, Egevad LL, ISUP Grading Committee. The 2005 International Society of Urological Pathology (ISUP) consensus conference on Gleason grading of prostatic carcinoma. Am J Surg Pathol. 2005;29(9):1228–42.
36. Vollmer RT. Tumour length in prostate cancer. Am J Clin Pathol. 2008;130:77–82.
37. Epstein JI, Herawi M. Prostate needle biopsies containing prostatic intraepithelial neoplasia or atypical foci suspicious for carcinoma: implications for patient care. J Urol. 2006;175(3 Pt 1): 820–34.
38. Merrimen JL, Jones G, Walker D, Leung CS, Kapusta LR, Srigley JR. Multifocal high grade prostatic intraepithelial neoplasia is a significant risk factor for prostatic adenocarcinoma. J Urol. 2009;182(2):485–90; discussion 490.
39. Srigley JR, Merrimen JL, Jones G, Jamal M. Multifocal high-grade prostatic intraepithelial neoplasia is still a significant risk factor for adenocarcinoma. Can Urol Assoc J. 2010;4(6):434.
40. Moore CK, Karikehalli S, Nazeer T, Fisher HA, Kaufman Jr RP, Mian BM. Prognostic significance of high grade prostatic intraepithelial neoplasia and atypical small acinar proliferation in the contemporary era. J Urol. 2005;173(1):70–2.
41. Salomon L, Azria D, Bastide C, Beuzeboc P, Cormier L, Cornu F, et al. Comité de Cancérologie de l'AFU. Recommandations en onco-urologie : cancer de la prostate. Prog Urol. 2010;20: S217–51.
42. Walz J, Graefen M, Chun FK, Erbersdobler A, Haese A, Steuber T, Schlomm T, Huland H, Karakiewicz PI. High incidence of prostate cancer detected by saturation biopsy after previous negative biopsy series. Eur Urol. 2006;50(3):498–505.
43. Prostate. In: Edge SB, Byrd DR, Compton CC, editors. AJCC cancer staging manual. 7th ed. New York: Springer; 2010. p. 461–2.
44. Lavery HJ, Brajtbord JS, Levinson AW, Nabizada-Pace F, Pollard ME, Samadi DB. Unnecessary imaging for the staging of low-risk prostate cancer is common. Urology. 2011;77(2):274–8.
45. Lizée D, Ouzzane A, Villers A. Cancer de la prostate: diagnostic et bilan d'extension. EMC – Urologie. 2012;5(2):1–8. [Article 18-560-A-12].
46. D'Amico AV, Whittington R, Malkowicz SB, Schultz D, Blank K, Broderick GA, et al. Biochemical outcome after radical prostatectomy, external beam radiation therapy, or interstitial radiation therapy for clinically localized prostate cancer. JAMA. 1998;280(11):969–74.
47. D'Amico A, Altschuler M, Whittington R, Kao G, Malkowicz SB, Wein A. The use of clinical parameters in an interactive statistical package to predict pathological features associated with local failure after radical prostatectomy for prostate cancer. Clin Perform Qual Health Care. 1993;1(4):219–22.
48. D'Amico AV, Moul J, Carrol PR, Sun L, Lubeck D, Chen MH. Cancer specific mortality after surgery or irradiation for patients with clinically localized prostate cancer managed during the prostate specific antigen era. J Clin Oncol. 2003;21:2163–72.

Chapter 4
Treatment of the Prostate Cancer

Said Abdallah Al-Mamari and Salim Said Al-Busaidy

The treatment of prostate cancer is a very broad subject where many aspects have to be taken into consideration. Apart from urological surgeons, it involves many specialists from other fields such as medical and radiotherapeutic oncologists, pathologists, radiologists, anaesthetists, geriatricians and specialized nurses. Sometimes, the expertise of a psychologist is also required to assist patients and families receiving unfortunate news.

After the histopathological grading and tumour staging have been defined, a *multidisciplinary expert team* plan the treatment based on whether curative or palliative. The possible benefits and risks as well as the patient's ability to tolerate the treatment are carefully considered in the context of the internationally accepted guidelines. *The treating urologist is the team leader who decides the final treatment which can be quite challenging, requiring flexibility and mature judgement.*

4.1 Primary Treatment (Fig. 4.1)

4.1.1 Localized Disease

This includes *all the tumours not extending beyond the prostate capsule, that is, cT1-T2, N0, M0 disease.* The proposed treatment modalities differ according to D'Amico risk groups' stratification.

S.A. Al-Mamari (✉)
Urology Department, The Royal Hospital, Muscat, Oman
e-mail: sabdal67@yahoo.com

S.S. Al-Busaidy
Senior Consultant and HOD, Urology Department, The Royal Hospital, Muscat, Oman
e-mail: salimalbusaidy@hotmail.com

S.A. Al-Mamari, S.S. Al-Busaidy (eds.), *Urological Cancer Management*,
DOI 10.1007/978-3-319-16301-7_4

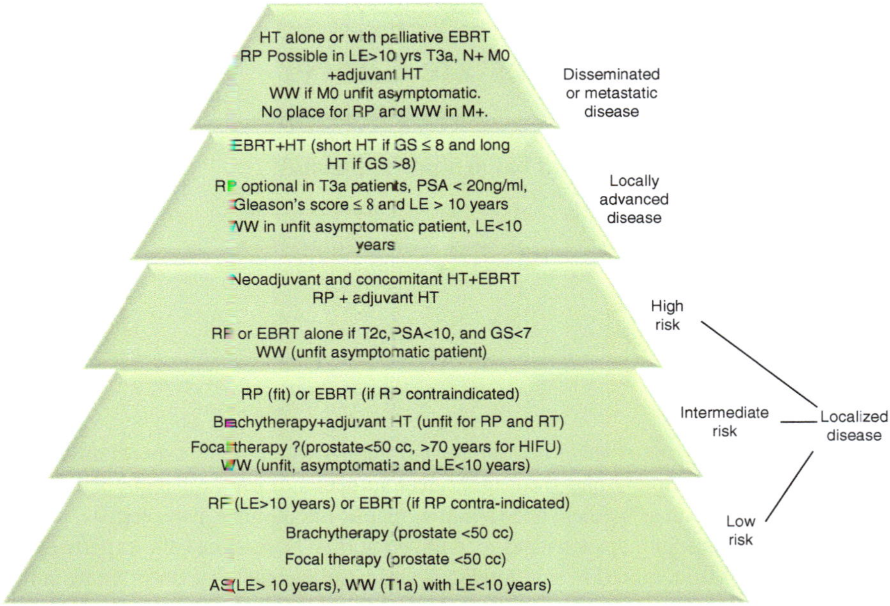

Fig. 4.1 Pyramid of the primary treatment of the prostate cancer

4.1.1.1 Low-Risk Patients

cT1–cT2a, Gleason's score (GS) <7 and PSA ≤ 10 ng/ml.

Observation

Two strategies apply when deciding not to treat the patient actively: watchful waiting (WW) and active surveillance (AS).

Watchful Waiting (WW)

Watchful waiting (WW) is proposed for *patients with T1a* (tumour seen in ≤5 % of tissues resected) *with <10 years life expectancy (LE). The principle of a WW strategy is simply to leave the patient 'alone' as long as he is asymptomatic, and to wait for the disease to eventually become symptomatic or metastatic where only palliative treatment will be offered* [1]. The reason for advocating WW is the expected indolent course of the low risk disease with a short life expectancy. The rationale is *not to endanger a patient's life with a major curative treatment and not to lower his quality of life (QoL).*

> WW may also be proposed to unfit asymptomatic patients at any stage of the disease, except for metastatic disease.

Active Surveillance (AS)

Active surveillance (AS) or active monitoring is indicated for patients with > *10-year life expectancy. The tumour behaviour is closely monitored and when treatment is initiated, it will be with a curative intent.* This strategy avoids over treating indolent tumours and prevents treatment-related complications in the younger age group [2]. During AS, it is recommended to repeat [3]:

- The PSA every 3-6 months for the PSADT calculation,
- A DRE every 6-12 months, and
- The TRUS-guided biopsy between 3-18 months after the first set to rule out undergrading of the tumour.

AS should not be considered when there is more than 50 % prostate cancer (PC) involving any needle biopsy core or more than 3 positive cores in the 12-core protocol [4] or >3 mm of tumour in a core [5].

Pathologists at Johns Hopkins Hospital recommend including the intervening normal prostatic tissue when there are two or more malignant foci in one core by measuring the entire stretch between the extreme ends of the most far apart cancer foci. This was shown to be a better predictor of organ-confined disease and surgical margin positivity in subsequent prostatectomy specimens [6].

AS appears to be the only indication for repeat biopsies after a positive one and before any curative therapy.

In a large retrospective study, patients primarily on AS have shown a *43 % 10-year treatment-free survival, but 100 % 10-year PC-specific survival* [7]. However, a great number of patients requested active treatment only because of anxiety, although objective signs of progression often had not indicated a need to shift to radical treatment.

Active Treatment

Radical Prostatectomy

Radical prostatectomy (RP*)* is *an option for T1a* in younger patients with long life expectancy.

RP is the standard for all other stages of the low risk D'Amico group (T1b–c and T2a, GS <7 and PSA ≤10 ng/ml) if life expectancy is >10 years [3, 8].

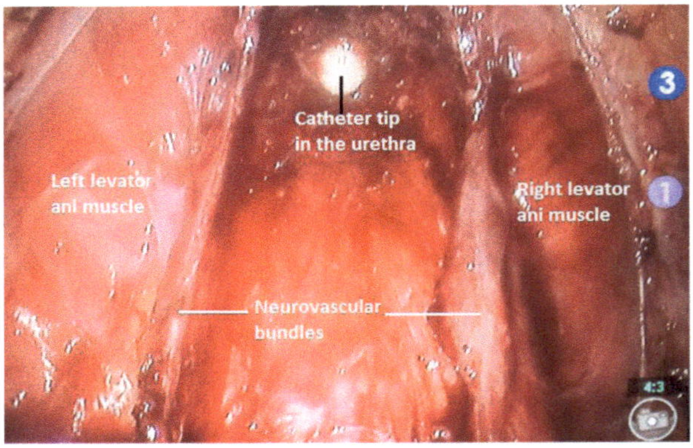

Fig. 4.2 RALP: View of the bilaterally preserved neurovascular bundles before urethro-vesical anastomosis

However, RP requires a patient's informed consent with regard to the complications, especially the possibility of unfavourable outcomes on erectile function and urinary continence [8]. Recently, a very large retrospective study comparing RP with radiotherapy (RT) and observation confirmed the superiority of RP in the overall survival in men with >10 years LE [9].

The techniques of performing RP may be by open surgery (perineal or retropubic), standard laparoscopic prostatectomy (LP) (transperitoneal or extraperitoneal) or robotic assisted laparoscopic prostatectomy (RALP) (also transperitoneal or extraperitoneal). No superiority was found in the oncological or functional outcomes in any of the approaches in one meta-analysis [10]. Another meta-analysis has suggested the superiority of RALP compared to LP and open procedures in terms of positive surgical margins and perioperative complications [11]. *Neurovascular bundles (NVB) preservation is the rule in all low-risk, sexually active patients, in order to prevent or minimize the complications on erectile function and urinary continence. The proposed nerve-preserving techniques consist either of an intrafascial or an interfascial dissection, with the latter appearing to be a better compromise between the functional and oncological outcomes* [12].

The advent of robotic-assisted laparoscopic surgery has brought a substantial contribution to the nerve-preserving techniques (Fig. 4.2). However, it is worth remembering that the da-Vinci robot is still unavailable in many parts of the world, and its high cost may continue to be an obstacle for a large number of institutions, especially in developing countries. On the other hand, the learning curve and technical difficulties of LP continue to challenge many surgeons despite its successful introduction by early pioneers more than 15 years ago [13, 14]. Finally, supporters of the open RP are not yet convinced by the superiority of the novel techniques and the former operation remains the preferred technique in few institutions, including in advanced countries [15].

Extended pelvic lymph nodes dissection (ePLND) with no frozen biopsy study is only optional in low risk cancers, because the nodal disease risk is very low (<7 %) [16].

This degree of risk does not justify the increased morbidity: lymphocoele, lymphoedema, deep venous thrombosis, pulmonary embolism, ureteral injury, obturator nerve injury, iliac vessels injury etc. [17, 18].

Major surgery is contraindicated in patients in the anaesthetic categories of ASA 3 and 4 according to the classification adopted by the American Society of Anesthesiologists in 1963 and last approved in 2014 (Table 4.1) [19].

Table 4.1 ASA physical status classification system [19], last approved by the ASA House of Delegates on October 15, 2014

ASA Physical status classification	Definition	Examples, including, but not limited to:
ASA I	A normal healthy patient	Healthy, nonsmoking, no or minimal alcohol use
ASA II	Mild systemic disease	Mild diseases only with substantive functional limitations. Examples include (but not limited to): current smoker, social alcohol drinker, pregnancy, obesity (30<BMI<40), well-controlled DM/HTN, mild lung disease
ASA III	Severe systemic disease	Substantive functional limitations; one or more moderate to severe diseases. Examples include (but not limited to): poorly controlled DM or HT, COPD, morbid obesity (BMI≥40), active hepatitis, alcohol dependence or abuse, implanted pacemaker, moderate reduction of ejection fraction, ESRD undergoing regularly scheduled dialysis, premature infant PCA<60 weeks, history (>3 months) of MI, CVA, TIA, CAD/stents.
ASA IV	Severe systemic disease that is a constant threat to life	Examples include (but not limited to): recent (<3 months) MI, CVA, TIA, or CAD/stents, ongoing cardiac ischaemia or severe valve dysfunction, severe reduction of ejection fraction, sepsis, DIC, ARD or ESRD not undergoing regularly scheduled dialysis
ASA V	A moribund person who is not expected to survive without the operation	Examples include (but not limited to): ruptured abdominal/thoracic aneurysm, massive trauma, intracranial bleed with mass effect, ischemic bowel in the face of significant cardiac pathology or multiple organ/systemic dysfunction
ASA VI	A declared brain-dead person whose organs are being removed for donor purposes	

Reproduced with permission from the American Society of Anesthesiologists, 1061 American Lane, Schaumburg, Illinois 60173

The mention 'E' is added if the surgery is performed in emergency basis, for example, '3E'. Class 5 per se is an emergency and is therefore usually '5E'. Organ retrieval in brain-dead patients (class 6) is also done urgently

External Beam Radiation Therapy

External Beam Radiation Therapy (EBRT) is another option. *Its indications parallel those of RP, but will be recommended only when RP is contraindicated or cannot be performed, because it is associated with multiple complications (interstitial radiation: cystitis, proctitis).* In conventional EBRT, a total dose of *64 Grays (Gy)* is delivered in multiple small fractions of 1.2–2 Gy each. Newer methods have been developed to minimize the side effects of EBRT, allowing higher fractionated and total doses *(≥74 Gy) to be given.* These include the following:

- *Intensity modulated radiotherapy IMRT, now considered as the gold standard.*
- Three-dimensional conformal radiotherapy 3D-CRT.
- Use of tridimensional conformational technique with intensity modulation (RCMI) permits higher dose and hypofractionating. RCMI allows for the irradiation of larger pelvic volumes including the whole prostate and lymph node (LN) areas without increasing toxicity [20].

Contraindications of EBRT

Absolute contraindications include previous pelvic radiation, Crohn's disease and active procto-colitis. Relative ones are presence of voiding difficulty and a recent history of transurethral resection of the prostate (TURP). It is advised to wait 6–8 weeks after a TURP to minimize the risk of urethral stricture which would be aggravated by EBRT.

Low-Dose Rate Transperineal Brachytherapy

Low-dose rate transperineal brachytherapy (from the Greek word *βραχυς*, pronounced brachys, which means 'short' or 'brief'): 140 Gy Iodide (^{125}I) or Iridium (^{192}Ir) or 120 Gy Palladium (^{103}Pd) radioisotopes are the most frequently used seeds in permanent interstitial prostatic brachytherapy. Brachytherapy can be considered in patients with a *cancer volume ≤50 ml, with less than 50 % of biopsy scores involved with cancer, and an International Prostate Symptom Score (I-PSS) ≤12 (mild to moderate urinary symptoms).*

Contraindications of Brachytherapy

A prostate volume >50 ml, the presence of a median lobe, a history of TURP and coexisting voiding difficulty. The presence of a median lobe increases the risk of a postimplantation urinary retention and a history of TURP increases the risk of incontinence [21]. Herein a modified TURP technique was recently proposed for men with moderate lower urinary tract infection (LUTS) prior to brachytherapy, in an attempt to prevent the traditional TURP-related complications [22].

Brachytherapy alone (154 Gy) is recommended for low risk patients, that is, GS 3 + 4 and a PSA <15 ng/ml [23], *but not for intermediate risk patients because the probability of biochemical failure is higher than with RP or RT* [24]. Neoadjuvant hormonal therapy prior to brachytherapy should not be initiated as it was shown to be associated with an increased risk of overall mortality [25].

The American expert panel has added a further perspective and concluded [26]:

'AS, interstitial prostate brachytherapy, EBRT, and RP are all appropriate monotherapy options for the low-risk group of patients, and the preference of one to another should be made on an individual patient basis'.

4.1.1.2 Intermediate Risk Patients

cT2b, GS 7 or PSA >10 and ≤20 ng/ml. There is no place here for WW, unless the patient is asymptomatic and unfit for any curative treatment. Also AS is not an option for any GS ≥7 or any PSA ≥10 ng/ml.

The treatment may be RP or EBRT, while brachytherapy and hormonal treatment are possible alternatives for patients unfit for the former treatment options.

In intermediate risk group, the probability of nodal involvement is estimated to be around 10–25 %. *It is therefore recommended to perform bilateral pelvic lymphnode dissection (PLND) aiming at clearing the obturator fossa as well as the internal and external iliac lymph nodes (LN) chains* [27]. A more extensive PLND (with ≥10 LN removed) has been shown to positively affect the biochemical relapse (BCR)-free survival in patients with intermediate- and high-risk prostate cancers [28]. NVB preservation may be bilateral, but is not recommended when extracapsular extension is suspected (T3a).

A bilateral PLND which should include the ilio-obturators, internal and external iliac groups of LNs up to the bifurcation of the common iliac *vessels is recommended in all intermediate and high risk groups. It is optional in low risk group. Frozen section is not recommended anymore* [3].

The limits of standard PLND and extended PLND (ePLND) are given in Table 4.2. However, the nomenclature varies according to publishing centres and a more detailed nomenclature was recently proposed including a limited, a standard, an extended and a superextended PLND [29] (Fig. 4.3).

In intermediate risk patients, EBRT can be given alone with an increased dose (>81Gy) or combined with a short course of hormonal therapy (HT). HT or androgen deprivation therapy (ADT) may be started 2 months before EBRT (70 Gy) and

Table 4.2 Anatomical limits of standard PLND and ePLND

	Standard PLND	Extended PLND (ePLND)
Proximal	Common iliac vessels bifurcation	Aortic bifurcation
Lateral	Genitofemoral nerve	Same
Medial	Bladder wall	Same
Distal	Inguinal ligament	Same
Posterior	Obturator nerve	Hypogastric vessels and pelvic floor

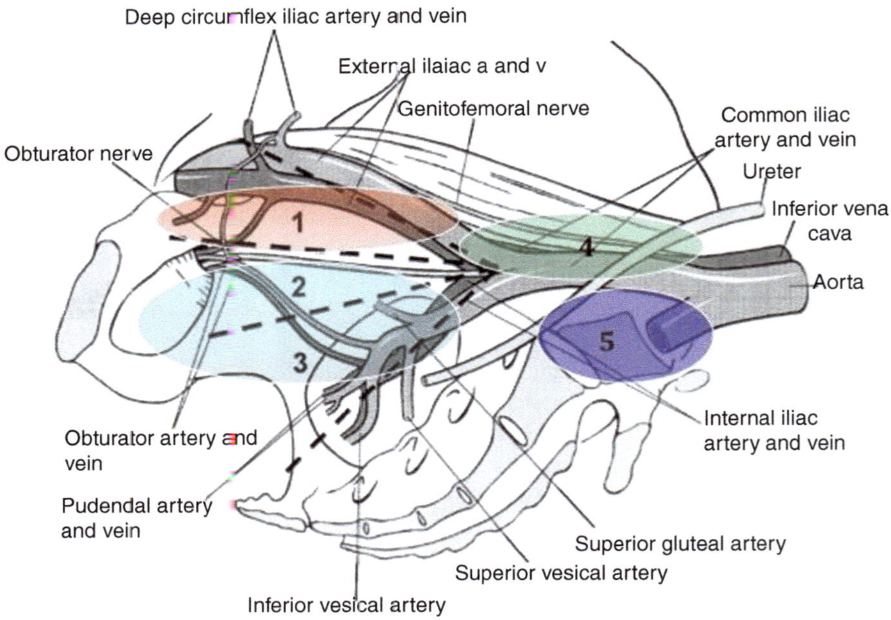

Fig 4.3 Proposed new nomenclature of pelvic lymph nodes dissection (PLND) [29]: Limited PLND (area 1): posteriorly up to the obturator nerve (corresponds to the classical standard PLND). Standard PLND (areas 1–3): deeper below the obturator nerve onto the internal iliac vessels (corresponds to the classical ePLND). Extended PLND (areas 1–4): proximally up to the aortic bifurcation. Superextended PLND (areas 1–5): deeper to the presacral region. *A* artery, *V* vein (By Ploussard et al. *European Urology*, January 2014; Reproduced and translated with permission from Elsevier)

continued for a total of 4–6 months. This *neoadjuvant and concomitant treatment* has been shown to be associated with significantly decreased disease-specific mortality and increased overall survival in the intermediate risk group, as opposed to lower risk group [30]. The benefit of pelvic LN radiation has not been demonstrated [31].

4.1.1.3 High Risk Patients

cT2c or PSA >20 ng/ml or GS >7: As with the intermediate risk group, there is no place for AS. *Despite the lack of consensus, a combination therapy may be recommended in high risk patients, and would consist of neoadjuvant hormonal treatment and concomitant hormonal therapy with EBRT*. This has been shown to result in an increased overall survival rate which was summarized in a review of several prospective randomized trials [32]. *These studies demonstrated that RP + adjuvant HT was associated with a lower cancer-specific mortality compared with EBRT + adjuvant HT* [33]. In highly selected patients with T2c, PSA <10 and GS <7, RP or RT alone remains a possible option, however very close posttreatment follow-up is required. Indeed, many researchers have suggested that this tumour is considered as an intermediate risk rather than the traditional high risk tumour based solely on the T2c status [34]. *HT may be a first line treatment option for palliation of patients with a short LE and a localized but more extensive or poorly differentiated PC* [26].

> If controversy and doubt exist about the benefits of neoadjuvant HT prior to EBRT, it is nonetheless generally agreed that *there is no place for neoadjuvant HT prior to RP for localized PC whatever the prognostic group* [35–39].

The Role of Focal Therapies

These therapeutic options are still under evaluation and it is necessary to inform patients who are offered these treatments about the limited data available for long-term (≥10 years) outcomes [8]. Two modalities are discussed:

High Intensity Focused Ultrasound (HIFU)

This causes tissue damage by thermal effects and cavitation. Temperatures over 65 °C result in coagulative necrosis. The procedure is performed utilizing transrectal ultrasound (U/S)-guidance under spinal or general anaesthesia. It is frequently preceded by a TURP to prevent the risk of urinary retention induced by the immediate cavitation and flare-up of the prostatic gland provoked by the ultrasound [40].

The qualifying criteria for this treatment are: *patients >70 years with LE ≥7 years, T1-T2N0M0, GS ≤7 (3 + 4), PSA ≤15, prostate volume <50 cc and limited tumour volume* (less than 4 out of 6 zones involved) [41]. Disease relapse is diagnosed by a *PSA value ≥Nadir + 2*. Patients with *any sign of progression* should be considered for *salvage radiotherapy*.

> Note: *Nadir* is derived from an Arabic word (نظير) which means 'opposed to'. It was first used in astronomy to refer to the lowest point of a star or a planet in the sky, as opposed to its highest level, the *zenith*, also from Arabic etymology. It is used here to refer to *the lowest level of the PSA in the follow-up after a treatment with curative intent*.

Cryotherapy

This is based on the principle of freezing and thawing the prostate in cycles using cryoneedles guided by transrectal ultrasonography. Temperatures of minus 40 ° C are reached under general anaesthesia. The insertion of a urethral warmer is mandatory to avoid thermal injury. The indications include *lower and intermediate risks tumours with volume <40 ml. The most commonly encountered complication is erectile dysfunction which occurs in 50–90 % of patients.* Other complications include urinary incontinence, bladder neck obstruction, recto-urethral fistulae and perineal pain [42].

4.1.2 Locally Advanced Disease

This includes tumours extending through the prostatic capsule and eventually invading the bladder neck or the seminal vesicles, that is, T3a-b, N0, M0.

(a) WW remains an option even for T3 patients unfit for local treatment, with a GS <7, and a life expectancy <10 years.
(b) *Combination of RT and HT (or ADT) is now considered as the standard of care for locally advanced PC*, as this has shown significant improvement in the 10-year survival compared with either RT or HT alone [43]. In this setting it has been suggested that patients with a lower GS (≤8) *could* have short-term HT (6 months). However those with a higher GS *must* be given a long-term HT (preferably ≥ 2 years if tolerated) because of the demonstrated better survival rate [44].
(c) RT alone is another option as primary treatment for T3 patients when LE is 5–10 years.
(d) For patients unfit for RT, long-term hormonal treatment alone can be recommended especially for symptomatic T3b patients, with high PSA >25–50, and PSA DT <1 year.
(e) RP is optional for T3a patients, PSA <20 ng/ml, biopsy Gleason's score ≤ 8 and LE >10 years, but *surgery must be non-nerve preserving with pelvic LN dissection*. The patient must be informed about the *increased possibility of adjuvant HT* in the follow-up because of an increased risk of positive surgical margins (PSM), unfavourable histology and positive lymph nodes in the final histopathology specimen. Similarly *adjuvant or salvage EBRT might also be indicated* when there are adverse pathological findings in the prostatectomy specimen (seminal vesicles invasion, PSM, or extraprostatic extension). This strategy was credited for the reductions in biochemical recurrences, local recurrence and clinical progression documented in earlier studies [45–47], however the patients should be informed on the uncertain impact of adjuvant EBRT on subsequent metastases and overall survival [48].

> As with localized PC, *neoadjuvant HT is not indicated prior to RP for locally advanced disease.*

4.1.2.1 Modalities of Hormonal Therapy

Complete (or Combined) Androgen Blockade (CAB)

The simplest way to achieve a CAB is by the combination of a bilateral orchiectomy with the use of anti-androgens. Another strategy includes a lutenizing hormone agonist such as leuprolide or goserelin and an androgen-receptor agonist such as flutamide, nilutamide and bicalutamide. The first group of drugs suppresses the secretion of testicular androgens and the second group inhibits the action of circulating androgens on their receptors. *Presently CAB is not recommended in locally advanced disease because of very poor survival benefit (<5 %) compared with anti-androgen monotherapy* [3].

Bicalutamide (Casodex®) 150-mg Monotherapy

Bicalutamide (Casodex) 150-mg monotherapy has also been shown to have a better posttreatment IIEF-5 score than CAB and could be considered as the treatment for locally advanced prostate cancer in patients concerned by their sexual function [49]. Bicalutamide 150 mg, either as monotherapy or adjuvant therapy to RP or EBRT, has also been shown to improve the progression-free survival (PFS) in patients with locally advanced prostate cancer, *but not in patients with localized disease* who have demonstrated no clinically or statistically significant improvement and even an unfavourable survival trend compared with WW. Bicalutamide 150 mg also showed benefit in the overall survival (OS) of patients with locally advanced disease as an adjuvant therapy to EBRT [50].

Continued or Intermittent Treatment

The latter aims at improving the side effect profile.

Short or Long

Short or long in combination with EBRT.

Side Effects of Hormonotherapy
Hot flashes, erectile dysfunction and loss of libido, gynaecomastia, cognitive functions impairment and mood disorders, anaemia, fatigue, pseudometabolic syndrome (gain of weight, insulin-resistance), osteopenia. *Osteopenia seems to be the most worrisome side effect of hormonotherapy as it may lead to spontaneous fractures*. The specific mortality of hip fracture at one year is 37.5 % and this complication alone contributes to an estimated 39-month loss in prostate cancer life expectancy [51].

4.1.3 Disseminated or Metastatic Disease

This is defined by disease extension to pelvic organs (other than seminal vesicles) or wall (i.e. T4), or any N+ or any M+.

Once more, WW is still acceptable for *M0 asymptomatic patients, with PSA <50 ng/ml and PSA DT >12 months;* however, very close follow-up is required. M+ patients are not suitable for WW.

RP is an option for N+, M0 and ≤T3a patients with LE >10 years. However, RP in this setting must be followed by early adjuvant hormonotherapy [8].

RT indications parallel those of RP, but a combination with androgen deprivation therapy (ADT) for 3 years is mandatory.

The benefit of adjuvant HT in pN1 patients remains controversial and survival has not been substantiated in a recent study [52].

HT is the standard adjuvant therapy in N+ disease with more than one positive LN, after RP or RT. In M0 disease, HT should not be used as monotherapy for patients fit for surgery or radiotherapy. It is the standard option for M+ disease where there is no place for WW and RP. Here RT can have a palliative option, in combination with androgen deprivation, to alleviate local cancer symptoms.

All patients with M+ disease should be offered *bilateral orchidectomy* as an alternative to continuous luteinizing hormone-releasing hormone (LHRH) agonist therapy (Goserelin or Zoladex®, leuprorelin and triptorelin). During the initial 1–2 weeks of LHRH-agonist therapy, a biochemical and, sometimes, a clinical '*flare*' can occur. This may be dangerous especially in presence of vertebral metastases whose flare may compress the spine with neurological consequences. Anti-androgen treatment using cyproterone acetate, diethylstilbestrol, flutamide or nilutamide should be initiated prior to/and concomitant with LHRH-agonist in the first 2 weeks to prevent this adverse event. Ketoconazole is also effective in this setting. LHRH-antagonists (Degarelix) are new drugs reported to cause a more rapid reduction in testosterone levels avoiding the testosterone-induced flare, and to be more effective at maintaining testosterone within castrate levels [53] (Table 4.3).

Novel drugs have not yet been recommended for primary treatment: Orteronel (TAK-700), galeterone (TOK-700), enzalutamide (MDV3100, Xtandi®) and ARN-509.

One should appreciate that with the general population's increasing LE, it is commonly recommended to overlook the patient's *chronological age* and consider the *biological or physiological age* which takes into account the patient's general condition, life style and the presence or absence of comorbidities. The Oncological University Center of Toulouse (IUCT-O) has proposed a theoretical projected estimate of the specific PC mortality which showed that if cardiovascular causes of mortality were delayed in the future, *this shift would unmask the PC specific mortality.* In other words, it implies that in future many patients will qualify for active PC treatment at an age presently considered as being too old. Conversely, the delay in PC mortality would increase deaths from other causes, deepening the masking effect on the PC specific mortality. This is referred to as 'competitive mortality theory' (Fig. 4.4a–c).

Table 4.3 Drugs used in hormonotherapy for PC

Surgical castration (the 'gold standard')	*Bilateral orchidectomy*. Subcapsular orchidectomy, also called *testicular pulpectomy*, has the advantage of leaving behind the tunica albuginea which gives the patient the psychological satisfaction of 'still having something to palpate in the scrotum'. Replacing the testes by size-matched silicon prostheses can serve the same purpose
Androgen synthesis inhibitors	Old drugs: Aminogluthetimide, ketoconazole (Nizoral)
	Newer drug: CYP 17 blockers: Abiraterone (Zytiga®)
Anti-androgens	These drugs block androgens by competitively binding to their receptors:
	Steroidal: Cyproterone acetate (Androcur)
	Nonsteoidal: Flutamide (Eulexin®), *bicalutamide* (Casodex®), nilutamide (Nilandron®).
	Newer drugs : Enzalutamide (Xtandi®, MDV3100)
Inhibitors of LHRH	Lutenizing hormone releasing hormone (LHRH)-agonists: Goserelin (Zoladex®), *leuprolide* (Lupron®, Eligard®), triptorelin (Trelstar®), histrelin (Vantas®)
	LHRH-antagonists: Degarelix (Firmagon®), abarelix, cetrorelix
Estrogens	Diethylstilbestrol diphosphate: Fosfetrol (Honvan®)

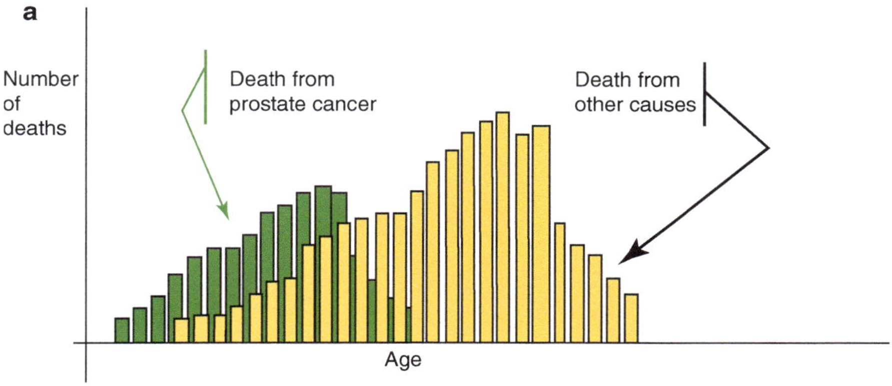

Fig. 4.4 (**a**–**c**) Competitive mortality theory between death from PC and other diseases. (**a**) Mortality from prostate is in competition with mortality from other causes. Therefore the specific mortality from PC is the result of various evolutions. (**b**) Decrease in mortality from cardiovascular may "unmask" the specific mortality from PC, causing the latter to increase. (**c**) Conversely a delay in the mortality from PC may deepen the masking effect through increased mortality from other causes (**a**–**c**: By P. Grosclaude, Tarn Cancers Registry, IUCT-O, Toulouse, F-31059, France. Reproduced and translated with permission)

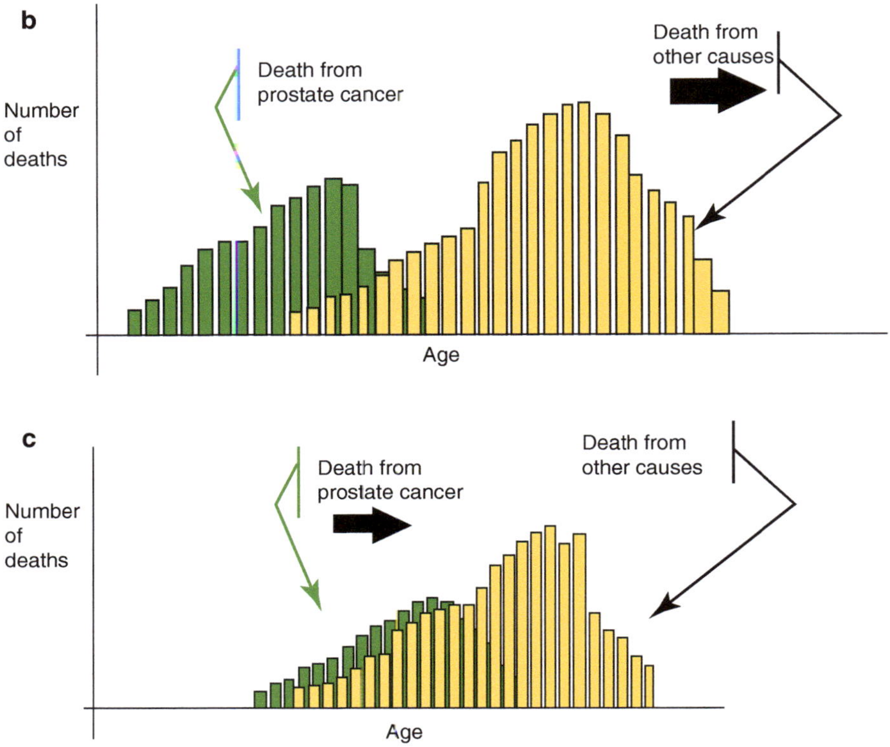

Fig. 4.4 (continued)

Take-Home Message: Role of the Various Primary Treatment Modalities in PC

Watchful waiting	*Standard in T1a with GS <7, LE <10*
	Optional in asymptomatic T3 GS <7, LE <10 years unfit for local treatment
	Optional asymptomatic M0, N+ with PSA <50 ng/ml, PSA DT >12 months (very close follow-up)
Active surveillance	This requires a regular follow-up of the patient with repeat PSA every 3–6 months for PSADT calculation, DRE every 6–12 months and TRUS-guided biopsy between 3 and 18 after the first set to rule out undergrading of the tumour
	All T1a when LE >10
	T1b-T2b with PSA <10, GS <7, ≤2 positive biopsies and ≤50 % cancer in each biopsy, patients LE <10 years, patients LE >10 years (informed about lack of survival data beyond 10 years), patients refusing treatment-related complications

Radical prostatectomy	*Standard treatment for organ-confined disease (T1a-T2c) with LE >10. Best indication for T1a when GS ≥7*
	Optional for T3a patients with PSA <20, GS ≤8 and LE >10. Increased risk of PSM, positive LN and unfavourable histology. Hence adjuvant RT or HT possibly needed
	Optional for N+ patients <T4 and LE >10 years, combined with adjuvant RT or HT
	No place in M+ patients
External beam radiation therapy	T1a in younger patients with long LE and GS >7.
	All organ-confined disease (T1c–T2c) with LE >10 unfit for surgery and accepting related complications. Unfit patients with LE 5–10 and GS >7 (combined with adjuvant HT
	T3 with LE >5–10 years. Escalating dose and adjuvant HT
	Optional in N+ with LE >10, combined with 3 years HT
	Local symptoms alleviation in M+. No curative intent
Brachytherapy	Low risk d'Amico group with prostate volume ≤50 ml and IPSS ≤12
Hormone therapy (ADT)	*As monotherapy:*
	Standard option in M+ disease and mandatory in symptomatic patients
	In organ-confined disease except T1a: palliation for symptomatic patients unfit for RP and RT. But avoid anti-androgens.
	In T3b-T4 with PSA >50 and PSA DT <1 year for patient unfit for RT
	In N+ for patients unfit for local therapies
	Combination of radiotherapy and HT (or ADT) is now considered as the standard of care for locally advanced PC. HT may be provided in a short (6 months) or long term protocol (≥2 years) respectively in patients with lower GS (≤8) or higher GS.
	Adjuvant therapy: *Standard N+ with more than one LN positive after RP or RT as primary treatment.*
	Neoadjuvant therapy: *No place prior to RP. Controversial place prior to/and concomitant with EBRT in high risk localized disease.*
Ablative therapies	These less invasive procedures are proposed for localized disease. They are still under evaluation, but have shown promising results.
	HIFU: patients >70 years with LE ≥7 years, T1-T2N0M0, GS ≤7 (3 + 4), PSA ≤15, prostate volume <50 cc and limited tumour volume (less than 4 zones involved out of 6)
	Cryotherapy: lower and intermediate risks tumour with volume <40 ml

4.2 Follow-up Management

The follow-up of a patient after a curative intent primary treatment is based upon the prognostic risk factors of the tumour, the initial treatment and the patient's conditions. It basically consists of a clinical examination and repeated total serum-PSA measurements. *The F/T PSA-ratio is not indicated and imaging investigations are only justified in case of biochemical failure or symptomatic patients.*

The correlation between the time to biochemical recurrence and the PSA doubling time (PSADT) with the site of recurrence and the PC specific mortality has been known for some time. *A late biochemical recurrence (BR) (>3 years) or a longer PSADT (>6 months) is associated with local disease recurrence and an earlier BR or a shorter PSADT suggests distant metastatic progression with increased risk of PC specific mortality* [54, 55].

The first PSA estimation after curative treatment should not be performed before 3 months because the 3-day half-life normally makes the marker become undetectable only 4–6 weeks after RP [56].

- The *definition of biological failure or relapse* depends on the primary treatment:
  - *After RP,* a first PSA is checked at 3 months and should then be repeated every 6 months for 3–5 years, then annually for 10–15 years. *Any PSA >0.2 ng/ml is regarded as a sign of possible residual or recurrent disease and must be confirmed by a repeat test* [57].
  - *After ERBT and brachytherapy, any PSA rising more than 2 ng/ml above the nadir* (Phoenix criteria) has to be considered as a sign of possible persistent or recurrent disease [58]. *A PSA value of less than 0.5 ng/ml following RT or brachytherapy is an indicator of good prognosis* [59–61], *but it may take up to 2 years post-RT for the PSA to reach the nadir (if no adjuvant HT is given), and even 5–6 years after brachytherapy* [62].
  - *After HIFU,* a PSA nadir ≤0.2 ng/ml correlates to a favourable oncological outcome [63], and the biochemical failure is determined as per the 'Stuttgart definition': *PSA nadir + 1.2 ng/ml* [64]. This justifies repeat transrectal ultrasound-guided prostatic (TRUS) biopsy to confirm disease recurrence and plan salvage therapy.
  - *After cryotherapy*: The target PSA nadir is ≤0.5 ng/ml, although levels of ≤1.0 ng/ml with stable readings are also considered as acceptable [65]. Biochemical recurrence is defined as an increase in PSA *of ≥0.2 ng/ml over the nadir* [66] or an absolute level of 0.5–1.0 ng/ml after repeat cryoablation [67].
  - *After hormonal treatment*: Three prognostic groups can be defined 6–9 months after ADT according to the serum PSA level: favourable (PSA <0.2 ng/ml), intermediate (0.2–0.4 ng/ml) and unfavourable (>0.4 ng/ml) [68].

TRUS-guided prostatic biopsy after either RP or EBRT is useful only if it will affect the treatment plan.

Imaging Modalities European Expert panel recommends *avoidance of CT, MRI investigations and isotope bone scans for detecting metastases in asymptomatic patients when the serum PSA levels are less than 20 ng/ml. But a bone scan should be considered in symptomatic patients (bone pain) irrespective of the serum PSA levels* [69]. When justified by symptoms and/or biochemical failure, various imaging tools should be used according to the extent of the suspected therapeutic failure:

- Local failure: there are studies suggesting that *multiparametric MRI (mp-MRI)* may be a better alternative to choline-PET in the detection and mapping of locally recurrent PC both after RP and RT. MRI can define recurrences early enough to allow for focal salvage treatments to be performed [70]. *mp-MRI is now the preferred imaging modality after either RP, EBRT, brachytherapy or focal therapies* (HIFU and cryotherapy)

– Distant metastasis: isotope bone scan, ^{18}F-sodium-fluoride Positron Emission Tomography-Tomodensitometry (FNa PTE-TDM*), fluoro-choline-PET-TDM and whole body MRI (Fig. 4.5) are all possible imaging means. Axial skeleton MRI has been proven superior to isotope bone scintigraphy for metastasis detection in high risk patients with sensitivity and specificity of 100 and 88 %, respectively* [71]. The corresponding values of technetium-99 m bone scintigraphy in the same study were only 46 and 42 %, respectively; 100 % specificity was achieved by the triple combination of axial skeleton MRI-Isotope bone scan-Targeted X ray. *^{18}F-Fluoro-desoxy-glucose (18F-FDG) PET-TDM is not indicated for PC because glucose uptake by the prostatic cancer cells is poor.*

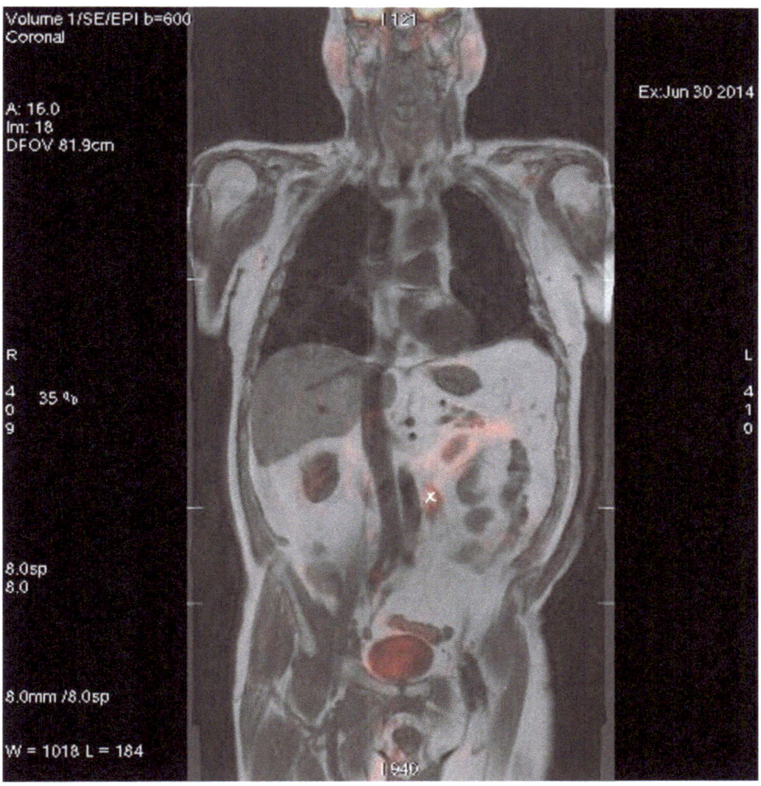

Fig. 4.5 Whole body MRI with images fusion between an anatomical T1-weighted sequence and a diffusion sequence. This study was performed for the disease-extent investigation of a PC and revealed a left paraaortic LN (**x**) (Courtesy of S. Novellas, Radiology, Arnault-Tzanck Institute, Saint-Laurent- du- Var and CHU Nice, Nice, France)

Take-Home Message: Follow-Up Modalities After Curative Treatment and Definition of Biochemical Failure/Relapse

A late biochemical failure (>3 years) or a longer PSADT (>6 months) is associated with a local recurrence and an early failure or a shorter PSADT is suggestive of a distant metastasis and an increased risk of PC specific mortality. Criteria to define BR depend on the primary treatment:

After RP	Any *PSA >0.2 ng/ml.* Needs to be confirmed by a repeat test.
Radiotherapy (either EBRT or Brachytherapy)	Any *PSA rising more than 2 ng/ml above the nadir* (Phoenix criteria)
	Nadir value <0.5 mg/ml is a favourable sign, but the nadir may take very long time to be reached (2 years for EBRT, up to 5–6 years for brachytherapy).
HIFU	PSA nadir + 1.2 ng/ml ('Stuttgart definition')
Cryotherapy	Increase in PSA of ≥0.2 ng/ml over the nadir, or absolute level of 0.5–1.0 ng/ml for repeat cryoablation
Hormonotherapy	There is no definition of biochemical relapse since this is not a curative intent treatment. However three prognostic groups may be defined 6–9 months after the initiation of ADT: favourable (PSA <0.2 ng/ml), intermediate (0.2–0.4 ng/ml) and unfavourable (>0.4 ng/ml).

Imaging investigations are justified only in case of biochemical failure and in symptomatic patients. Their choice depends on the local or distant nature of the disease.

Local failure	*mp-MRI*
Distant failure	*Fluoro-choline-PET-TDM*, FNa PTE-TDM, isotope bone scan, *whole body MRI. 18F-FDG-PET-TDM is not indicated.*
	Imaging investigations for bony metastases are not recommended in asymptomatic patients with PSA <20 ng/ml.
	But to consider an isotope bone scan in symptomatic patients (bone pain) irrespective of the serum PSA level.

4.3 Treatments of Relapse

It is always necessary to first categorize a relapse into either a purely *local* or *distant* one. Three commonly used parameters can help in this distinction: the initial pathological features, the time elapsed from the initial curative treatment (RP and RT) to the relapse and the PSADT. Poorly differentiated tumour (GS ≥7), an early PSA relapse and a short PSA DT (<6 months) are all signs of distant metastases, while positive surgical margins, late occurrence of biochemical failure (>12 months), PSADT >10 months and GS ≤7 are suggestive of local failure [72]. Apart from those predictive criteria, repeat imaging studies (MRI pelvis, CT chest and abdomen) are important to restage the disease when salvage therapy is contemplated with curative intent (e.g. RT after primary RP).

Defining whether the relapse is local or distant is necessary to guide the urologist in selecting the appropriate treatment:

- *Presumed local recurrence after RP: Salvage radiation therapy (SRT)* with at least 64–66 Gy is indicated, *preferably before the PSA has risen above 0.5 ng/ml* [73], because the effectiveness of EBRT *is greatest when given early with lower PSA levels.* Furthermore, an increase in pre-SRT PSA also directly correlates with an increase in the SRT dose required to achieve a given biochemical progression-free survival. This results in an increase in severe late toxicity [48, 74, 75]. LE <10 years can justify active surveillance (AS) with the possibility of giving HT should the patient become symptomatic.
- *Presumed local failure after RT – Salvage RP can be offered in selected patients after confirmation of the local nature of the recurrence*: PSA kinetics, repeat positive biopsy of the prostate and imaging (MRI or choline-PET) are helpful in ruling out distant metastases. In this setting *non-nerve-sparing surgery* is recommended and the procedure should be performed only *in experienced centres* because of the *high risk of incontinence* (21–90 %) and other complications, for example, bleeding, rectal injury, urethro-vesical anastomotic strictures etc. [76]. *Salvage cryoablation* is offered to patients unfit for surgery [66]. AS can also be offered to patients with LE <10 years, while contemplating the possibility of HT later.
- *Presumed distant metastases after either RP or RT:* There is no role for local therapies except for palliation. *Early HT* (<4 months) may be offered as it has some survival benefit compared to delayed HT [77]. However, conflicting results have been published in different studies [78]. One controversial question remains unanswered: *does the sole presence of LN metastases or asymptomatic bony or soft tissue metastases justify the side effects of long-term HT?* The latest opinion suggests initiating HT in symptomatic patients only.
- *Relapse after HT*: This is referred to as *castration-resistant prostate cancer (CRPC)* which can be metastatic (mCRPC) or not. It is diagnosed by a *PSA progression in three consecutive readings despite a documented castration level of testosterone defined as <32 ng/dl* (normal level is 500–600 ng/dl or 17.3–20.8 nmol/l). Another definition is the appearance of two or more bony lesions on a bone scan or a soft tissue mass. CRPC often affects elderly patients and the decision whether to provide further cancer-targeted treatment or not has *to be individualized for each case and debated in a multidisciplinary approach* with an input from medical and radiation oncologists, urologists, geriatric physicians, nurses, psychologists and social workers. If adopted, further treatment is staged in three steps:

  1. *Anti-androgen withdrawal once PSA progression is documented.* This may produce some response 4–6 weeks after discontinuation of flutamide and bicalutamide (Casodex®). The phenomenon of anti-androgen withdrawal

syndrome was first described for *flutamide* over 20 years ago. A decrease in serum PSA level after the removal of the drug is often associated with clinical improvement [79]. Similar phenomena were described later on with other anti-androgen drugs: Bicalutamide, cyproterone acetate and more recently with abiraterone acetate [80] and enzalutamide [81]. This phenomenon is attributed to androgen receptor mutation in which the drugs paradoxically stimulate rather than inhibit; however, the exact mechanism has not been clarified [82].

2. *Second-line hormonal manipulation: Abiraterone* (Zytiga) and *enzalutamide* (MDV3100) (Xtandi®).
3. *Cytotoxic therapy: This is reserved only for metastatic CRPC.*
   - First line: Docetaxel (Taxotere®) at 75 mg/m^2 every 3 weeks (significant survival benefit). If the docetaxel is contra-indicated, mitoxantrone + prednisolone or hydrocortisone can be proposed.
   - Second line: Combination of cabazitaxel (Jevtana®) and abiraterone (Zytiga®).

Take-Home Message: Treatment of Relapse

This depends on the local or distant nature of the relapse and on the primary treatment.	
The *initial pathological features*, the *time to BR* and the *PSADT* are the three commonly used predictive factors to suggest the local or distant nature of the recurrence.	
Local failure after RP	Salvage radiation therapy (SRT) with at least 64–66 Gy, *preferably before PSA has risen above 0.5 ng/ml*
Local failure after RT	A non-nerve-sparing salvage RP can be offered in selected patients after good confirmation of the local nature of the failure. To be reserved for experienced centres only because of high risk of complications (incontinence, etc.).
	Salvage cryoablation for patients unfit for surgery
	AS in asymptomatic patients with LE <10 years, with possible HT later on when indicated
Presumed distant failure after either RP or RT	Early HT (<4 months). But this is a controversial recommendation and many authors would advise to start HT later on when the symptoms occur
Failure after HT (CRPC)	CRPC is defined by *a PSA progression in three consecutive readings despite a documented castration level of testosterone defined as <32 ng/dl.* Can be metastatic (mCRPC) or not. Further management is discussed in a multidisciplinary approach and treatment eventually proceeds in three steps: Anti-androgen withdrawal Second-line hormonal manipulation: Abiraterone and enzalutamide
	Cytotoxic drugs only for mCRPC: First-line Docetaxel, second line cabazitaxel and abiraterone

4.4 Palliative Management of CRPC Patients

The mere goal of the treatment is to improve the patient's quality of life (QoL) and to control pain. No attempt should be made to hypothetically prolong the patient's life with additional hormonal manipulation which will only worsen his condition by additional side effects [8]. Patients with non-metastatic CRPC should not be offered systemic chemotherapy or immunotherapy outside the context of a clinical trial [83].

When skeletal metastasis is documented, *biphosphonates such as zoledronic acid (Zometa®, Zomera®, Aclasta® or Reclast®)* are indicated to prevent osseous complications; however, beware of the known side effect of *osteonecrosis of the jaw (ONJ) occurring in 0.85 % of patients* [84]. *Denosumab (an anti-RANKL antibody)* has been shown to have a better efficacy than zoledronic acid in the prevention of osseous events; however, it has also been incriminated in jaw osteonecrosis [85].

Radionuclides (strontium-89, radium-223), EBRT, cementoplasty with poly-methyl methacrylate (PMMA) and analgesic agents can also be considered early on in the management of painful osseous metastases. Cementoplasty is also indicated when an immediate bone structure consolidation is needed especially in osteolytic lesions to prevent a pathological fracture. It helps also to provide a rapid pain regression and mobility improvement [85]. The alpha-emitting radium-223 has a shorter radiation range (≤100 μm) which reduces damage to surrounding healthy tissues resulting in a more localized effect compared to the beta-emitting strontium-89 and samarium-153 (several millimetres radiation range) [86, 87]. Therefore, bone marrow suppression (cytopenias) is less common with Ra-223 and this radionuclide is now recommended by the American expert panel for docetaxel-naive patients with symptomatic bony metastases, good PS and with no visceral metastases [88].

Docetaxel-based chemotherapy is the standard care for symptomatic mCRPC patients, with good performance status [8, 88].

Combined with prednisolone, Docetaxel is associated with improved patient survival and QoL with moderate toxic side effects. The combination of abiraterone and prednisolone is the second choice, while ketoconazole + steroid, mitoxantrone or radionuclide therapy *is an option for patients who do not want or cannot tolerate the standard therapies* [88, 89]. The very recent multinational AFFIRM trial which enrolled over 1,000 men with mCRPC men from Europe and North America after failure of docetaxel has shown significant benefit in improving the patients' overall survival when given enzalutamide over placebo [90]. Cabazitaxel + prednisolone is another proposed combination for patients after docetaxel failure due to the proven survival benefit. Sipuleucel-T is an autologous drug (vaccine) used as immunotherapy for asymptomatic or minimally symptomatic docetaxel-naïve patients and has also shown survival benefit [91]. However, the particular toxicity risk of cabazitaxel and sipuleucel-T should be discussed with the patient. Other vaccines being tried include GVAX-PCa, viral prostate vaccines (ProstVac VF, or PSA-TRICOM and Ad5-PSA), DNA-based vaccines (DNA-PAP and DNA-PSA) and gene-mediated cytotoxic immunotherapy (through intratumoural delivery of an adenovirus encoding the Herpes simplex virus enzyme thymidine kinase) [92]. Bevacizumab, estramustine and sunitinib should not be offered because of the excessive toxicity without obvious clinical benefit [89].

Take-Home Message: Palliative Management of CRPC Patients

The treatment aims only at improving the patient's quality of life (QoL) and at controlling pain.	
Skeletal metastases: prevention of pathological fractures	*Biphosphonates (zoledronic acid) or denosumab (an anti-RANKL antibody).* Beware of jaw osteonecrosis. Cementoplasty with polymethyl methacrylate (PMMA)
Skeletal metastases: prevention of pain	Radionuclides (strontium-89, radium −223), EBRT, cementoplasty with polymethyl methacrylate (PMMA) and analgesic agents. ^{223}Ra is preferred to ^{89}Sr because of a shorter radiation range and a consequently less healthy-tissue damage and bone marrow suppression
Symptomatic mCRPC patients with good performance	*Docetaxel + prednisolone: Standard care because it* improves patient's survival and QOL with moderate toxicity risk
	Second choice: Abiraterone + prednisolone
	Ketoconazole + steroid, mitoxantrone or radionuclide therapy is other possible option.
mCRPC patients after failure of docetaxel	Cabazitaxel + prednisolone or enzalutamide
Minimally symptomatic or asymptomatic patients with no prior docetaxel	Sipuleucel-T
Currently, no place for bevacizumab, estramustine or sunitinib	

References

1. Albertsen PC, Hanley JA, Gleason DF, Barry MJ. Competing risk analysis of men aged 55 to 74 years at diagnosis managed conservatively for clinically localized prostate cancer. JAMA. 1998;280:975–80.
2. Staerman F, Peyromaure M, Irani J, Gaschignard N, Mottet N, Soulié M, et al. Place de la surveillance active dans le cancer de la prostate à faible risque de progression. Prog Urol. 2011;21:448–54.
3. Salomon L, Bastide C, Beuzeboc P, et al. Les membres du CCAFU. Recommandations en onco-urologie 2013 du CCAFU: Cancer de la prostate. Prog Urol 2013; 23(Suppl 2):S69–101.
4. Patel MI, DeConcini DT, Lopez-Corona E, Ohori M, Wheeler T, Scardino PT. An analysis of men with clinically localized prostate cancer who deferred definitive therapy. J Urol. 2004;171(4) 1520–4.

5. Bastian PJ, Carter BH, Bjartell A, Seitz M, Stanislaus P, Montorsi F, et al. Insignificant prostate cancer and active surveillance: from definition to clinical implications. Eur Urol. 2009;55:1321–30.
6. Karram S, Trock BJ, Netto GJ, Epstein JI. Should intervening benign tissue be included in the measurement of discontinuous foci of cancer on prostate needle biopsy? Correlation with radical prostatectomy findings. Am J Surg Pathol. 2011;35:1351–5.
7. van den Bergh RC, Roemeling S, Roobol MJ, Aus G, Hugosson J, Rannikko AS, Tammela TL, Bangma CH, Schröder FH. Outcomes of men with screen-detected prostate cancer eligible for active surveillance who were managed expectantly. Eur Urol. 2009;55(1):1–8.
8. Mottet N, Bastian PJ, Bellmunt J, et al. Guidelines on prostate cancer. The European Association of Urology. 2014. http://uroweb.org/wp-content/uploads/1607-Prostate-Cancer_LRV3.pdf#
9. Sun M, Sammon JD, Becker A, Roghmann F, Tian Z, Kim SP, Larouche A, Abdollah F, Hu JC, Karakiewicz PI, Trinh QD. Radical prostatectomy vs radiotherapy vs observation among older patients with clinically localized prostate cancer: a comparative effectiveness evaluation. BJU Int. 2014;113(2):200–8.
10. Moran PS, O'Neill M, Teljeur C, Flattery M, Murphy LA, Smyth G, et al. Robot- assisted radical prostatectomy compared with open and laparoscopic approaches: a systematic review and meta- analysis. Int J Urol. 2013;20:312–21.
11. Tewari A, Sooriakumaran P, Bloch DA, Seshadri-Kreaden U, Hebert AE, Wiklund P. Positive surgical margin and perioperative complication rates of primary surgical treatments for prostate cancer: a systematic review and meta-analysis comparing retropubic, laparoscopic, and robotic prostatectomy. Eur Urol. 2012;62(1):1–15.
12. Al-Mamari SA, Quintens H, Mentine N, Burté C, Rouyer N, Jacob G, Amiel J. RALP: comparison of the oncological and functional outcomes of the intrafascial and the interfascial approaches. Prog Urol. 2015;25:54–61.
13. Schuessler WW, Schulam PG, Clayman RV, et al. Laparoscopic radical prostatectomy: initial short-term experience. Urology. 1997;50:854–7.
14. Guillonneau B, Vallencien G. Laparoscopic radical prostatectomy: initial experience and preliminary assessment after 65 operations. Prostate. 1999;39:71–5.
15. Barré C. Open radical retropubic prostatectomy. Eur Urol. 2007;52:71–80.
16. Partin AW, Mangold LA, Lamm DM, Walsh PC, Epstein JI, Pearson JD. Contemporary update of prostate cancer staging nomograms (Partin Tables) for the new millennium. Urology. 2001;58:843–8.
17. Keegan KA, Cookson MS. Complications of pelvic lymph node dissection for prostate cancer. Curr Urol Rep. 2011;12(3):203–8.
18. Briganti A, Chun FK, Salonia A, Suardi N, Gallina A, Da Pozzo LF, Roscigno M, Zanni G, Valiquette L, Rigatti P, Montorsi F, Karakiewicz PI. Complications and other surgical outcomes associated with extended pelvic lymphadenectomy in men with localized prostate cancer. Eur Urol. 2006;50(5):1006–13.
19. New Classification of Physical Status. Anesthesiology. 1963; 24:111. http://www.asahq.org/search?q=asa%20physical%20status%20classification%20system
20. Riou O, Regnault de la Mothe P, Azria D, Ailleres N, Dubois JB, Fenoglietto P. Simultaneous integrated boost plan comparison of volumetric- modulated arc therapy and sliding window intensity-modulated radiotherapy for whole pelvis irradiation of locally advanced prostate cancer. J Appl Clin Med Phys. 2013;14:4094.
21. Chen AB, D'Amico AV, Neville BA, Earle CC. Patient and treatment factors associated with complications after prostate brachytherapy. J Clin Oncol. 2006;24(33):5298–304.
22. Brousil P, Hussain M, Lynch M, Laing RW, Langley SE. Modified TURP for men with moderate LUTS prior to brachytherapy is safe and feasible. BJU Int. 2014. doi: 10.1111/bju.12798. [Epub ahead of print].
23. Nag S, Beyer D, Friedland J, Grimm P, Nath R. American Brachytherapy Society (ABS) recommendations for transperineal permanent brachytherapy of prostate cancer. Int J Radiat Oncol Biol Phys. 1999;44:789–99.

24. D'Amico AV, Whittington R, Malkowicz SB, Schultz D, Blank K, Broderick GA, et al. Biochemical outcome after radical prostatectomy, external beam radiation therapy, or interstitial radiation therapy for clinically localized prostate cancer. JAMA. 1998;280(11):969–74.
25. Dosoretz AM, Chen MH, Salenius SA, Ross RH, Dosoretz DE, Katin M, et al. Mortality in men with localized prostate cancer treated with brachytherapy with or without neoadjuvant hormone therapy. Cancer. 2010;116(4):837–42.
26. Thompson I, Thrasher JB, Aus G, Burnett AL, Canby-Hagino ED, Cookson MS, D'Amico AV, Dmochowski RR, Eton DT, Forman JD, Goldenberg SL, Hernandez J, Higano CS, Kraus SR, Moul JW, Tangen CM, AUA Prostate Cancer Clinical Guideline Update Panel. Guideline for the management of clinically localized prostate cancer 2007 update. J Urol. 2007;177(6):2106–31.
27. Heidenreich A, Ohlmann CH, Polyakov S. Anatomical extent of pelvic lymphadenectomy in patients undergoing radical prostatectomy. Eur Urol. 2007;52:29–37.
28. Schiavina R, Manferrari F, Garofalo M, Bertaccini A, Vagnoni V, Guidi M, Borghesi M, Baccos A, Morselli-Labate AM, Concetti S, Martorana G. The extent of pelvic lymph node dissection correlates with the biochemical recurrence rate in patients with intermediate- and high-risk prostate cancer. BJU Int. 2011;108(8):1262–8.
29. Ploussard G, Briganti A, de la Taille A, et al. Pelvic lymph node dissection during robot-assisted radical prostatectomy: efficacy, limitations, and complications—a systematic review of the literature. Eur Urol. 2014;65:7–16.
30. Jones CU, Hunt D, McGowan DG, Amin MB, Chetner MP, Bruner DW, et al. Radiotherapy and short- term androgen deprivation for localized prostate cancer. N Engl J Med. 2011;365:107–18.
31. Peneau M, Villers A, Molinie V, Theis D, Soulié M. Indications de la lymphadénectomie ilio-obturatrice dans le cancer de prostate cliniquement localisé. Prog Urol. 2004;14:287–94.
32. Roach M. Neoadjuvant hormonal therapy in men being treated with radiotherapy for localized prostate cancer. Rev Urol. 2004;6 Suppl 8:S24–31.
33. Lee JY, Cho KS, Kwon JK, Jeh SU, Kang HW, Diaz RR, Ham WS, Koom WS, Keum KC, Choi YD. A competing risk analysis of cancer-specific mortality of initial yreatment with radical prostatectomy versus radiation therapy in clinically localized high-risk prostate cancer. Ann Surg Oncol. 2014;21(12):4026–33.
34. Furubayashi N, Nakamura M, Hishikawa K, et al. Radical prostatectomy as radical cure of prostate cancer in a high-risk group: a single-institution experience. Mol Clin Oncol. 2013;1(2):337–42.
35. Soloway MS, Pareek K, Sharifi R, Wajsman Z, McLeod D, Wood Jr DP, et al. Neoadjuvant androgen ablation before radical prostatectomy in cT2bNxMo prostate cancer: 5- year results. J Urol. 2002;167:112–6.
36. Klotz LH, Goldenberg SL, Jewett MA, Fradet Y, Nam R, Barkin J, et al. Long- term followup of a randomized trial of 0 versus 3 months of neoadjuvant androgen ablation before radical prostatectomy. J Urol. 2003;170:791–4.
37. Aus G, Abrahamsson PA, Ahlgren G, Hugosson J, Lundberg S, Schain M, et al. Three- month neoadjuvant hormonal therapy before radical prostatectomy: a 7- year follow- up of a randomized controlled trial. BJU Int. 2002;90:561–6.
38. Schulman CC, Debruyne FM, Forster G, Selvaggi FP, Zlotta AR, Witjes WP. 4- year follow-up results of a European prospective randomized study on neoadjuvant hormonal therapy prior to radical prostatectomy in T2-3N0M0 prostate cancer. European Study Group on Neoadjuvant Treatment of Prostate Cancer. Eur Urol. 2000;38:706–13.
39. Van Poppel H. Neoadjuvant hormone therapy and radical prostatectomy: the jury is still out. Eur Urol 2001; 39:10–4. Prezioso D, Lotti T, Polito M, Montironi R. Neoadjuvant hormone treatment with leuprolide acetate depot 3.75 mg and cyproterone acetate, before radical prostatectomy: a randomized study. Urol Int 2004; 72:189–95.
40. Rebillard X, Soulié M, Chartier-Kastler E, Davin JL, Mignard JP, Moreau JL, et al. High-intensity focused ultrasound in prostate cancer; a systematic literature review of the French Association of Urology. BJU Int. 2008;101:1205–13.

41. Salomon L, Azria D, Bastide C, Beuzeboc P, Cormier L,Cornu F, et al. Comité de Cancérologie de l'AFU. Recommandations en onco- urologie: cancer de la prostate. Prog Urol 2010; 20:S217–51.
42. Finley DS, Pouliot F, Miller DC, Belldegrun AS. Primary and salvage cryotherapy for prostate cancer. Urol Clin North Am. 2010;37:67–82.
43. Quero L, Wong-Hee-Kam S, Rivera S, Hennequin C. Association of radiotherapy and hormonotherapy in locally advanced prostate cancer. Bull Cancer. 2012;99 Suppl 1:S30–6.
44. Bolla M, de Reijke TM, Van Tienhoven G et al. EORTC Radiation Oncology Group and Genito-Urinary Tract Cancer Group. Duration of androgen suppression in the treatment of prostate cancer. N Engl J Med. 2009; 360(24):2516–27.
45. Bolla M, Van Poppel H, Collette L, Van Cangh P, Vekemans K, Da Pozzo L, et al. European Organization for Research and Treatment of Cancer. Postoperative radiotherapy after radical prostatectomy: a randomised controlled trial (EORTC trial 22911). Lancet 2005;366:572–8.
46. Wiegel T, Bottke D, Steiner U, Siegmann A, Golz R, Störkel S, et al. Phase III postoperative adjuvant radiotherapy after radical prostatectomy compared with radical prostatectomy alone in pT3 prostate cancer with postoperative undetectable prostate- specific antigen: ARO 96-02/ AUO AP 09/95. J Clin Oncol. 2009;27:2924–30.
47. Thompson Jr IM, Tangen CM, Paradelo J, Lucia MS, Miller G, Troyer D, et al. Adjuvant radiotherapy for pathological T3N0M0 prostate cancer significantly reduces risk of metastases and improves survival: long- term follow up of a randomized clinical trial. J Urol. 2009;181:956–62.
48. Thompson IM, Valicenti RK, Albertsen P, Davis BJ, Goldenberg SL, Hahn C, Klein E, Michalski J, Roach M, Sartor O, Wolf Jr JS, Faraday MM. Adjuvant and salvage radiotherapy after prostatectomy: AUA/ASTRO Guideline. J Urol. 2013;190(2):441–9.
49. Kang YJ, Kim KH, Lee KS. Efficacy of bicalutamide 150-mg monotherapy compared with combined androgen blockade in patients with locally advanced prostate cancer. Korean J Urol. 2014;55(5):315–20.
50. Iversen P, McLeod DG, See WA, Morris T, Armstrong J, Wirth MP, Casodex Early Prostate Cancer Trialists' Group. Antiandrogen monotherapy in patients with localized or locally advanced prostate cancer: final results from the bicalutamide Early Prostate Cancer programme at a median follow-up of 9.7 years. BJU Int. 2010;105(8):1074–81.
51. Mg O, Ricchiuti V, Conrad W, Resnick MI. Skeletal fractures negatively correlate with overall survival in men with prostate cancer. J Urol. 2002;168:1005–7.
52. Wong YN, Freedland S, Egleston B, Hudes G, Schwartz JS, Armstrong K. Role of androgen deprivation therapy for node- positiveprostate cancer. J Clin Oncol. 2009;27:100–5.
53. Crawford ED, Hou AH. The role of LHRH antagonists in the treatment of prostate cancer. Oncology (Williston Park). 2009;23(7):626–30.
54. Hancock SL, Cox RS, Bagshaw MA. Prostate specific antigen after radiotherapy for prostate cancer: a reevaluation of long-term biochemical control and the kinetics of recurrence in patients treated at Stanford University. J Urol. 1995;154(4):1412–7.
55. Freedland SJ, Humphreys EB, Mangold LA, Eisenberger M, Partin AW. Time to prostate specific antigen recurrence after radical prostatectomy and risk of prostate cancer specific mortality. J Urol. 2006;176(4 Pt 1):1404–8.
56. Mn S, Aj S, Klein EA. Natural history of biochemical recurrence after radical prostatectomy: risk assessment for secondary therapy. Eur Urol. 2007;51:1175–84.
57. Soulié M, Beuzeboc P, Cornud F, Eschwege P, Gaschignard N, Grosclaude P, et al. Comité de Cancérologie de l'Association Française d'Urologie. Recommandations 2007 en onco- urologie. Cancer de la prostate. Prog Urol 2007;17:1157–230.
58. Roach 3rd M, Hanks G, Thames HJR, Schellhammer P, Shipley WU, et al. Defining biochemical failure following radiotherapy with or without hormonal therapy in men with clinically localized prostate cancer: recommendations of the RTOG- ASTRO Phoenix Consensus Conference. Int J Radiat Oncol Biol Phys. 2006;65:965–74.
59. Nelson CP, Rubin MA, Strawderman M, Montie JE, Sanda MG. Preoperative parameters for predicting early prostate cancer recurrence after radical prostatectomy. Urology. 2002;59:740–6.

60. Ray ME, Thames HD, Levy LB, Horwitz EM, Kupelian PA, Martinez AA, Michalski JM, Pisansky TM, Shipley WU, Zelefsky MJ, Zietman AL, Kuban DA. PSA nadir predicts biochemical and distant failures after external beam radiotherapy for prostate cancer: a multi-institutional analysis. Int J Radiat Oncol Biol Phys. 2006;64(4):1140–50.
61. Palma D, Tyldsley S, Blood P, Liu M, Morris J, Pickles T. Prostate cohort outcomes initiative: pretreatment PSA velocity as a predictor of disease outcome following radical radiation therapy. Int J Radiat Oncol Biol Phys. 2007;67:1425–9.
62. Grimm PD, Blasko JC, Sylvester JE, Meier RM, Cavanagh W. 10 year biochemical (PSA) control of prostate cancer with 125I brachytherapy. Int J Radiat Oncol Biol Phys. 2001;51:31–40.
63. Ganzer R, Rogenhofer S, Walter B, Lunz JC, Schostak M, Wieland WF, Blana A. PSA nadir is a significant predictor of treatment failure after high-intensity focussed ultrasound (HIFU) treatment of localised prostate cancer. Eur Urol. 2008;53(3):547–53.
64. Blana A, Brown SC, Chaussy C, Conti GN, Eastham JA, Ganzer R, et al. High- intensity focused ultrasound for prostate cancer: comparative definitions of biochemical failure. BJU Int. 2009;104:1058–62.
65. Cytron S, Greene D, Witzsch U, Nylund P, Bjerklund Johansen TE. Cryoablation of the prostate: technical recommendations. Prostate Cancer Prostatic Dis. 2009;12(4):339–46.
66. De La Taille A, Benson MC, Bagiella E, Burchardt M, Shabsigh A, Olsson CA, et al. Cryoablation for clinically localized prostate cancer using an argon-based system: complication rates and biochemical recurrence. BJU Int. 2000;85:281.
67. Bahn DK, Lee F, Badalament R, Kumar A, Greski J, Chernick M. Targeted cryoablation of the prostate: 7-year outcomes in the primary treatment of prostate cancer. Urology. 2002;60(2 Suppl 1):3.
68. Salomon L, Bastide C, Beuzeboc P, et al. Les membres du CCAFU. Recommandations en onco-urologie 2013 du CCAFU: Cancer de la prostate. Prog Urol, 2013;23(Suppl 2): S69–101. p. 20.
69. Mottet N, Bastian PJ, Bellmunt J, et al. Guidelines on prostate cancer. The European Association of Urology. 2014. p. 133–4. Available from http://uroweb.org/wp-content/uploads/1607-Prostate-Cancer_LRV3.pdf#.
70. Flavio B, Valeria P. Multiparametric MRI for recurrent prostate cancer post radical prostatectomy and postradiation therapy. Biomed Res Int. 2014;2014:316272.
71. Lecouvet FE, Geukens D, Stainier A, et al. Magnetic resonance imaging of the axial skeleton for detecting bone metastases in patients with high-risk prostate cancer: diagnostic and cost-effectiveness and comparison with current detection strategies. J Clin Oncol. 2007;25(22):3281–7.
72. Buskirk SJ, Pisansky TM, Schild SE, MacDonald OK, Wehle MJ, Kozelsky TF, et al. Salvage radiotherapy for isolated prostate specific antigen increase after radical prostatectomy: evaluation of prognostic factors and creation of a prognostic scoring system. J Urol. 2006;176:985–90.
73. Stephenson AJ, Scardino PT, Kattan MW, Pisansky TM, Slawin KM, Klein EA, et al. Predicting the outcome of salvage radiation therapy for recurrent prostate cancer after radical prostatectomy. J Clin Oncol. 2007;25:2035–41.
74. Ohri N, Dicker AP, Trabulsi EJ, Showalter TN. Can early implementation of salvage radiotherapy for prostate cancer improve the therapeutic ratio? A systematic review and regression meta-analysis with radiobiological modelling. Eur J Cancer. 2012;48(6):837–44.
75. King CR. The timing of salvage radiotherapy after radical prostatectomy: a systematic review. Int J Radiat Oncol Biol Phys. 2012;84(1):104–11.
76. Heidenreich A, Richter S, Thuer D, Pfister D. Prognostic parameters, complications, and oncologic and functional outcome of salvage radical prostatectomy for locally recurrent prostate cancer after 21st- century radiotherapy. Eur Urol. 2010;57:437–43.
77. Newling DW. Early versus late androgen deprivation therapy in metastatic disease. Urology. 2001;58(2 Suppl 1):50–5.
78. Keating NL, O'Malley AJ, McNaughton-Collins M, Oh WK, Smith MR. Use of androgen deprivation therapy for metastatic prostate cancer in older men. BJU Int. 2008;101(9):1077–83.

79. Kelly WK, Scher HI. Prostate specific antigen decline after antiandrogen withdrawal: the flutamide withdrawal syndrome. J Urol. 1993;149(3):607–9.
80. Gauthier H, Bousquet G, Pouessel D, Culine S. Abiraterone acetate withdrawal syndrome: does it exist? Case Rep Oncol. 2012;5(2):385–7.
81. Phillips R. Prostate cancer: an enzalutamide antiandrogen withdrawal syndrome. Nat Rev Urol. 2014;11(7):366.
82. Miyamoto H, Rahman MM, Chang C. Molecular basis for the antiandrogen withdrawal syndrome. J Cell Biochem. 2004;91(1):3–12.
83. Hoff AO, Toth BB, Altundag K, et al. Osteonecrosis of the jaw in patients receiving intravenous bisphosphonate therapy. J Clin Oncol. 2006;24(Suppl):8528.
84. Fizazi K, Carducci M, Smith M, Damio R, Brown J, Karsh L, et al. Denosumab versus zoledronic acid for treatment of bone metastases in men with castration- resistant prostate cancer: a randomised, double- blind study. Lancet. 2011;377:813–22.
85. Anselmetti GC. Osteoplasty: percutaneous bone cement injection beyond the spine. Semin Intervent Radiol. 2010;27(2):199–208.
86. Saylor PJ, Armstrong AJ, Fizazi K, Freedland S, Saad F, Smith MR, Tombal B, Pienta K. New and emerging therapies for bone metastases in genitourinary cancers. Eur Urol. 2013;63(2):309–20.
87. McDevitt MR, Sgouros G, Finn RD, Humm JL, Jurcic JG, Larson SM, Scheinberg DA. Radioimmunotherapy with alpha-emitting nuclides. Eur J Nucl Med. 1998;25(9):1341–51.
88. Cookson MS, Roth BJ, Dahm P, Engstrom C, Freedland SJ, Hussain M, Lin DW, Lowrance WT, Murad MH, Oh WK, Penson DF, Kibel AS. Castration-resistant prostate cancer: AUA guideline. J Urol. 2013;190(2):429–38.
89. Basch E, Loblaw DA, Oliver TK et al. Systemic Therapy in Men With Metastatic Castration-Resistant Prostate Cancer: American Society of Clinical Oncology and Cancer Care Ontario Clinical Practice Guideline. J Clin Oncol. 2014;32(30):3436–48.
90. Merseburger AS, Scher HI, Bellmunt J, et al. Enzalutamide in European and North American men participating in the AFFIRM trial. BJU Int. 2014. doi:10.1111/bju.12898. [Epub ahead of print].
91. Ouzaid I, Ravery V. Sipuleucel-T: a prostate cancer vaccine: “instructions for use” for urologists. Prog Urol. 2011;21(9):595–8.
92. Geary SM, Salem AK. Prostate cancer vaccines: update on clinical development. Oncoimmunology. 2013;2(5):e24523.

Part II
Urinary Bladder Tumours

Said Abdallah Al-Mamari and Salim Said Al-Busaidy

Introduction

Bladder cancer (BC) or bladder tumour (BT) is the second most common urological malignancy after PC. In this study we will mainly consider transitional cell carcinoma (TCC) and only a brief account will be given for the other pathological entities. Several points differentiate BT from PC in a clinical point of view. Many etiological factors have been consistently linked to BT with smoking being the most frequent. There is no serum marker used in the diagnosis nor in the follow-up of this tumour. BT is rarely asymptomatic and often produces early symptoms with haematuria being the most frequent. There is no watchful waiting in this tumour as it is capable of rapid progression with fatal issue. Surveillance applies here only after the tumour has been totally resected endoscopically and is limited to low-grade non-muscle invasive tumours. Localized muscle-invasive tumours are ideally addressed by a radical cystectomy or a radiation therapy and chemotherapy is used for metastatic disease.

Chapter 5
Epidemiology, Pathology, Aetiological Factors, Prevention, Screening, Symptoms, and Signs

Said Abdallah Al-Mamari and Salim Said Al-Busaidy

5.1 Epidemiology

Urinary bladder cancer (or tumour) (BC or BT) had an estimated worldwide incidence of 430,000 new cases in 2012 comprising 330,000 men and 100,000 women approximately [1]. The associated specific mortality was 165,000 [1] in the world and 55,200 in the European Union and the United States alone [2].

Contrary to PC, Caucasian Americans are more likely to develop BC than African Americans [3].

The male-to-female ratio is generally reported to be 5:3 and *approximately 75 % of newly diagnosed urinary BCs are noninvasive*.

The estimated annual cost of treatment of BC is 3.4 billion dollars in the United States [4].

It mostly affects elderly patients with the *majority of them presenting at an age of 60 plus* [5, 6]; however, many studies of subjects aged 40 years or younger have been published [7, 8]. *The younger age group is associated with low-grade disease and a relatively good prognosis*.

Unlike PC, bladder cancers must generally be treated rapidly once diagnosed regardless of the clinical stage because of the possibility of a rapidly progressive disease with lethal consequences.

S.A. Al-Mamari (✉) • S.S. Al-Busaidy
Urology Department, The Royal Hospital, Muscat, Oman
e-mail: sabdal67@yahoo.com; salimalbusaidy@hotmail.com

S.A. Al-Mamari, S.S. Al-Busaidy (eds.), *Urological Cancer Management*,
DOI 10.1007/978-3-319-16301-7_5

5.2 Histopathology

It is consistent with transitional cell carcinoma (TCC) in 90 % of cases [9]. The majority of urothelial cancers are found in their pure form, but they are known to show variant histological features or divergent differentiation such as the squamous or glandular types as well as carcinosarcomas and micropapillary tumours. The second most commonly encountered histopathological type in developed countries is *squamous cell carcinoma* (*SCC*) seen in approximately 2.7 %, followed by *adenocarcinoma* (1 %). These two types are more common in developing countries. Rarer types of primary bladder tumours are seen including lymphomas, leiomyosarcomas, rhabdomyosarcomas, and small cell (neuroendocrine) carcinomas. Secondary bladder malignancies can occur either by direct invasion from a local cancer such as a PC in men, or a cervical cancer in women, or as metastases from a distant primary. Neurofibromas, pheochromocytomas, and myomas are well-known benign tumours which also affect the bladder.

5.3 Aetiological Factors

The most commonly incriminated aetiological factor for TCC is smoking which accounts for 50 % of the cases. A large retrospective study conducted in the United States and published in 2011 revealed the incidence rates of 177.3, 119.8, and 39.8 per 100,000 person-years seen in current, former, and never smokers, respectively [10].

The incriminated carcinogenic agents contained in the tobacco smoke are aromatic amines (benzidine, 4-aminobiphenyl, 2-naphthylamine, 4-chloro-o-toluidine) and polycyclic aromatic hydrocarbons which are filtered by kidneys and excreted in the urine. As tobacco advertising is being banished in most Western countries, the geography of smoking will possibly move from developed to developing countries, with the probable increase in bladder cancer incidence in these communities in the next decades [11].

5.3.1 *Occupational Exposure*

Occupational exposure to the aromatic amines, polycyclic aromatic hydrocarbons, as well as chlorinated hydrocarbons contained in dyes, paint, and petroleum products is the second most common risk factor in BC [12].

5.3.2 *Genetic Susceptibility*

The most frequently altered gene in humans, p53, nicknamed the *guardian of human genome*, has been described for a long time [13]. Indeed p53 tumour suppression gene mutations or overexpressions have been widely studied in relation to different tumour types, and these anomalies were shown to be associated with an unfavourable prognosis in urothelial carcinomas [14]. Inherited genetic factors, such as the genetic slow acetylator *N*-acetyltransferase (NAT2) variants and glutathione S-transferase mu 1 (GSTM1) null genotypes, have been established as risk factors in BC, and the risk of BC is reported to be twofold higher in first-degree relatives of BC patients [12]. A recent study has suggested genetic predisposition in relation to the urea transporter (UT) gene SLC14A (*SLC14A1*) which is associated with renal urine concentration, thus with the concentration of carcinogens in contact with urothelial surfaces [15]. This would support the old "*urogenous contact hypothesis*" which associates the development of bladder cancer with prolonged exposure of the urothelium to carcinogens in urine. Conversely it suggests that increasing urine production (with higher fluid intake) and voiding frequently can reduce the risk of BC. Another supporting fact for this theory is the commonly encountered, but not yet fully researched, localization of TCC in the region just above the ureteral meatus and the posterior wall as opposed to the anterior wall. This area is where carcinogen-containing urine is believed to stagnate longer during the patient's sleep in the normal supine position.

5.3.3 Dietary Factors

Increased fluid intake has protective effects by diluting the carcinogens and increasing micturition. Arsenic contained in water and trihalomethanes have been suggested as possible causative factors for bladder cancer. However, the relationship with coffee and alcohol is controversial [12].

5.3.4 Environmental Pollution

These include air pollution and ionizing radiation.

5.3.5 Medical Conditions and Drugs

Cyclophosphamide (alkylating agent), pioglitazone (antidiabetic drug of the thiazolidinedione class), and EBRT for PC have been incriminated. Squamous cell carcinoma is generally associated with chronic infections, especially *Schistosoma haematobium*, a parasitic agent commonly encountered in the Nile, Congo, Niger, and other areas in the Middle East, India, Far East, and South America. The pathogenesis is triggered by the *Schistosoma* eggs which cause a *chronic irritation* of the bladder mucosa, giving rise to *fibrosis*, proliferation, hyperplasia, and metaplasia of the normal bladder transitional epithelium. This results in the development of squamous or adenomatous variants and finally malignant transformation. Other possible mechanisms which may cause this transformation include the production of *nitrosamines* from secondary chronic urinary bacterial super infections and *urinary stasis*.

This leads to a high concentration of endogenous carcinogens and *raised urinary beta-glucuronidase levels* originating from miracidia and adult schistosomes which liberate carcinogenic amines in the urine [16]. The endemic bilharzia infection in Egypt has resulted in the country recording the highest incidence of BC in the world (37.1 per 100,000 males) [17]. Other risk factors for pure squamous cell carcinoma include chronic inflammation due to long-term indwelling catheters or bladder calculi and recurrent urinary tract infections. Adenocarcinoma of the bladder is generally reported to occur from urachal origin. Malignant transformation of the neobladder occurring as late as 15–40 years following a substitution enterocystoplasty is another cause for this histological type [18].

The most commonly encountered risk factors associated with bladder leiomyosarcoma are cyclophosphamide therapy and hereditary retinoblastomas whether treated with cyclophosphamide or not. The acrolein, a cytotoxic metabolite of cyclophosphamide excreted in the urine, was incriminated as a possible causative agent [19]; also the loss of the retinoblastoma protein (RB) gene and P53 factor was suggested in leiomyosarcoma associated with hereditary retinoblastoma [20]. Therefore, it appears that treating retinoblastoma with cyclophosphamide potentiates the risk. Other abnormalities in tumour suppressor genes including p21 and p16 have also been suggested.

5.4 Prevention and Screening

Prevention should involve avoiding all carcinogenic agents, especially smoking. Patients known to be at increased risk, especially those with a past history of schistosomiasis, enterocystoplasty, or exposure to carcinogenic agents, should undergo regular cystoscopies based on an established protocol to detect early changes. This has been suggested by a small population study of patients suffering from aristolochic acid nephropathy after ingestion of Chinese herbs-containing slimming pills. Biannual screening cystoscopies and biopsies proved to be effective in preventing deaths [21].

5.5 Symptoms and Signs

The most prominent symptom of bladder tumour is *haematuria*. This is reported to occur in approximately ¾ of cases of bladder cancer [22]. Conversely it has been shown that investigations of *frank haematuria* have led to the diagnosis of a urological malignancy in 10 % of patients aged <50 years and 34.5 % of those aged >50 years. *Microscopic haematuria* has led to a malignant diagnosis in 7.5 % of patients aged >50 years and *in none aged <50 years* [23]. This study with 381 patients has raised doubt about the benefit of fully investigating *younger patients* presenting with microscopic haematuria.

Classically haematuria associated with bladder and kidney diseases has been described as *total*, which means it is observed during the entire urinary stream, i.e. from the beginning until the end of micturition.

The severity of the haematuria depends on the bleeding epithelial surface and the importance of the tumour-induced neo-vasculature. It can be *continuous or intermittent*, *microscopic* (incidentally detected by laboratory means), or more often *gross or macroscopic*. This haematuria is also *painless*, except when associated with clot retention. This fact helps differentiate it from urinary infections or stone-associated haematuria which is painful. In more severe cases, the patient can present with clot retention, anaemia, or uremic syndrome; the latter is usually associated with a muscle-invasive tumour encroaching the ureteric orifices and causing obstruction by infiltration or compression. Rarely patients can present with bone pain due to metastases.

Unlike PC, BC is very rarely asymptomatic. When a BC is "incidentally" discovered during a cystoscopic procedure, it is often possible to discover retrospectively that the patient had forgotten or overlooked an episode of mild haematuria or find that microscopic haematuria was missed in previous investigations. Moreover, being an unpredictable feature, one negative microscopic haematuria result does not exclude the possibility of a urological malignancy. Microscopic haematuria should be defined as "*three or more red blood cells per high-power field*" and repeated two or three times by properly collecting the specimens, as recommended by the AUA expert panel [24]. This panel also recommends a prompt evaluation for renal parenchymal disease and referral to a nephrologist when the microscopic haematuria consists of red cell casts or predominantly dysmorphic red blood cells with associated significant proteinuria and/or renal failure.

Bladder irritation syndrome with symptoms of suprapubic pain, frequency, urgency, and burning micturition in the absence of urinary tract infection (UTI) is another potential way a bladder neoplasm may present, especially if carcinoma in situ. Studies have reported that this occurs in 20 % of cases [25].

Take-Home Message: Epidemiology, Pathology, Aetiology, and Symptoms of BC

Epidemiology	430,000 new cases in the world in 2012: 330,000 men and 100,000 women
	Approximately 75 % of newly diagnosed UBTs are noninvasive
	Majority of patients ≥60 years at presentation
	Younger patients ≤40 years have generally a low-grade disease and a relatively good prognosis
Pathology	*TCC* found in 90 %, then squamous cell carcinoma and adenocarcinoma
Aetiological factors	*Smoking* accounts for 50 % of cases
	Occupational exposure (to aromatic amines, polycyclic aromatic hydrocarbons, and chlorinated hydrocarbons contained in dyes, paint, and petroleum products)
	Medical conditions and drugs (schistosomiasis, recurrent UTI, long-term indwelling catheter, cyclophosphamide, EBRT, etc.)
	Possible genetic susceptibility, dietary factors, environmental pollution, etc.
Symptoms	*Haematuria* is found in approximately ¾ of cases of BC. Conversely BC will be diagnosed in 10 % of patients aged <50 years and in 34.5 % of those aged >50 years presenting with gross haematuria
	Bladder irritation syndrome is especially associated with CIS

References

1. Ferlay J, Soerjomataram I, Ervik M, Dikshit R, Eser S, Mathers C, Rebelo M, Parkin DM, Forman D Bray, F. GLOBOCAN 2012. v1.0, cancer incidence and mortality worldwide: IARC Cancer Base no. 11 [Internet]. Lyon: International Agency for Research on Cancer; 2013. Available from: http://globocan.iarc.fr
2. Ferlay J, Steliarova-Foucher E, Lortet-Tieulent J, et al. Cancer incidence and mortality patterns in Europe: estimates for 40 countries in 2012. Eur J Cancer. 2013;49:1374–403.
3. American Cancer Society. Cancer facts and figures 2014. Atlanta: American Cancer Society; 2014. p. p. 22.
4. Brown ML, Riley GF, Schussler N, et al. Estimating health care costs related to cancer treatment from SEER-Medicare data. Med Care. 2002;40:IV-104–17.
5. Gupta P, Jain M, Kapoor R, Muruganandham K, Srivastava A, Mandhani A. Impact of age and gender on the clinicopathological characteristics of bladder cancer. Indian J Urol. 2009;25(2):207–10.
6. Siegel R, Naishadham D, Jemal A. Cancer statistics, 2012. CA Cancer J Clin. 2012;62: 10–29.
7. Yossepowitch O, Dalbagni G. Transitional cell carcinoma of the bladder in young adults: presentation, natural history and outcome. J Urol. 2002;168(1):61–6.
8. Poletajew S, Walędziak M, Fus L, et al. Urothelial bladder carcinoma in young patients is characterized by a relatively good prognosis. Ups J Med Sci. 2012;117(1):47–51.
9. Fleshner NE, Herr HW, Stewart AK, Murphy GP, Mettlin C, Menck HR. The National Cancer Data Base report on bladder carcinoma. The American College of Surgeons Commission on Cancer and the American Cancer Society. Cancer. 1996;78(7):1505–13.

10. Freedman ND, Silverman DT, Hollenbeck AR, Schatzkin A, Abnet CC. Association between smoking and risk of bladder cancer among men and women. JAMA. 2011;306:737–45 [Published correction appears in JAMA. 2011;306:2220].
11. Ploeg M, Aben KK, Kiemeney LA. The present and future burden of urinary bladder cancer in the world. World J Urol. 2009;27:289–93.
12. Burger M, Catto JWF, Dalbagni G, et al. Epidemiology and risk factors of urothelial bladder cancer. Eur Urol. 2013;63(1):234–41.
13. Lane DP. p53, guardian of the genome. Nature. 1992;358:15–6.
14. Sarkis AS, Dalbagni G, Cordon-Cardo C, Zhang ZF, Sheinfeld J, Fair WR, Herr HW, Reuter VE. Nuclear overexpression of p53 protein in transitional cell bladder carcinoma: a marker for disease progression. J Natl Cancer Inst. 1993;85(1):53–9.
15. Rafnar T, Vermeulen SH, Sulem P, et al. European genome-wide association study identifies SLC14A1 as a new urinary bladder cancer susceptibility gene. Hum Mol Genet. 2011;20: 4268–81.
16. Zaghloul MS. Bladder cancer and schistosomiasis. J Egypt Nat Cancer Ins. 2012;24(4): 151–9.
17. Ferlay J, Bray F, Pisani P, Parkin DM. GLOBOCAN 2002: cancer incidence, mortality and prevalence worldwide, IARC CancerBase No. 5, version 2.0. Lyon: IARC Press; 2004.
18. Quinta A, Carvalho AP, Oliveira M, Oliveira C, Ribeiro Santos A. Bladder adenocarcinoma 41 years after augmentation enterocystoplasty for tuberculosis. Arch Esp Urol. 2013;66(2):231–3.
19. Tanguay C, Harvey I, Houde M, Srigley JR, Têtu B. Leiomyosarcoma of urinary bladder following cyclophosphamide therapy: report of two cases. Mod Pathol. 2003;16:512–4.
20. Bléoo SL, Godbout R, Rayner D, Tamimi Y, Moore RB. Leiomyosarcoma of the bladder in a retinoblastoma patient. Urol Int. 2003;71:118–21.
21. Zlotta AR, Roumeguere T, Kuk C, et al. Select screening in a specific high-risk population of patients suggests a stage migration toward detection of non-muscle-invasive bladder cancer. Eur Urol. 2011;59:1026–31.
22. Cummings KB, Barone JG, Ward WS. Diagnosis and staging of bladder cancer. Urol Clin North Am. 1992;19:455–65.
23. Sultana SR, Goodman CM, Byrne DJ, Baxby K. Microscopic haematuria urological investigation using a standard protocol. Br J Urol. 1996;78:691–8.
24. Grossfeld GD, Wolf Jr JS, Litwan MS, et al. Asymptomatic microscopic hematuria in adults: summary of the AUA best practice policy recommendations. Am Fam Physician. 2001;63:1145–54.
25. Pfister C, Roupret M, Wallerand H, Davin JL, Quintens H, Guy L, et al. Recommandations du CCAFU 2010: Tumeurs urothéliales. Prog Urol. 2010;20:S255–74.

Chapter 6
Investigations

Said Abdallah Al-Mamari and Salim Said Al-Busaidy

6.1 Primary Diagnosis of Bladder Cancer

- *Urine cytology* is highly sensitive in detecting high-grade tumours. Its sensitivity is as high as *90 % in the presence of CIS*; however, it is low in lower-grade tumours [1]. It should be requested in cases of irritable bladder syndrome after excluding urinary tract infection and stones. To date, there is no urinary marker validated for bladder tumour detection in routine practice despite extensive research on hyaluronic acid, telomerase, BCLA-4, BTA TRAK test, bladder tumour antigen STAT test, fluorescence in situ hybridization (FISH), ImmunoCyt test, nuclear matrix protein (NMP)22, etc. [2].
- *Suprapubic full bladder ultrasound* has a sensitivity ranging from 61 to 84 % for tumours >5 mm [3]. It is also very useful in detecting bladder stones which could be associated with a bladder irritation syndrome. In obese patients or whenever the bladder cannot be kept full for any reason, a transrectal approach is a valuable alternative to the suprapubic route.
- *When US is negative and there is a strong clinical suspicion of a bladder tumour*, it is recommended to perform *flexible cystoscopy* under local anaesthesia on an outpatient basis after excluding urine infection [3].
- However, *when the US findings are highly suggestive of a bladder tumour*, flexible cystoscopy becomes just optional preferring to proceed directly to *rigid cystoscopy ± TURBT* under general anaesthesia on an inpatient basis.

S.A. Al-Mamari (✉)
Urology Department, The Royal Hospital, Muscat, Oman
e-mail: sabdal67@yahoo.com

S.S. Al-Busaidy
Senior Consultant and HOD, Urology Department, The Royal Hospital, Muscat, Oman
e-mail: salimalbusaidy@hotmail.com

S.A. Al-Mamari, S.S. Al-Busaidy (eds.), *Urological Cancer Management*,
DOI 10.1007/978-3-319-16301-7_6

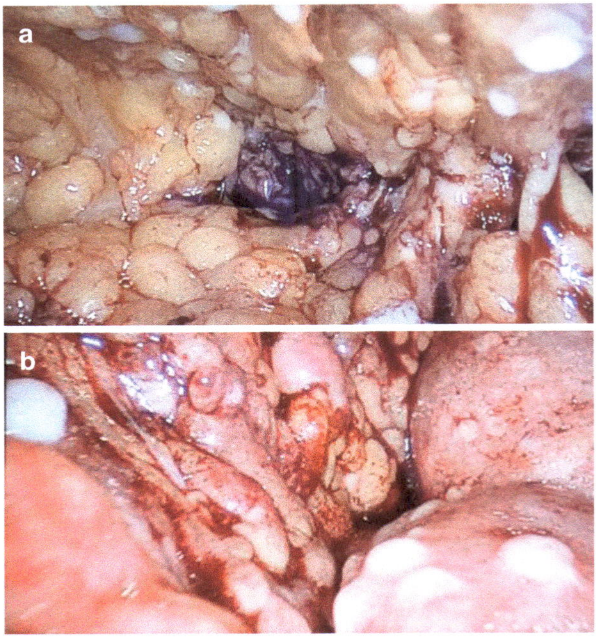

Fig. 6.1 (**a**, **b**) Laparoscopic views of peritoneal carcinomatosis with the characteristic numerous white nodules on both parietal and visceral peritoneum (This was seen 2 months after a history of bladder perforation during resection of a tumour which turned out to be a high-grade MIBT)

- *In the presence of frank haematuria*, if diagnostic cystoscopy is technically difficult or contraindicated, a *CT scan combined with urine cytology* is an acceptable alternative to reach the diagnosis.
- *TURBT*: Before the procedure, urine infection has to be ruled out. *Mapping and numbering the lesions is mandatory* for future follow-up and should provide an accurate record of the tumours in relation to *the prostatic urethra and ureteric orifices. The details should include the size and shape of the tumours and if pedunculated or sessile*. The resection has to be as complete as possible and deep to the muscle layer, in order to obtain adequate material for correct staging. Absence of muscle in the resected specimen is associated with downstaging and may expose the patient to a high risk of residual disease with early recurrence especially in high-grade pT1 tumours. It has been shown that the resection of *large-size and high-grade tumours* and the *seniority of the performing surgeon* are independent factors associated with the presence of detrusor muscle in the resected specimens [4]. Junior surgeons are more likely to perform incomplete resection but also to perforate the vesical wall especially when the tumour is located at the bladder dome. This adverse event may be followed by a dramatic peritoneal carcinomatosis especially in high-grade urothelial tumours and in non-urothelial carcinomas (Fig. 6.1a, b).

  A bimanual examination performed under general anaesthesia when the patient's abdominal, perineal, and pelvic musculature is fully relaxed, before and after the TURBT, may be helpful for an initial assessment of the clinical stage. Large muscle-invasive tumours which are palpable before the resection are usually not felt after the procedure.

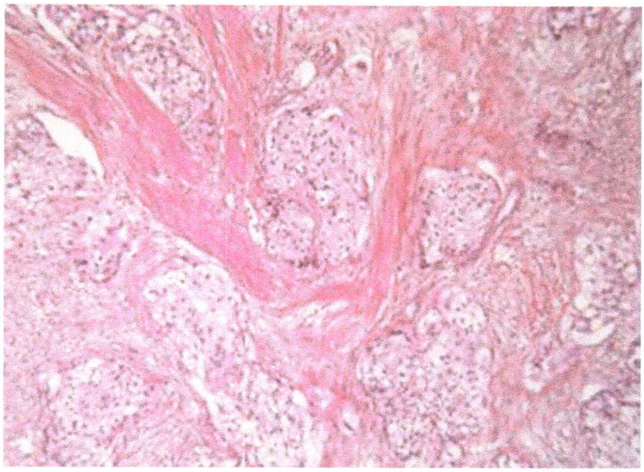

Fig. 6.2 TURBT specimen showing islands of tumour invading the muscle layer, i.e. a pT2 stage (Courtesy of A. Durlach, Pol Bouin Laboratory, University Hospital of Reims, France)

- *Random biopsies* performed on normal-looking bladder mucosa to detect CIS are not recommended since the chances of a positive result are very low (<2 %) [3]. *However, biopsies are indicated when urine cytology is positive or in the presence of mucosal lesions suggestive of CIS.*
- The use of *hexaminolevulinate* (Hexvix®) fluorescence has been shown to improve detection of Ta, T1, and CIS lesion, thereby improving the quality of the resection with a positive impact on the recurrence-free survival rate [5, 6].
- The *confirmatory diagnosis* is obtained by a histopathological study of the TURBT specimens or the tumour biopsy. This is performed using H&E staining and reported according to different classifications:
  - WHO 1973: Grade 1 well differentiated, grade 2 moderately differentiated, and grade 3 poorly differentiated. This is gradually being replaced by the most recent classification below.
  - WHO 2004: Low-grade and high-grade tumours.

The next priority for the pathologist is *to assess muscle invasion and categorize the disease as* muscle-invasive (MIBT) (Fig. 6.2) or non-muscle-invasive bladder tumour (NMIBT).

6.1.1 Novel Biological Parameters

- *Substaging T1 (T1a, T1b, and T1c) by evaluating the extension and depth of the lamina propria invasion has a good prognostic value*: T1a = superficial invasion of lamina propria, T1b = invasion into the muscularis mucosa (MM), and T1c = invasion beyond the MM but not to the muscularis propria [7, 8]. Although not yet included in the current TNM classification, this substaging is recommended by the American expert panel in order to differentiate a simple microinvasion just beyond the basement membrane from a deeper invasion where the possibility of understaging is greater [9].

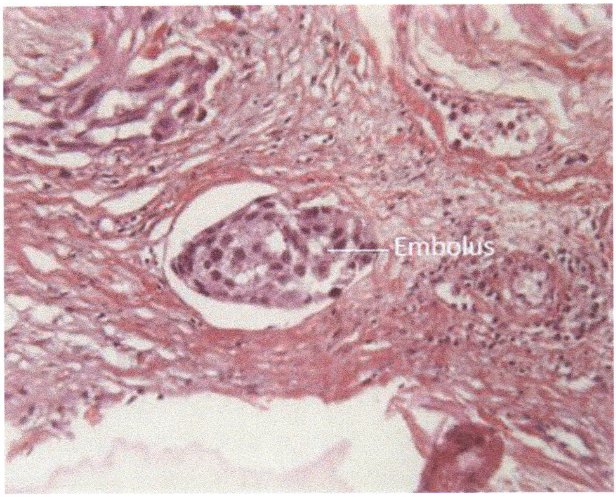

Fig. 6.3 Microphotograph of a TURBT specimen showing lymphovascular invasion (Courtesy of A. Durlach, Pol Bouin Laboratory, University Hospital of Reims, France)

- *Lymphovascular invasion* in T1 correlates with disease progression and metastases [10] (Fig. 6.3). Its presence in either T1 or T2 TURBT or radical cystectomy specimens is a strong predictor of frequent recurrences and a shorter survival rate [11]. However, its mention in the histopathological report (HPR) for T2 disease is only considered optional by the European expert panel [12].
- *Urothelial carcinoma subtypes*: Several studies have identified three major molecular subtypes of urothelial carcinoma which carry important prognostic difference and various responses to conventional chemotherapy. Depending on the authors, these subtypes were named basal, luminal, and p53-like tumours [13] or urobasal, genomically unstable, and squamous cell carcinoma-like [14].
- *Study of the fibroblast growth factor receptor 3 (FGFR3) mutation or overexpression status*: FGFR3 mutation has been found in the majority of low-grade NMIBT and in a minority of MIBT. However, in the latter there were an additional number of tumours harbouring FGFR3 overexpression, and about half of the cases of MIBT showed either FGFR3 mutation or overexpression [15]. Therefore, FGFR3 was suggested to be a promising target for therapy in bladder cancer [16].

The tumour staging is categorized according to the 2010 AJCC classification [17] (Table 6.1).

At the time of diagnosis, it has been estimated that *75–85 % of all urothelial bladder tumours are non-muscle invasive and that 60–70 % will recur within the first year after TURBT, but only 10–20 % will progress to become muscle invasive or/and metastasize* [3]. *It is this progression risk which is assessed by classifying the NMIBT as low-, intermediate-, or high-risk tumours* (see below).

Table 6.1 2010 AJCC staging for bladder tumours [17]

Primary tumour (T)	
Tx	Primary tumour cannot be assessed
T0	No evidence of primary tumour
Ta	Non-invasive papillary carcinoma
Tis	Carcinoma in situ: "flat tumour"
T1	*Tumour invades subepithelial connective tissue*
T2	*Tumour invades muscularis propria*
pT2a	Tumour invades superficial muscularis propria (inner half)
pT2b	Tumour invades deep muscularis propria (outer half)
T3	*Tumour invades perivesical tissue*
pT3a	Microscopically
pT3b	Macroscopically (extravesical mass)
T4	*Tumour invades any of the following: prostatic stroma, seminal vesicles, uterus, vagina, pelvic wall, abdominal wall*
T4a	Tumour invades prostatic stroma, uterus, vagina
T4b	Tumour invades pelvic wall, abdominal wall
Regional lymph nodes (N)	
Nx	Regional lymph nodes[a] cannot be assessed
N0	No regional lymph node spread
N1	Single lymph node metastasis in the true pelvis (hypogastric, obturator, external iliac, or presacral lymph node)
N2	Multiple lymph node metastases in the true pelvis
N3	Metastasis to the common iliac lymph nodes
Distant metastasis (M)	
M0	No distant metastasis
M1	Distant metastasis
Anatomic stages/prognostic groups	
Stage 0a	Ta, N0, M0
Stage 0is	Tis, N0, M0
Stage I	T1, N0, M0
Stage II	T2a or T2b, N0, M0)
Stage III	T3a or T3b or T4a, N0, M0
Stage IV	T4b, N0, M0 or any T, N1–3, M0 or any T, any N, M1

Used with the permission of the American Joint Committee on Cancer (AJCC), Chicago, Illinois. The original source for this material is the *AJCC Cancer Staging Manual*, Seventh Edition (2010), published by Springer Science and Business Media LLC, www.springer.com

[a]Regional lymph nodes include both primary and secondary drainage regions. All other nodes above the aortic bifurcation are considered distant lymph nodes

6.1.2 Progression Risk Factors

Traditionally, after *staging* and *grading* their infantries, strong armies were defined as those who could recruit larger *numbers* of soldiers to increase the *size* of their troops or who needed *less time* to prepare for new battles and those who were capable of *deep* penetration beyond the enemy lines.

These military principles also apply to the progression risk factors and aggressiveness of the BC.

- Tumour *stage*: T1 is more prone to progress than Ta.
- Tumour *grade*: High grade is more prone than low grade. *CIS must always be considered as high-grade tumour, while Ta is more often regarded as low grade.*
- Tumour *number*.
- Tumour *size*.
- *Time* (in months) elapsed between the first tumour resection and the first recurrence.
- The *depth* of lamina propria infiltration. This helps to differentiate between T1a and T1b.

Based on the abovementioned factors, three risk groups were defined in NMIBT (similar to the d'Amico groups described for PC) [18, 19]:

- *Low risk: solitary low-grade Ta, <3 cm, seen for the first time and not recurring on subsequent follow-up at 3 months.* Carries a 7.1 % progression risk at 5 years and a 4.3 % mortality risk at 10 years.
- *Intermediate risk: multifocal and/or recurrent low-grade Ta (pTa G1–2) or first-time-seen single high-grade Ta (pTaG3) or low-grade T1 (pT1G2).* Carries 17.4 % progression risk at 5 years and 12.8 % mortality at 10 years.
- *High risk: recurrent pTaG3, multifocal or recurrent pT1G2 in less than 6 months, first-time-seen pT1G3, any CIS.* Carries 41.6 % progression risk at 5 years and 36.1 % mortality at 10 years.

Following a combined analysis of several trials of the European Organization for Research and Treatment of Cancer (EORTC), a Belgian and Dutch study has proposed a practical way to easily calculate the short- and long-term risks of recurrence and progression for superficial bladder cancers [20] (Tables 6.2a and 6.2b).

Table 6.2a Weights used to calculate the recurrence and progression scores

Factor	Recurrence	Progression
Number of tumours		
Single	0	0
2–7	3	3
≥8	6	3
Tumour size		
<3 cm	0	0
≥3 cm	3	3
Prior recurrence rate		
Primary	0	0
≤1 rec/year	2	2
>1 rec/year	4	2
T category		
Ta	0	0
T1	1	4
CIS		
No	0	0
Yes	1	6
Grade (1973 WHO)		
G1	0	0
G2	1	0
G3	2	5
Total score	*0–17*	*0–23*

Reproduced from Sylvester et al. [20], with permission from Elsevier

Table 6.2b Probability of recurrence and progression according to total score

Recurrence score	**Prob recurrence**	**Prob recurrence**
	1 year (95 % CI)	**5 years (95 % CI)**
0	15 % (10 %, 19 %)	31 % (24 %, 37 %)
1–4	24 % (21 %, 26 %)	46 % (42 %, 49 %)
5–9	38 % (35 %, 41 %)	62 % (58 %, 65 %)
10–17	61 % (55 %, 67 %)	78 % (73 %, 84 %)
Progression score	**Prob progression**	**Prob progression**
	1 year (95 % CI)	**5 years (95 % CI)**
0	0.2 % (0 %, 0.7 %)	0.8 % (0 %, 1.7 %)
2–6	1.0 % (0.4 %, 1.6 %)	6 % (5 %, 8 %)
7–13	5 % (4 %, 7 %)	17 % (14 %, 20 %)
14–23	17 % (10 %, 24 %)	45 % (35 %, 55 %)

Reproduced from Sylvester et al. [20], with permission from Elsevier

6.2 Disease Extension Investigations

6.2.1 Computed Tomography (CT) Scan

Classically all cases of haematuria used to be investigated with the combination of intravenous urography or pyelography (IVP or IVU) and cystoscopy. Now *CT is the standard imaging for defining a locally advanced or disseminated BC, but should not be automatically requested if it is a non-muscle-invasive bladder tumour (non-MIBT)*. The selective indication for CT scan in non-MIBT includes high-grade or large-size tumours (>3 cm) [21] (Fig. 6.4a, b). It is also recommended to perform *an excretory-phase CT urography (Uroscanner) to exclude synchronous upper urinary tract tumours. In the presence of multifocal or high-risk tumours, the Uroscanner should be repeated every 2 years, because of an increased risk of developing metachronous upper urinary tract tumours. This risk was revealed by a large study of 1,500 patients which also showed that all patients with metachronous upper urinary tract tumours had a previous recurrent primary superficial bladder tumour* [22].

In the presence of a muscle-invasive bladder tumour (MIBT), a CT of the chest, abdomen, and pelvis (C-A-P) is the standard means of defining the extent of the disease. The aim of the study is to accurately assess the upper urinary tract, the perivesical fat, and the pelvic organs around the bladder including the prostate and seminal vesicles in males, and the vagina, uterus and ovaries in females. The study also defines the regional LNs and detects distant metastases. Any LN above 8 mm in diameter is by definition considered to be suspicious.

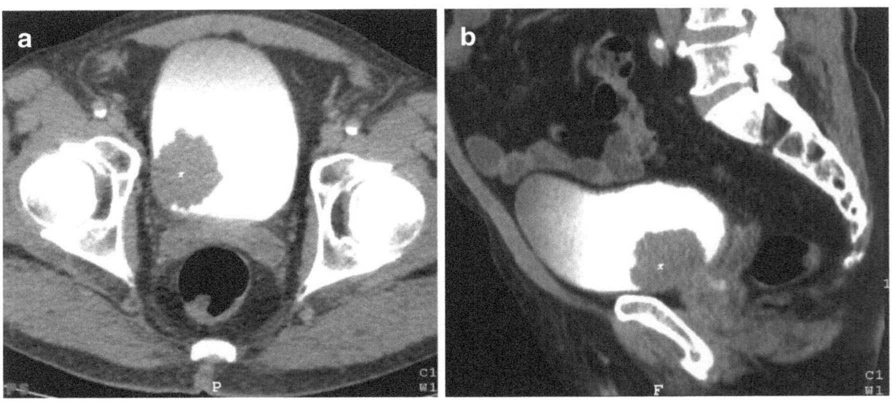

Fig. 6.4 (**a**, **b**) Excretory phase of transverse and sagittal CT of the bladder showing a large tumour (x) (Courtesy of S. Novellas, Radiology, Arnault-Tzanck Institute, Saint-Laurent-du-Var and CHU Nice, Nice, France)

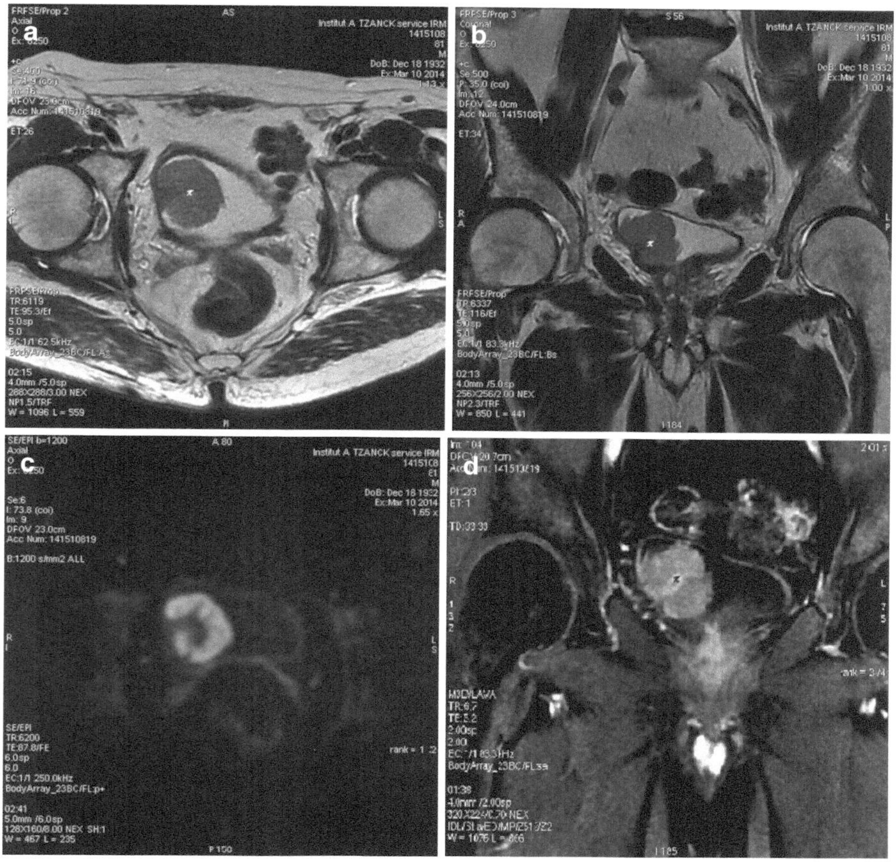

Fig. 6.5 (**a**–**d**) cT1 bladder tumour in T2-weighted MRI (**a**, **b**), in diffusion phase (**c**), and after gadolinium injection (**d**) (Courtesy of S. Novellas, Radiology, Arnault-Tzanck Institute, Saint-Laurent-du-Var and CHU Nice, Nice, France)

6.2.2 MRI

Contrary to the investigations of PC, MRI in BC is *only indicated when IV-iodinated contrast media are contraindicated*. It is not superior in detecting pelvic LNs; however, it can be helpful when there is a suspicion of tumour infiltration of the pelvic organs or bones since it is known to have a very high positive predictive value (Figs. 6.5a, d and 6.6a–d).

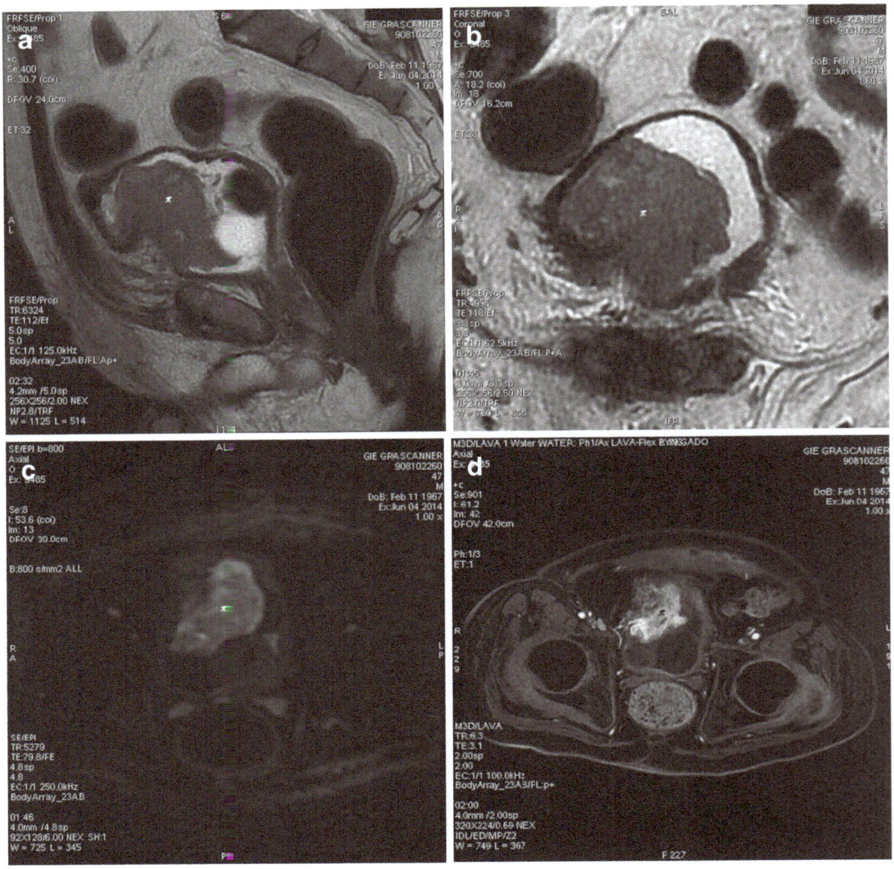

Fig. 6.6 (**a–d**) cT3 bladder tumour in T2-weighted MRI (**a**, **b**), in diffusion phase (**c**), and after gadolinium injection (**d**) (Courtesy of S. Novellas, Radiology, Arnault-Tzanck Institute, Saint-Laurent- du- Var and CHU Nice, Nice, France)

6.2.3 The Positron Emission Tomodensitometry

A combination of ^{18}F-FDG PET with TDM, has not been recommended for the evaluation of urothelial carcinoma; however, available data suggest that this examination could be used to assess primary bladder tumours and nodal disease with very good sensitivity and specificity.

6.2.4 Bone Scan

Bone scan is indicated only when there are symptoms suggesting bony metastases.

Take-Home Message: Investigations of BC

Patient presenting with irritable bladder syndrome or mild haematuria	First rule out UTI, then request *urinary cytology* and perform a *full bladder US* which may be normal or reveal bladder growths or stones.
	If US is negative but there is a clinical suspicion (recurrent history, old patient, smoker, etc.), perform an ambulatory *flexible cystoscopy*.
	If US is suggestive of a BT, the flexible cystoscopy is only optional and an inpatient-based *rigid cystoscopy + eventual TURBT* may be directly performed under general anaesthesia.
Patient presenting with frank haematuria	If diagnostic cystoscopy is technically difficult, arrange *CT scan combined with urine cytology.*
TURBT technique	*Mapping and numbering* the lesions is mandatory. The lesions must be removed *completely and deeply up to the muscular layer.*
	Random biopsies are not recommended in normal-looking bladder mucosa. They are indicated when urine cytology is positive or in presence of lesions suggestive of CIS.
	The use of *hexaminolevulinate (Hexvix®) fluorescence* improves detection of Ta, T1, and CIS lesion.
Tumour grading	Pathologists are now using the 2004 WHO classification which categorize the disease in *low-grade and high-grade tumours.*
	They are also differentiating the disease into *NMIBT and MIBT.*
Progression risk factors (i.e. from a NMIBT to a MIBT)	*Tumours stage, grade, numbers, size, time between two recurrences, and depth of lamina propria infiltration*
Progression risk groups	*Low risk (7.1 % progression risk at 5 years)*: solitary low-grade Ta, < 3 cm, seen for the first time and not recurring on subsequent follow-up at 3 months
	Intermediate risk (17.4 % progression risk at 5 years): multifocal and/or recurrent low-grade Ta (pTa G1–2) or first-time-seen single high-grade Ta (pTaG3) or low-grade T1 (pT1G2)
	High risk (41.6 % progression risk at 5 years): recurrent pTaG3, multifocal or recurrent pT1G2 in less than 6 months, *first-time-seen pT1G3, any CIS*
Disease extension investigations	*CT is the standard means for assessing locally advanced and disseminated BC* but to be requested only in MIBT and high-grade/high-volume (>3 cm) NMIBT. Uroscanning at the time of primary diagnosis and in the future follow-up is essential to rule out synchronous and metachronous upper tract TCC.
	For MIBT the CT study should include the chest, abdomen, and pelvis regions. MRI is indicated when CT is contraindicated, and PET-FDG is optional.
	Isotope bone scan: only for symptoms of skeletal metastasis

References

1. Lokeshwar VB, Habuchi T, Grossman HB, Murphy WM, Hautmann SH, Hemstreet GP, et al. Bladder tumour markers beyond cytology: international consensus panel on bladder tumour markers. Urology. 2005;66:35–63.
2. Mowatt G, Zhu S, Kilonzo M, Boachie C, Fraser C, Griffiths TR, et al. Systematic review of the clinical effectiveness and cost effectiveness of photodynamic diagnosis and urine biomarkers (FISH, ImmunoCyt, NMP22) and cytology for the detection and follow-up of bladder cancer. Health Technol Assess. 2010;14:1–331.
3. Pfister C, Roupret M, Wallerand H, et al. Recommandations en Onco-Urologie 2010: tumeurs urothéliales. Prog Urol. 2010;20:S255–74.
4. Mariappan P, Zachou A, Grigor KM. Detrusor muscle in the first, apparently complete transurethral resection of bladder tumour specimen is a surrogate marker of resection quality, predicts risk of early recurrence, and is dependent on operator experience. Eur Urol. 2010; 57:843–9.
5. Kausch I, Sommerauer M, Montorsi F, Stenzl A, Jacqmin D, Jichlinski P, et al. Photodynamic diagnosis in non-muscle-invasive bladder cancer: a systematic review and cumulative analysis of prospective studies. Eur Urol. 2010;57:595–606.
6. Witjes JA, Redorta JP, Jacqmin D, Sofras F, Malmstrom PU, Riedl C, et al. Hexamino levulinate-guided fluorescence cystoscopy in the diagnosis and follow-up of patients with non-muscle-invasive bladder cancer: review of the evidence and recommendations. Eur Urol. 2010;57:607–14.
7. Younes M, Sussman J, True LD. The usefulness of the level of the muscularis mucosae in the staging of invasive transitional cell carcinoma of the urinary bladder. Cancer. 1990;66:543.
8. Lee JY, Joo HJ, Cho DS, Kim SI, Ahn HS, Kim SJ. Prognostic significance of substaging according to the depth of lamina propria invasion in primary T1 transitional cell carcinoma of the bladder. Korean J Urol. 2012;53(5):317–23.
9. Gorin MA, Ayyathurai R, Soloway MMS. Transurethral management of urothelial carcinoma of the bladder. AUA Update Series. 2011; Lesson 23: 30. p. 10. http://www.auanet.org/content/cme/references/updateseries/updateseries1123.pdf#
10. Cho KS, Seo HK, Joung JY, Park WS, Ro JY, Han KS, Chung J, Lee KH. Lymphovascular invasion in transurethral resection specimens as predictor of progression and metastasis in patients with newly diagnosed T1 bladder urothelial cancer. J Urol. 2009;182(6):2625–31.
11. Streeper NM, Simons CM, Konety BR, Muirhead DM, Williams RD, O'Donnell MA, et al. The significance of lymphovascular invasion in transurethral resection of bladder tumour and cystectomy specimens on the survival of patients with urothelial bladder cancer. BJU Int. 2009;103:475–93.
12. Witjes JA, Compérat E, Cowan NC et al. Guidelines on muscle-invasive and metastatic bladder cancer. ©European Association of Urology. Limited update. 2014, page 17. http://www.24hmb.com/voimages/web_image/upload/file/20140626/78131403773860416.pdf#
13. Choi W, Porten S, Kim S, et al. Identification of distinct basal and luminal subtypes of muscle-invasive bladder cancer with different sensitivities to frontline chemotherapy. Cancer Cell. 2014;25(2):152–65.
14. Sjödahl G, Lövgren K, Lauss M, et al. Toward a molecular pathologic classification of urothelial carcinoma. Am J Pathol. 2013;183(3):681–91.
15. Tomlinson DC, Baldo O, Harnden P, et al. FGFR3 protein expression and its relationship to mutation status and prognostic variables in bladder cancer. J Pathol. 2007;213(1):91–8.
16. Gust M, McConkey DJ, Awrey S, et al. Fibroblast growth factor receptor 3 is a rational therapeutic target in bladder cancer. Mol Cancer Ther. 2013;12(7):1245–54.
17. Urinary bladder. In: Edge SB, Byrd DR, Compton CC, Fritz AG., Greene FL, Trotti A, editors. AJCC cancer staging manual. 7th ed. New York: Springer; 2010. p. 497–505.

18. Irani J, Bernardini S, Bonnal JL, et al. Tumeurs urothéliales : recommandations du Comité de cancérologie de l'Association française d'urologie. Prog Urol. 2004;14:959–96.
19. Babjuk M, Burger M, Zigeuner R et al. EAU Guidelines on Non-Muscle-Invasive Urothelial Carcinoma of the Bladder: Update 2013. Eur Urol. 2013;64:639–53.
20. Sylvester RJ, van der Meijden AP, Oosterlinck W, Witjes JA, Bouffioux C, Denis L, Newling DW, Kurth K. Predicting recurrence and progression in individual patients with stage Ta T1 bladder cancer using EORTC risk tables: a combined analysis of 2596 patients from seven EORTC trials. Eur Urol. 2006;49(3):466–77.
21. Pfister C, Rouprêt M, Neuzillet Y, et al. Les membres du CCAFU. Recommendations en Onco-Uologie 2013 du CCAFU: Tumeurs de la vessie. Prog Urol, 2013;23(suppl. 2):S105–S125.
22. Millan-Rodríguez F, Chéchile-Toniolo G, Salvador-Bayarri J, Huguet-Pérez J, Vicente-Rodríguez J. Upper urinary tract tumours after primary superficial bladder tumours: prognostic factors and risk groups. J Urol. 2000;164:1183–7.

Chapter 7
Treatment

Said Abdallah Al-Mamari and Salim Said Al-Busaidy

The treatment mainly depends on whether the tumour is muscle-invasive or not.

7.1 Non-MIBC (or Non-MIBT)

Every non-MIBT has to be treated, and unlike PC, surveillance only applies after the primary treatment (i.e. TURBT) has been completed. The surveillance protocol can only be followed once the tumour has been 'completely removed' and the histopathology has revealed no muscle invasion. The purpose of surveillance is to detect as earlier as possible any recurrence or progression. If only recurrence is detected, TURBT is repeated. However, if progression is seen, further active management must be offered which may include a partial or total cystectomy.

7.1.1 Primary Treatment

This involves performing a TURBT under general anaesthesia, with the purpose of removing the entire tumour for both diagnostic and curative purposes. As mentioned above, topography of the lesions has to be mapped and documented (number, size, location), and *the resection must include the muscle layer at the base of the tumour* in order to get an accurate assessment of the tumour and depth of penetration. A complete TURBT is the first therapeutic step of non-MIBT and may indeed

S.A. Al-Mamari (✉)
Urology Department, The Royal Hospital, Muscat, Oman
e-mail: sabdal67@yahoo.com

S.S. Al-Busaidy
Senior Consultant and HOD, Urology Department, The Royal Hospital, Muscat, Oman
e-mail: salimalbusaidy@hotmail.com

S.A. Al-Mamari, S.S. Al-Busaidy (eds.), *Urological Cancer Management*,
DOI 10.1007/978-3-319-16301-7_7

be the only active management, being merely combined with cystoscopic surveillance for *low-risk tumours* [1].

According to the European expert panel, the HPR of a non-MIBT should mention the following elements: location of the sample, the grade of each lesion, the depth of tumour invasion, the eventual presence of CIS, the presence of detrusor muscle, the lymphovascular invasion and any eventual unusual histology [2].

Expert panels recommend a second TURBT to be done within 2–6 weeks in the following circumstances [2, 3]:

- After an incomplete initial procedure (large-size or multiple lesions)
- If there is no muscle in the initial resection, except for Ta G1 and primary CIS
- In all T1 tumours
- In all G3 tumours, except primary CIS

A primary CIS is defined as an *isolated CIS* with no previous or concurrent papillary tumours and no previous CIS. Other clinical forms of CIS are *secondary* (during the follow-up of a papillary or exophytic tumour), *concurrent* (coexisting with an exophytic urothelial tumour) and *recurrent* (repeat occurrence of CIS after initial treatment) [4, 5]. All these forms can be either focal or diffuse [5].

During a primary cystoscopic evaluation or a TURBT procedure, biopsy of the prostatic urethra is indicated when [2]:

- There is bladder neck tumour.
- There is presence or suspicion of CIS.
- There is positive cytology without evidence of tumour in the bladder.
- There are visible abnormalities of the prostatic urethra.

The standard surveillance remains *routine cystoscopy* also referred to as *check cystoscopy*, often combined with *urine cytology*. In view of the economical issues and the invasive nature of this examination, other methods of surveillance have been suggested. However, none of the imaging techniques nor the numerous urinary tumour markers have been proven to be effective in replacing cystoscopy on the basis of diagnostic performances [1].

The follow-up schedule for NMIBT is [3]:

- Low-risk tumours: cystoscopy at 3, 6 and 12 months and then yearly for 5 years
- Intermediate risk: cystoscopy + urine cytology at 3, 6 and 12 months and then yearly for 10 years
- High risk: cystoscopy + urine cytology at 3, 6 and 12 months and then yearly for life

7.1.2 Adjuvant Intravesical Instillations

For *intermediate- or high-risk tumours*, intravesical instillation of cytotoxic or immunotherapeutic agents is combined with TURBT.

7.1.2.1 Cytotoxic Agents

Thiotepa was the first drug to be proposed for this indication. The drawback of this cheap alkylating agent is the possibility of its absorption through the urothelium because of its low molecular weight (189 kDa) with the resultant risk of myelosuppression. Now the most commonly used is *mitomycin C* (Ametycine®), a DNA synthesis inhibitor antibiotic which has a larger molecular weight (329 kDa). Other drugs are the deoxycytidine analogue *gemcitabine* and the intercalating agents Adriamycin (doxorubicin), epirubicin and valrubicin.

Mitomycin C (MMC, Ametycine®) can be instilled in the operating theatre early *after TURBT* once its contraindications are ruled out (bleeding, bladder perforation). The instillation is performed ideally *within the first 6 h, or not later than 24 h, post-operatively*. This technique is reported to reduce the recurrence risk by 12–39 %, either for uni- or multifocal tumour [4]. More traditionally MMC is instilled remote from the time of TURBT when the recommended schedule is weekly instillations of 40 mg Ametycine® diluted in 100 ml of saline for 6–8 weeks. This may or may not be followed by one instillation monthly [4]. The technique of instillation is simple: The patient is prescribed a urine alkaliniser and has fluid restriction 8 h prior to the procedure. A Foley catheter is introduced per urethra and the bladder is completely emptied. Then the diluted MMC is instilled into the bladder with the patient in supine position, and the catheter removed immediately. The patient is requested not to micturate during the treatment. He is instructed to change his position every 20 min (supine → left lateral → prone → right lateral) to allow the drug to impregnate all the bladder walls. After 2 h he is allowed to pass urine into the toilet and to resume high fluid intake.

The treatment is generally well tolerated, and possible side effects are chemical cystitis and dermatitis. Very rarely systemic effects may occur when the drug is accidentally absorbed into the bloodstream.

A recent meta-analysis has shown that *gemcitabine is more active with a lower toxicity profile than mitomycin for intermediate-risk tumours* [6]. In the next few years, it may be recommended as the standard treatment by expert panels if further corroborative evidence becomes available.

7.1.2.2 Intravesical Immunotherapy

This involves the use of the *Bacillus Calmette and Guérin (BCG) vaccine*, which is a living attenuated form of the *Mycobacterium tuberculosis* and exists in many strains. Historically, these have been divided into early strains (Japan, Birkhaug,

Russia and Brazil) and late strains developed after 1931 (Pasteur, Danish, Glaxo, Tice and Connaught) [7]. Nowadays, Tice (a substrain developed from the French Pasteur strain) and Connaught are the most commonly used BCG strains for intravesical immunotherapy, and a very recent study has revealed the superiority of the latter in preventing recurrences [8].

Intravesical BCG is contraindicated in the immediate post-operative period to avoid the risk of serious complications related to the living bacillus. *The interval should not be less than 15 days*. Several studies have demonstrated more than one benefit gained by maintenance treatment with BCG: It reduces the frequency of the recurrences and has a significant role in preventing the disease progression [9]. However, *the indication of BCG is generally limited to high-grade non-MIBT*, as cytotoxic agents, e.g. mitomycin C, have a proven efficacy against low-grade recurrent tumours and have less side effects.

Absolute contraindications of intravesical immunotherapy include inborn or acquired immune deficiency (diabetes mellitus, renal failure under hemodialysis, long-course corticosteroid treatment), active tuberculosis, a history of systemic reaction to BCG therapy and a history of radiotherapy to the bladder.

BCG instillation must be postponed when the following are present: insufficient time has lapsed since the TURBT (<2 weeks), macroscopic haematuria, unexplained fever and untreated bacterial infection of the urinary tract [1].

> The improper use of BCG therapy is very dangerous for the patient and may be hazardous for the health care providers as well. It is therefore essential to re-emphasise some important points of the technique, and although the detailed information provided below is fastidious, it has a direct bearing on the patient's care.

Product Preparation

Cautious preparations using mask, glasses and gloves are mandatory. Usual rules of asepsis are to be observed. Those handling the drug must not be immunocompromised. All consumables have to be considered as potentially infectious and must be properly discarded for incineration.

Patient Preparation

The patient must be well informed about the indications, the technique and the possible side effects. Urine has to be sent for culture and the negative result confirmed. The blood tests to be performed are full blood count, creatinine, urea and electrolytes, liver function tests and enzymes, i.e. transaminases and gamma-glutamyl transferase. Additionally, PSA should be requested in men because of the reported elevation which occurs in upto 40% of patients after intravesical BCG instillation [10]. Anteroposterior chest X-ray should be performed. Fluid intake should be reduced 8 h before to minimise the diuresis and allow good intravesical concentration of the product and an oral urinary alkaliniser prescribed.

Instillation Technique

Strictly aseptic and atraumatic bladder catheterisation is essential. *If catheterisation is difficult resulting in urethral bleeding, the procedure must be abandoned* because subsequent BCG infiltration could cause sepsis with serious complications. The bladder has to be emptied initially, then the BCG suspension is instilled slowly and the catheter is removed straight away. The patient must remain supine during the first 15 min, and the suspension should be kept intravesically for at least 2 h. When allowed to urinate, the patient must do so in a sitting position to prevent any urine spilling onto his body or on the toilet seat. Overhydration is recommended during the first 48 h after each instillation.

Dosage and Protocol

The following details refer to the Connaught strain (ImmuCyst®); however, Tice strain (TheraCys®) is also available at a strength of 81 mg:

- Induction:

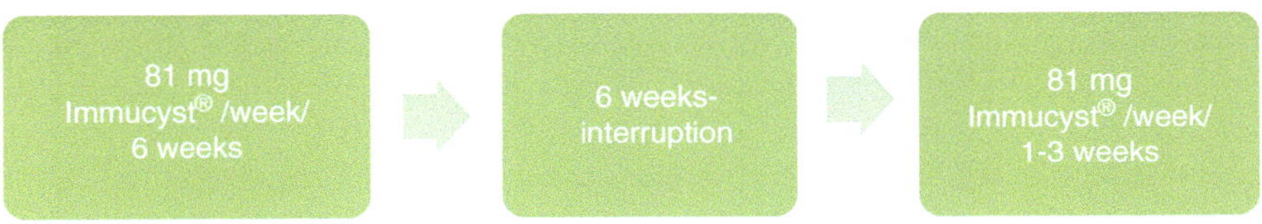
81 mg
Immucyst® /week/
6 weeks
6 weeks-
interruption
81 mg
Immucyst® /week/
1-3 weeks

Subtotal$_1$: 9 instillations

- Lamm's maintenance treatment (SWOG) [9]:

Wait 6 months after the
induction
Immucyst 81 mg® /week/ 3
weeks. To be repeated 6
monthly upto 36 months

Subtotal$_2$: 18 instillations

The total number of instillations is 9 + 18 = *27* for a total drug cost of approximately *1955 euros.*

Because of the side effects, only 16 % of the patients can tolerate the complete treatment [8]. On the other hand, the interest in the BCG maintenance therapy has been questioned due to differences in the published results on the efficacy on recurrence and tumour progression when comparing the maintenance and non-maintenance groups [11].

Many alternatives have been proposed to Lamm's protocol, mainly by reducing the dose or prolonging the break period between two instillations: A Spanish study has shown no significant difference in recurrence and progression rates between the standard dose group (81 mg) and a ⅓ (one third) dose (27 mg) group with significantly less side effects in the latter [12]. Despite criticism for the lack of randomisation in this study, *it still has merit in suggesting that BCG maintenance doses could be reduced for the intermediate-risk group without jeopardising the oncological outcomes.*

A recent meta-analysis has demonstrated that maintenance treatment was associated with a better progression-free survival but produced more side effects. Also *the standard maintenance dose was superior to the reduced dose*, and the combination of BCG with mitomycin C or interferon α-2b did not result in significant oncologic improvement compared to BCG alone [13].

The Lamm (or SWOG) maintenance treatment protocol is actually the most utilised therapy because it is based on a randomised study of a large cohort population (550 patients).

Side Effects of BCG Instillation

These are often minor causing the irritable bladder syndrome (increased urinary frequency, urgency and dysuria) sometimes accompanied by transient low-grade fever and haematuria. They generally respond to a symptomatic treatment and don't require admission. In <1–3 % however severe systemic manifestations (high fever, uraemia, jaundice, asthenia, hypotension and septic shock) may occur within hours or days after the BCG instillation, requiring admission and rarely even intensive care treatment [14, 15]. If bacteraemia from the live vaccine occurs through a urothelial breach, e.g. during traumatic catheterisation [16], the clinical aftermath will depend on the patient's immunological status, and symptoms may occur hours, days, months or even years later [15, 17].

Summary of the Side Effects

- Allergy: skin manifestations (rash) and joints pain.
- Inflammatory syndrome: transient fever and asthenia.
- Others: urinary tract infection, haematuria, increased urinary frequency, dysuria, bladder contracture, symptomatic granulomatous prostatitis and/or epididymo-orchitis, ureteral obstruction and renal abscess.
- Systemic reaction to the BCG (rare but serious): fever ≥39.5 °C lasting for at least 12 h or ≥38.5 °C lasting for at least 48 h and/or visceral involvement (essentially the lung and/or the liver). Disseminated BCGitis has been recognised over many years manifesting as granulomatous infiltration in the lungs, liver and/or bone marrow [15]. Potentially lethal complications such as sepsis and shock are very rare events.

Prophylactic Measures to Prevent or Minimise Side Effects

- Ofloxacine: One tablet 200 mg can be taken 6 h after the first post-procedure micturition and again 12 h later. This has been shown to significantly reduce class 2 (moderate) and class 3 (severe) side effects by 18.5 % without affecting the 12-month recurrence-free survival [18].
- Pre-emptive antituberculous drugs: These limit the stimulation of the immune reaction and could reduce the effectiveness of the antitumoural action.
- BCG dose reduction: During the maintenance period, the dose can be reduced to half or a third, but the standard dose must be maintained whenever possible for high-risk or multifocal tumours [19].

Management of Adverse Events

This depends on their seriousness [20]:

- Low-grade fever and irritative symptoms: They generally subside within 48 h and do not require any specific treatment, apart from antipyretics (paracetamol) and antispasmodics (butyl-hyoscine: Buscopan®). If the fever persists, urinary infection should be ruled out before starting a *2-week course of isoniazid.*
- Regional complications such as granulomatous prostatitis or epididymitis require a *3-month course of isoniazid with rifampicin.*
- Systemic infections such as granulomatous nephritis and abscesses, pneumonitis, hepatitis and osteomyelitis are treated with a *6-month course of the triple therapy isoniazid-rifampicin-ethambutol.*
- Life-threatening adverse events (either due to septicaemia or to immunoallergic reactions) may be delayed several months or even few years after the end of BCG therapy and require *urgent treatment with antituberculous drugs and prednisolone*.

Note: Initial encouraging reports of bladder instillations combining BCG and interferon alpha-2b as a second-line therapy after first-line failure with BCG alone [21, 22] have not been confirmed in a recent meta-analysis [13]; however, the controversy is as yet not concluded.

7.1.3 Radical Cystectomy (RC)

RC is considered optional in high-risk T1 (high-grade, multifocal, large-size) tumours and in carcinoma in situ. It should be considered for all T1 tumours unresponsive to intravesical therapy; however, the possibility of performing a partial cystectomy should be considered initially if the tumour is suitably located (bladder dome). It is also recommended if CIS does not completely respond to a course of BCG induction and six maintenance instillations [23].

Take-Home Message: Treatment of NIMBT and MIBT

Primary treatment	*TURBT, complete and deep to the muscle layer*
	Second TURBT to be done within 2–6 weeks in the following cases: After an incomplete initial procedure (large-size or multiple lesions) If there is no muscle in the initial resection, except for Ta G1 and primary CIS In all T1 tumours In all G3 tumours, except primary CIS
Follow-up after primary treatment	Low-risk tumours: cystoscopy at 3, 6 and 12 months and then yearly for 5 years
	Intermediate risk: cystoscopy + urine cytology at 3, 6 and 12 months and then yearly for 10 years
	High risk: cystoscopy + urine cytology at 3, 6 and 12 months and then yearly for life
Adjuvant intravesical instillation (for intermediate- and high-risk groups)	*Cytotoxic agents for low-grade tumours*: now *mitomycin C* is mostly used. *Gemcitabine* is another promising drug
	Immunotherapy for high-grade tumours: uses mainly the *BCG vaccine* in different strains. The induction schedule followed by the Lamm maintenance protocol (SWOG) is more effective but has many side effects
Radical cystectomy	Optional in high-risk T1 (high-grade, multifocal, large-size) tumours and in carcinoma in situ
	Should be considered for all T1 unresponsive to intravesical therapy (a partial cystectomy is to be considered when tumour is favourably located)
	Recommended for a CIS when complete response is not reached after the BCG induction and six maintenance instillations
Localized MIBT	*Radical cystectomy (RC) is the treatment of choice. To be performed within 3 months of diagnosis and to include PLND* If no contraindication and technically possible, a substitution orthotopic entero-cystoplasty should follow the RC to preserve the bodily image. Otherwise, urinary derivations to be done through ileal conduit (incontinent, Bricker, or continent, Cock, Indiana, etc.) or direct urostomies
	Bladder-sparing strategies: *EBRT or brachytherapy for patients unfit for surgery*, partial cystectomy and TURBT with concomitant radio-chemotherapy for highly selected patients
	Neoadjuvant chemotherapy (cisplatin based) advised before either RC or EBRT
	Adjuvant chemotherapy not recommended outside clinical trials
	Neoadjuvant EBRT not recommended

Locally advanced	Neoadjuvant chemotherapy
	pT3 and pT4 N+ tumours with positive SM: to be included in clinical trial for adjuvant chemotherapy
Metastatic MIBT	*Two independent factors have a negative impact on the patient's survival: the altered G-C (PS >1) and the presence of visceral metastases*
	1st line: MVAC regimen equal to G-C protocol, but the latter has a better toxicity profile
	Patients ineligible for cisplatin (PS 2 or creatinine clearance <60 ml/min) can be proposed a gemcitabine monotherapy (overall survival limited to 1 year) or a combination gemcitabine-carboplatin
	2nd line: vinflunine (Javlor®)
	Unfit patients: Supportive treatment and pain management only. Zoledronic acid and denosumab if bony metastases

7.2 MIBT

EAU expert panel recommends the following information be contained in an HPR of an MIBT: the histological subtype, the depth of tumour invasion, the resection margins status including the eventual presence of CIS and the extensive lymph node representation. Optionally the report may also include the lymphovascular invasion status [24]. However, there are pitfalls that urologists should be aware of with regard to pathological studies of TURBT specimens:

- Pathologists consider any tumour crossing the basal membrane of the bladder mucosa and invading the lamina propria as infiltrating. Therefore, urologists must cautiously read the pathologist's report and not consider all the tumours that are reported to be infiltrating as muscle-invasive, i.e. mistake T1 for T2 tumours.
- Muscularis mucosae hyperplasia seen in chronic inflammation may be mistaken for the muscularis propria and give a false impression of muscular infiltration [25].
- The presence of a fatty tissue inside the tumour proliferation is not synonymous with pT3 stage (extra-vesical), since the fatty tissue has been also described in the muscular layer as well as in the deep layer of the lamina propria [26]. *Therefore, a reliable diagnosis of the pT3 stage can only be established in a cystectomy specimen* (Fig. 7.1).
- *It is impossible to differentiate the stages pT2a and pT2b in a TURBT specimen.*
- It is difficult to determine the stage for tumours developing inside a bladder diverticulum; due to the absence of a muscle layer, there are two possibilities in this setting: either pTa tumour or extra-vesical extension.

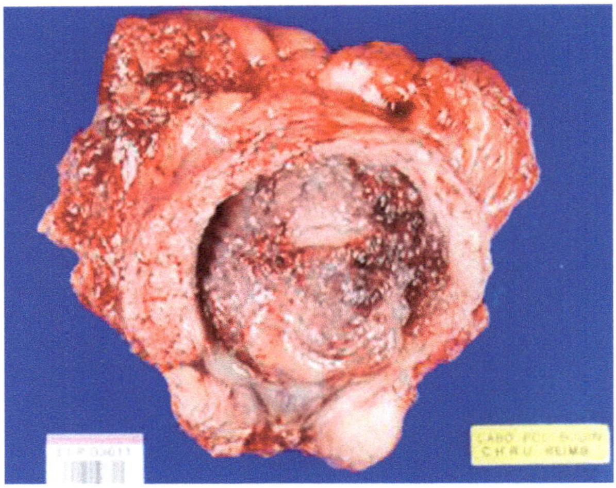

Fig. 7.1 A cystectomy specimen showing an exophytic and endophytic bladder carcinoma (Courtesy of A. *Durlach*, Pol Bouin Laboratory, University Hospital of Reims, France)

- A positive epithelial membrane antigen (EMA) result alone does not confirm its epithelial origin since this finding has also been associated with leiomyosarcoma [27–29]. Therefore, the morphological examination is of paramount importance.

The treatment options of MIBC depend on whether the disease is metastatic or not.

7.2.1 Non-metastatic MIBC

7.2.1.1 Radical Cystectomy

Radical cystectomy (RC) is the treatment of choice for non-metastatic urothelial MIBC (T2-T4a, cN0M0), as well as for non-urothelial bladder tumours and for non-MIBC with high risk of progression after failed conservative treatment. RC must include removal of regional lymph nodes. Despite the above indications, this procedure is considered optional in patients over the age of 80 years for whom an onco-geriatric assessment is important to weigh the advantages and the risks of major surgery. The decision to consider bladder-sparing treatment versus cystectomy in the geriatric population with invasive bladder cancer should be based on a validated score which considers tumour staging, comorbidities and perioperative mortality, such as the Charlson comorbidity index [30] (Table 7.1).

A statistically significant correlation exists between the diagnosis-to-cystectomy time interval and the final pathological stage, with *a delay of more than 3 months increasing the stage of the tumour and consequently reducing the rate of localised*

Table 7.1 Charlson comorbidity index

Scores	Age (years)	Comorbidities
0	<40	
1	41–50	Myocardial infarct, congestive heart failure, peripheral vascular disease, dementia, cerebrovascular disease, chronic lung disease, connective tissue disease, ulcer, chronic mild liver disease, uncomplicated diabetes
2	51–60	Hemiplegia, moderate or severe chronic kidney disease, diabetes with end organ damage, non-metastatic solid tumour, leukaemia, malignant lymphoma
3	61–70	Moderate or severe liver disease
4	71–80	
6		Metastatic tumour, AIDS (not just HIV positive)

By Charlson et al. [30], with permission from Elsevier)

Charlson comorbidity index: It is in reality a Charlson combined age-comorbidity index. Helps predicting the ten-year mortality for a patient considering his age and his eventual comorbid conditions The scores from corresponding age and associated comorbidities are summed to provide a total score. For example, a 65-year-old man with severe liver disease and localised prostate cancer has a score of 3 for his age (65 years old) + 3 for the severe liver disease + 2 for the non-metastatic solid tumour = 8. Charlson et al. found that the 10-year mortality rates for the different scores were 1 % for score 0, 3 % for score 1, 13 % for score 2, 21 % for score 3, 53 % for score 4 and 66% for score 5 [30]

bladder cancer from 81 to 52 %. Specifically, patients with an interval greater than 90 days were more likely to have pT3 or higher [31].

RC should always be done within 3 months of the diagnosis to minimise the risks of progression and disease-specific mortality.

An extended PLND has been proven to improve survival compared to the standard or limited PLND. It is aimed at removing the obturator, external iliac, internal iliac and distal common iliac LNs *up to the ureteric crossing*. This is reported to remove about 90 % of all potentially metastatic LNs. The drawback of LN dissection is the increased morbidity and mortality which may be improved by an experienced surgeon. *Extended PLND increases the duration of the operation, but not the complication rate when compared to the limited PLND.* Moreover, the prognosis is correlated to the total number of lymph nodes removed and to the extent of the excision as well as *the lymph node density (defined as the number of metastatic nodes/normal nodes) which is the most important prognosis factor* [32].

The standard technique is still an open radical cystectomy, but many centres of excellence have now published series of successful laparoscopic or robotic-assisted laparoscopic cystectomies with long-term oncological outcomes similar to the open surgery [33, 34]. A recent randomised study showed similar rates of perioperative complications and lengths of hospital stay among patients who underwent robot-assisted versus open surgery [35]. Whatever the technique, it should completely remove en bloc the bladder with the prostate and the seminal vesicles in men or the bladder with the uterus plus or minus the ovaries in women. Details of the technique are beyond the scope of this book. It is however common in many centres to preserve the uterus and ovaries in a select group of young females.

Whenever possible, radical cystectomy should be followed by a *substitution orthotopic enterocystoplasty* using detubularised ileal loop also called ileal neobladder (*Studer, Padua, Camey-2, Z-shaped or Ghoneim's technique*), which has the advantage of preserving the body image. However, a significant long-term complication rate (40.8 %) was reported in a high-volume institution including hydronephrosis, incisional hernia, small bowel obstruction, recurrent UTI, local tumour recurrence with subsequent obstruction and anastomotic stricture [36]. Megaloblastic macrocytic anaemia is a constant long-term complication of ileal neobladder and should be prevented by parenteral vitamin B12 therapy. The overall survival rate was estimated to be 65.5, 49.8 and 28.3 % at 5, 10 and 20 years, respectively [36].

Neobladder is contraindicated when there is urethral involvement or positive margins anywhere on the bladder specimen in either sex, bladder neck involvement in females or prostatic stroma extension in males. Other contraindications include senile, non-compliant or unmotivated patients (Table 7.2). In the presence of a multifocal tumour or CIS, a frozen section of the ureteral and urethral surgical margins is necessary before any reconstructive surgery [37].

When an orthotopic bladder replacement is contraindicated or when it cannot be performed, e.g. due to a short mesentery not allowing enough descent of a chosen ileal loop for a tension-free anastomosis with the urethra, incontinent or continent urinary diversion is performed. The ureters can be brought to the skin, either directly (*cutaneous urostomies*) or through a short ileal incontinent conduit (*Bricker*) or an

Table 7.2 General contraindications to continent urinary diversions

1. Chronic renal failure with serum creatinine exceeding 2 mg/dl without acute hydronephrosis. In doubtful cases percutaneous drainage is indicated preoperatively in an attempt to normalise renal function
2. Severe hepatic failure
3. Compromised intestinal function especially caused by radiation or inflammatory bowel disease
4. The presence of histologically proven cancer at the prostatic apex (male) or bladder neck (female)
5. Lack of patient motivation and/or intellect to follow a strict post-operative voiding regime, to accept possible incontinence (mainly nocturnal) in the early post-operative phase and sometimes in the long term
6. Pelvic floor disorders such as detrusor sphincter dyssynergia or neurourological diseases

By Nagele et al. [37], reproduced with permission from Elsevier ileal continent pouch (*Kock pouch*). The ureters can also be anastomosed to a larger segment which includes the caecum and part of the ascending colon using the ileal-caecal valve for continence and a short segment of the terminal ileum attached to the skin as a catheterisable conduit (*Indiana Pouch*). Rarer techniques aiming at preserving the body image consist of rectal or sigmoid enterocystoplasties, namely, *uretero-ileo-rectostomy or uretero-ileo-sigmoidostomy*.

Total urethrectomy is indicated along with radical cystectomy when there is a positive frozen section of the urethral surgical margin or when there is a massive infiltration of the prostatic urethra in men or the bladder neck and urethra in women.

7.2.1.2 Alternative to Radical Cystectomies

1. *Partial cystectomy* for TCC of the bladder has been described many years ago and has strict indications [38]: single-site muscle-infiltrating tumour, no evidence of in situ carcinoma, no trigonal or posterior urethra involvement and possibility to obtain at least a 1.5–2-cm negative surgical margin. Other indications include intra-diverticular tumours with no disease extension and localised urachal adenocarcinomas. The patient needs to be motivated in order to have a regular cystoscopic follow-up programme. A PLND is also performed for accurate staging. Any recurrence should prompt the decision for a radical cystectomy.
2. *TURBT with concomitant radio-chemotherapy* is a possible alternative option for a small T2 tumour (<3 cm). It implies the absence of an associated CIS and a complete and deep resection of the tumour which should be located far enough from the trigone and the ureteric meatus to allow for safe radiotherapy (12 fractions of 28 Gy).
3. *External beam radiation therapy (EBRT) alone is less effective than RC and should be considered only when the patient is unfit for cystectomy and chemotherapy*. It may still be offered to highly selected patients following a Dutch study which has shown that a *bladder-sparing strategy based on a combination of TURBT with EBRT and brachytherapy* with iridium (^{192}Ir) produced equivalent 5-year overall survival and 5- and 10-year disease-free survival rates to cystectomy [39]. The study group consisted of patients with *solitary, T1G3 or T2 bladder tumours, with a diameter <5 cm.*
4. *At present chemotherapy alone (after TURBT) using MVAC or CG is not recommended as primary therapy for localised bladder cancer.* However, there is an ongoing prospective multicentric trial in France called ReChiVe which includes patients with small and isolated T2a (<3 cm), with no associated CIS, aged ≥18 years and <75 years and having an ECOG PS ≤1. Selected patients undergo an 'optimal' resection of the tumour followed by MVAC chemotherapy. A cystoscopy performed one month after the end of the chemotherapy course allows early detection of nonresponders who are then offered radical cystectomy. Results of the 5-year disease-free survival rate with bladder preservation are awaited.

Table 7.3 ECOG performance status

Grade	Description
0	Fully active, able to carry on all pre-disease performance without restriction
1	Restricted in physically strenuous activity but ambulatory and able to carry out work of a light or sedentary nature, e.g. light house work, office work
2	Ambulatory and capable of all self-care but unable to carry out any work activities. Up and about more than 50 % of waking hours
3	Capable of only limited self-care, confined to bed or chair more than 50 % of waking hours
4	Completely disabled. Cannot carry on any self-care. Totally confined to bed or chair
5	Dead

By Oken et al. [41], with permission from Wolters Kluwer Health

7.2.1.3 Neo-adjuvant Chemotherapy

Neo-adjuvant chemotherapy has the dual purpose of clearing micrometastases which cannot be seen by imaging techniques and reducing the tumour bulk *before* curative surgery or EBRT is performed. A cisplatin-based combination chemotherapy has been shown to improve the overall survival by 5 % for grade 3 T2–T4a, cN0M0 tumours, before either RC or EBRT [40].

Readers should keep in mind that besides the contraindications of chemotherapy, i.e. renal failure with creatinine clearance <60 ml/min and poor performance status (PS) (Table 7.3) [41], *the challenge of neo-adjuvant chemotherapy is keeping the patient as fit as possible in preparation for the final definitive treatment*, i.e. RC or EBRT. Patients not responding to the chemotherapy should undergo surgery within 3 months.

7.2.1.4 Adjuvant Chemotherapy

Adjuvant is from the Latin verb *adjuvare* which means ‘to help, to aid’. Adjuvant Chemotherapy is done *after* surgery and aims theoretically at clearing tumoural cells or tissues left behind following incomplete surgery. Generally, it is not recommended after RC as it has not demonstrated a clear advantage; however, it may be suggested in a setting of research and clinical trials for pT3 and pT4 N+ tumours with positive surgical margins [3].

7.2.1.5 Neo-adjuvant EBRT

Is not recommended.

7.2.2 *Locally Advanced and Metastatic Bladder Cancer*

7.2.2.1 T4b

T4b is considered an incurable stage of BC and RC would be indicated only as a palliative measure for symptomatic disease (uncontrollable haematuria), but it will add to the patient's morbidity and worsen his or her quality of life. Neo-adjuvant chemotherapy has also been proven to be effective for locally advanced tumours (T3-T4 and/or N1-3), and as mentioned above, routine adjuvant cisplatin-based combination chemotherapy should be considered only in clinical trials for pT4 N+ patients.

7.2.2.2 For Metastatic Disease

The two independent factors which negatively impact on the patient's survival are the altered general condition (PS >1) and the presence of visceral metastases [42]. This is particularly important in first-line treatment where the fitness of the patient who is to receive cisplatin-based combination therapy is essential to improve his survival.

First-Line Therapy

A randomised study with over 400 patients has shown equivalent efficacy in global survival between the classical methotrexate-vinblastine-Adriamycin[1]-cisplatin (MVAC) and the newer gemcitabine-cisplatin (G-C) protocols; however, the latter has a better toxicity profile [43]. *Therefore, the tendency now is to consider the G-C protocol as the standard one.* A more recent study combining G-C with paclitaxel has shown a 4-month improvement in the overall survival among patients with bladder, but not with upper urinary tract, urothelial cancers when compared to G-C protocol [44]. Cisplatin-containing combination chemotherapy (G-C or MVAC) is associated with a median survival of up to 14 months and with a long-term disease-free survival in about 15 % of patients with N+ disease. Patients not eligible for cisplatin, i.e. with PS ≥2 or impaired renal function with creatinine clearance <60 ml/min, can be offered gemcitabine monotherapy with expected overall survival of less than 1 year or offered a combination gemcitabine-carboplatin.

Second-Line Therapy

Only *vinflunine* (Javlor®) has been validated for this use with an overall survival of 6.9 months compared to best supportive care alone [45]. The prognostic factors are liver metastasis, PS ≥1 and low haemoglobin (<10 g/dl). Unfit patients should be offered only supportive care. Zoledronic acid and denosumab are recommended to reduce and delay skeletal-related events (SREs) in metastatic bone disease.

---

[1] Adriamycin = doxorubicin

References

1. Irani J. Prise en charge des tumeurs de vessie n'infiltrant pas le muscle (TVNIM). Prog Urol. 2009;19:248–53.
2. Babjuk M, Burger M, Zigeuner R, et al. EAU Guidelines on Non-Muscle-Invasive Urothelial Carcinoma of the Bladder: Update 2013. Eur Urol. 64(2013), 639–53.
3. Pfister C, Rouprêt M, Neuzillet Y, et al. Les membres du CCAFU. Recommendations en Onco-Uologie 2013 du CCAFU: Tumeurs de la vessie. Prog Urol. 2013;23(suppl. 2):S105–25.
4. Babjuk M, Oosterlinck W, Sylvester R, Kaasinen E, Böhle A, Palou-Redorta J, Rouprêt M. EAU guidelines on non–muscle-invasive urothelial carcinoma of the bladder, the 2011 update. Eur Urol. 2011;59:997–1008.
5. Lamm D, Herr H, Jakse G, et al. Updated concepts and treatment of carcinoma in situ. Urol Oncol Semin Orig Invest. 1998;4(4–5):130–8.
6. Jones G, Cleves A, Wilt TJ, Mason M, Kynaston HG, Shelley M. Intravesical gemcitabine for non-muscle invasive bladder cancer. Cochrane Database Syst Rev. 2012;(1):CD009294.
7. Inamoto T, Azuma H. Immunotherapy of genitourinary malignancies. J Oncol. 2012;2012:397267.
8. Rentsch CA, Birkhäuser FD, Biot C, et al. Bacillus Calmette-Guérin strain differences have an impact on clinical outcome in bladder cancer immunotherapy. Eur Urol. 2014;66(1):677–88.
9. Lamm DL, et al. Maintenance Bacillus Calmette-Guerin immunotherapy for recurrent Ta T1 and carcinoma in situ transitional cell carcinoma of the bladder: a randomized South West Oncology Group study. J Urol. 2000;163:1124–9.
10. Leibovici D, Zisman A, Chen-Levyi Z, Cypele H, Siegel YI, Faitelovich S, Lindner A. Elevated prostate specific antigen serum levels after intravesical instillation of bacillus Calmette-Guerin. J Urol. 2000;164(5):1546–9.
11. Herr HW. Is maintenance Bacillus Calmette-Guérin really necessary? Eur Urol. 2008; 54:971–3.
12. Martinez-Pineiro JA, et al. Long-term follow-up of a randomized prospective trial comparing a standard 81 mg dose of intravesical bacillus Calmette-Guerin with a reduced dose of 27 mg in superficial bladder cancer. BJU Int. 2002;89:671–80.
13. Shimiao Z, et al. Optimal schedule of bacillus Calmette-Guérin for non-muscle-invasive bladder cancer: a meta-analysis of comparative studies. BMC Cancer. 2013;13:332.
14. Korać M, Milosević B, Lavadinović L, Janjić A, Brmbolić B. Disseminated BCG infection in patients with urinary bladder carcinoma. Med Pregl. 2009;62(11–12):592–5.
15. Steg A, Leleu C, Debré B, Boccon-Gibod L, Sicard D. Systemic bacillus Calmette-Guerin infection in patients treated by intravesical BCG therapy for superficial bladder cancer. Prog Clin Biol Res. 1989;310:325–34.
16. Frickmann H, Jungblut S, Hanke P, Bargon J. Tuberculosis induced by Bacillus Calmette-Guerin immuno-prophylaxis – case study. Pneumologie. 2004;58(11):773–6.
17. Nadasy KA, Patel RS, Emmett M, Murillo RA, Tribble MA, Black RD, Sutker WL. Four cases of disseminated Mycobacterium bovis infection following intravesical BCG instillation for treatment of bladder carcinoma. South Med J. 2008;101(1):91–5.
18. Neuzillet Y, Rouprêt M, Wallerand H, Pignot G, Larré S, Irani J, et al. Diagnosis and management of severe adverse events occurring during BCG therapy for non-muscle invasive bladder cancer (NMIBC). Prog Urol. 2012;22:989–98.
19. Oddens J, Brausi M, Sylvester R, Bono A, Van de Beek C, Van Andel G, et al. Final results of an EORTC-GU cancers Group randomized study of maintenance BCG in intermediate and high risk Ta. T1 papillary carcinoma of the urinary bladder: one third dose versus full dose and 1 versus 3 years of maintenance. Eur Urol. 2013;63:462–72.
20. Rischmann P, Desgrandchamps F, Malavaud B, Chopin DK. BCG intravesical instillations: recommendations for side-effects management. Eur Urol. 2000;37 Suppl 1:33–6.
21. Mohanty NK, Malhotra V, Nayak RL, Arora RP. Combined low-dose intravesical immunotherapy (BCG + interferon alpha-2b) in the management of superficial transitional cell carcinoma of the urinary bladder: a five-year follow-up. J Chemother. 2002;14(2):194–7.

22. Joudi FN, Smith BJ, O'Donnell MA. Final results from a national multicenter phase II trial of combination bacillus Calmette-Guerin plus interferon alpha-2B for reducing recurrence of superficial bladder cancer. Urol Oncol. 2006;24:344–8.
23. Pfister C, Roupret M, Wallerand H, Davin JL, Quintens H, Guy L, et al. Recommandations en Onco-Urologie 2010: tumeurs urothéliales. Prog Urol. 2010;20:S255–74.
24. Witjes JA, Comperat E, Cowan NC et al. EAU Guidelines on Muscle-invasive and metastatic Bladder Cancer. Summary of the 2013 guidelines. Eur Urol. 2014;65(4):778–92.
25. Paner GP, Ro JY, Wojcik EM, Venkataraman G, Datta MW, Amin MB. Further characterization of the muscle layers and lamina propria of the urinary bladder by systematic histologic mapping: implications for pathologic staging of invasive urothelial carcinoma. Am J Surg Pathol. 2007;31(9):1420–9.
26. Philip AT, Amin MB, Tamboli P, Lee TJ, Hill CE, Ro JY. Intravesical adipose tissue: a quantitative study of its presence and location with implications for therapy and prognosis. Am J Surg Pathol. 2000;24(9):1286–90.
27. Iwata J, Fletcher CD. Immunohistochemical detection of cytokeratin and epithelial membrane antigen in leiomyosarcoma: a systematic study of 100 cases. Pathol Int. 2000;50(1):7–14.
28. Kin T, Aizawa T, Namiki K, Noda K, Oyama H, Samesima T, Arai Y, Miki M. A case of epithelial membrane antigen-positive leiomyosarcoma of the urinary bladder. Hinyokika Kiyo. 2000;46(3):189–91.
29. Miettinen M. Immunoreactivity for cytokeratin and epithelial membrane antigen in leiomyosarcoma. Arch Pathol Lab Med. 1988;112(6):637–40.
30. Charlson ME, Pompei P, Ales KL, MacKenzie CR. A new method of classifying prognostic comorbidity in longitudinal studies: development and validation. J Chronic Dis. 1987; 40(5):373–83.
31. Chang SS, Hassan JM, Cookson MS, Wells N, Smith JR. Delaying radical cystectomy for muscle invasive bladder cancer results in worse pathological stage. J Urol. 2003;170:1085–7.
32. Larré S, Quintens H, Houede N, Comperat E, Roy C, Pignot G, et al. Benefit of bladder and upper urinary tract urothelial tumours lymph node dissection: review from the Bladder Cancer Committee of the French National Association of Urology. Prog Urol. 2012;22:380–7.
33. Collins JW, Tyritzis S, Nyberg T, Schumacher M, Laurin O, Khazaeli D, Adding C, Jonsson MN, Hosseini A, Wiklund NP. Robot-assisted radical cystectomy: description of an evolved approach to radical cystectomy. Eur Urol. 2013;64(4):654–63.
34. Snow-Lisy DC, Campbell SC, Gill IS, Hernandez AV, Fergany A, Kaouk J, Haber GP. Robotic and laparoscopic radical cystectomy for bladder cancer: long-term oncologic outcomes. Eur Urol. 2014;65(1):193–200.
35. Bochner BH, Sjoberg DD, Laudone VP, Memorial Sloan Kettering Cancer Center Bladder Cancer Surgical Trials Group. A randomized trial of robot-assisted laparoscopic radical cystectomy. N Engl J Med. 2014;371(4):389–90.
36. Hautmann RE, de Petriconi RC, Volkmer BG. 25 years of experience with 1,000 neobladders with long-term complications. J Urol. 2011;185(6):2207–12.
37. Nagele U, Sievert K-D, Merseburger AS, Anastasiadis AG, Stenzl A. Urinary diversion following cystectomy. EAU Update Ser. 2005;3(3):129–37.
38. Brannan W, Ochsner MG, Fuselier Jr HA, Landry GR. Partial cystectomy in the treatment of transitional cell carcinoma of the bladder. J Urol. 1978;119(2):213–5.
39. Van Der Steen-Banasik E, Ploeg M, Witjes JA, Van Rey FS, Idema JG, Heijbroek RP, et al. Brachytherapy versus cystectomy in solitary bladder cancer: a case control, multicentre. East-Netherlands study. Radiother Oncol. 2009;93(2):352–7.
40. Griffiths G, Hall R, Sylvester R, Raghavan D, Parmar MK, the International Collaboration of Trialists. International phase III trial assessing neoadjuvant cisplatin, methotrexate, and vinblastine chemotherapy for muscle-invasive bladder cancer: long-term results of the BA06 30894 trial. J Clin Oncol. 2011;29:2171–7.
41. Oken MM, Creech RH, Tormey DC, Horton J, Davis TE, McFadden ET, Carbone PP. Toxicity and response criteria of the Eastern Cooperative Oncology Group. Am J Clin Oncol. 1982;5:649–55.

42. Jessen C, Agerbaek M, Von Der Maase H. Predictive factors for response and prognostic factors for long-term survival in consecutive, single institution patients with locally advanced and/or metastatic transitional cell carcinoma following cisplatin based chemotherapy. Acta Oncol. 2009;48:411–7.
43. Von der Maase H, Sengelov L, Roberts JT, Ricci S, Dogliotti L, Oliver T, et al. Long-term survival results of a randomized trial comparing gemcitabine plus cisplatin, with methotrexate, vinblastine, doxorubicin, plus cisplatin in patients with bladder cancer. J Clin Oncol. 2005;23:4602–8.
44. Bellmunt J, Von der Maase H, Mead GM, Skoneczna I, De Santis M, Daugaard G, et al. Randomized phase III study comparing paclitaxel/cisplatin/gemcitabine and gemcitabine/cisplatin in patients with locally advanced or metastatic urothelial cancer without prior systemic therapy: EORTC Intergroup Study 30987. J Clin Oncol. 2012;30:1107–13.
45. Bellmunt J, Fougeray R, Rosenberg JE, Von der Maase H, Schutz FA, Salhi Y, et al. Long-term survival results of a randomized phase III trial of vinflunine plus best supportive care versus best supportive care alone in advanced urothelial carcinoma patients after failure of platinum-based chemotherapy. Ann Oncol. 2013;17.

Chapter 8
Non-urothelial Bladder Cancers

Said Abdallah Al-Mamari and Salim Said Al-Busaidy

Non-urothelial bladder cancers include squamous cell carcinoma, adenocarcinoma and the non-epithelial bladder tumours (NEBT).

Squamous cell carcinomas and adenocarcinomas are non-urothelial but epithelial cancers. Their pathology is often a high grade, and the patients generally present in an advanced stage. If any possibility of cure exists, surgery in the form of partial or radical cystectomy including excision of the urachus up to the umbilicus plus PLND may be attempted. EBRT is ineffective, and as yet there is no proven role for neoadjuvant or adjuvant chemotherapy.

Half-century ago, a study conducted in the United Kingdom examining 2,480 bladder tumours found only 40 non-epithelial tumours (1.6 %) [1]. Of these tumours, a minority were benign, e.g. pheochromocytoma and neurofibroma, and the majority were malignant, e.g. lymphoma, leiomyosarcoma, fibrosarcoma, fibroleiomyosarcoma, rhabdomyosarcoma and carcinosarcoma. The histopathological pattern has remained the same, lymphomas being most common followed by leimyosarcomas which are extremely rare. Only about 150 cases of urinary bladder leiomyosarcoma have been reported so far in the medical literature which limits the opportunity to study such patients and develop recognized guidelines. These tumours are generally moderately or poorly differentiated at presentation.

Bladder lymphomas are quite rare; however, secondary involvement from the disseminated disease is more common than the primary type. Furthermore, secondary bladder lymphomas have a very poor prognosis, and the advanced systemic disease is managed by the medical oncologist. Primary bladder lymphomas are mainly extranodal marginal zone B-cell lymphomas of the mucosa-associated lym-

S.A. Al-Mamari (✉)
Urology Department, The Royal Hospital, Muscat, Oman
e-mail: sabdal67@yahoo.com

S.S. Al-Busaidy
Senior Consultant and HOD, Urology Department, The Royal Hospital, Muscat, Oman
e-mail: salimalbusaidy@hotmail.com

S.A. Al-Mamari, S.S. Al-Busaidy (eds.), *Urological Cancer Management*,
DOI 10.1007/978-3-319-16301-7_8

phoid tissue (MALT) type; it is postulated that the aetiological cause of these tumours is due to chronic cystitis [2]. They have an indolent course, and radiotherapy alone is reported to be the treatment of choice with a favourable prognosis. Less commonly a high-grade diffuse large B-cell variety of this tumour is also seen which has a more aggressive course and is treated by a combination of chemo- and radiotherapy. Surgical resection may be beneficial for relieving irritative symptoms. In a study of 62 reported cases of primary bladder lymphomas, 22 patients received radiotherapy, 18 received chemotherapy and nine cases were treated with both. Only one patient underwent surgical treatment [3].

Take-Home Message: Non-urothelial BC

Non-urothelial BT	Radical cystectomy. Partial cystectomy in favourable anatomical locations. Apart from primary lymphomas, no consensus yet concerning NEBT because of their rarity

References

1. Cameron KM. Non-epithelial tumours of the bladder. Proc R Soc Med. 1963;56:930.
2. Horasanli K, Kadihasanoglu M, Aksakal OT, et al. A case of primary lymphoma of the bladder managed with multimodal therapy. Nat Clin Pract Urol. 2008;5:167–70.
3. Hayashi A, Miyakawa Y, Bokuda K, et al. Primary diffuse large B-cell lymphoma of the bladder. Inter Med. 2009;48:1403–6.

Part III
Upper Tract Urothelial Carcinomas

Kurian George

Introduction

Upper tract urothelial carcinomas (UTUC) are neoplasms arising from the upper urinary tract urothelium from the renal calyces to the distal ureter. Urothelial carcinoma of the renal pelvis was first reported by Rayer in the year 1841 [1]. UTUC is a rare malignancy commonly presenting with haematuria and the gold standard management for non-metastatic stages is radical nephroureterectomy with bladder cuff excision [2]. The progressive move toward nephron-sparing approaches initiated over the past decade for treatment of T1 renal cell carcinoma, even in the context of a normal contralateral kidney, has encouraged the development of organ-preserving techniques in the management of UTUC for selected cases. This transition has been initiated by data showing the substantial negative impact of chronic kidney disease (CKD) on cardiovascular events and overall mortality [3].

References

1. Rayer PFO. Traités des Maladies des Reins, Des Alterations De La Secretion Urinaire. Tome 3. Paris: J.B. Baillière, years 1839–41.
2. Roupret M, Babjuk E, Comperat R, et al. European guidelines on upper tract urothelial carcinomas: 2013 update. Eur Urol. 2013;63:1059–71.
3. Go AS, Chertow GM, Fan D, McCulloch CE, Hsu CY. Chronic kidney disease and the risks of death, cardiovascular events, and hospitalization. N Engl J Med. 2004;351:1296–305.

Chapter 9
Epidemiology, Risk Factors, Pathology and Tumour Staging

Kurian George

9.1 Epidemiology

In comparison with bladder urothelial cancers, upper tract urothelial tumours present at an older age, the mean being around 65 years. Upper tract urothelial carcinoma (UTUC) is a relatively rare malignancy with an annual incidence of only 1–4 cases per 100,000 population, constituting 5–10 % of all urothelial carcinomas [1–3].

9.2 Risk Factors

Tobacco smoking has been found to be an important risk factor for these tumours, which increases with increased consumption [4, 5]. Other risk factors include *long-term use of analgesics, especially phenacetin* [6, 7], *Balkan nephropathy* (degenerative interstitial nephropathy occurring in Balkan countries), papillary necrosis, stones, occupational exposure to petrochemicals, plastic materials, coal, asphalt, tar and thorium-containing contrast media [8, 9]. A history of previous lower urinary tract tumours also predisposes to upper urinary tract tumours [10]. Exposure to Aristolochic acid which is a component of certain Chinese herbal medicines has been noted to be significantly associated with an increased risk of UTUC. There is also a dose-dependent relationship between cumulative aristolochic acid exposure and end-stage renal disease (ESRD) risk [11, 12].

K. George
Senior Consultant, Urology Department, The Royal Hospital, Muscat, Oman
e-mail: kuriangeorge60@gmail.com

S.A. Al-Mamari, S.S. Al-Busaidy (eds.), *Urological Cancer Management*,
DOI 10.1007/978-3-319-16301-7_9

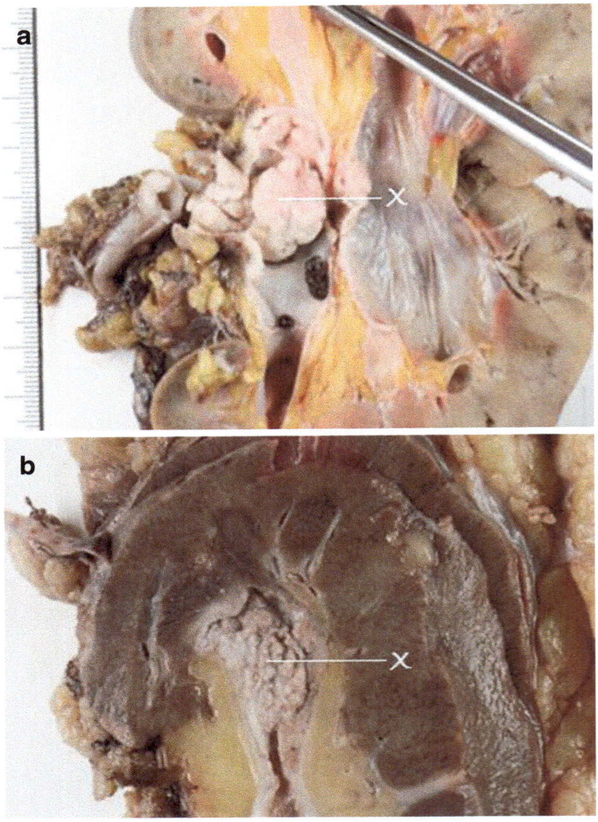

Fig 9.1 (**a, b**) Papillary TCC of the renal pelvis and upper calyx (*x*) (Courtesy of A. Durlach, Pol Bouin Laboratory, University Hospital of Reims, France)

The presence of upper urinary tract tumours also increases the risk of bladder cancer from 15 to 75 % over a 5-year period. Therefore, check cystoscopies at regular intervals are mandatory in these patients [13–15]. *Multicentricity is a characteristic of these tumours and recurrences are very common* [15, 16]. Synchronous bilateral upper tract urothelial tumours are rare and appear to have reduced in incidence (2 %) since the prohibition of phenacetin in the 1960s. Some familial syndromes, like Lynch syndrome, have been associated with the development of upper tract TCC [4]. The female-to-male ratio is 1:3–4.

9.3 Pathology

Grossly, these tumours may appear as a papillary (Fig. 9.1a, b), polypoid, infiltrating mass or an ulcerative lesion. The tumours may involve the renal parenchyma and thus mimic a primary renal tumour [17]. P63 immunoreactivity may be used to differentiate the two pathological entities: urothelial cancers are P63 positive and renal cell carcinomas (RCCs) are negative [18].

The histopathology of upper urinary tract urothelial tumours is similar to that of urothelial neoplasia of the urinary bladder (Table 9.1) [1]. The grading system used for upper tract neoplasms is also similar to that used for bladder tumours [17].

The tumour spread occurs:

1. By direct extension into the renal parenchyma or surrounding structures
2. Along the epithelial line in an antegrade or retrograde manner
3. Through lymphatic channels to the para-aortic, paracaval and ipsilateral common iliac and pelvic lymph nodes
4. By haematogenous route to the liver, lung and bone [4]

9.4 Tumour Staging

The 2010 AJCC cancer staging is the most commonly used [19] (identical to the UICC tumour classification) (Table 9.2).

Table 9.1 Histological classification of urothelial tumours of the upper urinary tract [4]

Benign lesions
Urothelial papilloma and inverted papilloma (rare)
Villous adenoma and squamous papilloma (rare)
Malignant lesions
Urothelial (transitional cell) carcinoma
Squamous cell carcinoma
Adenocarcinoma

Table 9.2 The 2010 AJCC staging for the renal pelvis and ureteric cancers [19]

Primary tumour (T)	
TX	Primary tumour cannot be assessed
T0	No evidence of primary tumour
Ta	Papillary noninvasive carcinoma
Tis	Carcinoma in situ
T1	Tumour invades subepithelial connective tissue
T2	Tumour invades the muscularis
T3	For renal only: Tumour invades beyond muscularis into peripelvic fat or the renal parenchyma
	For ureter only: Tumour invades beyond muscularis into periureteric fat
T4	Tumour invades adjacent organs or through the kidney into the perinephric fat

(continued)

Table 9.2 (continued)

Regional lymph nodes (N) (laterality does not affect the N classification)	
NX	Regional lymph nodes cannot be assessed
N0	No regional lymph node metastasis
NI	Metastasis in a single regional lymph node, 2 cm or less in greatest dimension
N2	Metastasis in a single regional lymph node, more than 2 cm but not more than 5 cm in greatest dimension, or multiple lymph nodes, none more than 5 cm in greatest dimension
N3	Metastasis in a regional lymph node, more than 5 cm in greatest dimension
Distant metastasis (M)	
M0	No distant metastasis
M1	Distant metastasis
Anatomic stage/prognostic groups	
Stage 0a	Ta N0 M0
Stage 0 is	Tis N0 M0
Stage I	T1 N0 M0
Stage II	T2 N0 M0
Stage III	T3 N0 M0
Stage IV	T4 N0 M0, or any T N1–3 M0, or any T, any N, M1

Used with the permission of the American Joint Committee on Cancer (AJCC), Chicago, Illinois. The original source for this material is the *AJCC Cancer Staging Manual*, Seventh Edition (2010), published by Springer Science and Business Media LLC, www.springer.com

Take-Home Message: Epidemiology and Etiology of UTUC

Incidence	*Rare, 5–10 % of all TCC*
Age at presentation	Older age than TCC bladder, at around 65 years
Etiological factor	*Mostly smoking*. Others: alcohol, phenacetin, Balkan nephropathy, occupational (petrochemicals), aristolochic acid (Chinese herb), etc.

References

1. Olgac S, Mazumdar M, Dalbagni G, et al. Urothelial carcinoma of the renal pelvis: a clinicopathologic study of 130 cases. Am J Surg Pathol. 2004;28:1545.
2. Green DA, Rink M, Xylinas E, et al. Urothelial carcinoma of the bladder and upper tract: disparate twins. J Urol. 2013;189:1214.
3. Gupta R, Paner GP, Amin MB. Neoplasms of the upper urinary tract: a review with focus on urothelial carcinoma of the pelvicalyceal system and aspects related to its diagnosis and reporting. Adv Anat Pathol. 2008;15:127.
4. Sagalowsky AI, Jarrett TW, Flanigan RC. Chapter 53. Urothelial tumours of the upper urinary tract and ureter. In: Partin AW, Peters CA, Kavoussi LR, Novick AC, editors. Campbell-Walsh urology. 10th ed. Philadelphia: Sanders; 2012. p. 1517–9.

5. McLaughlin JK, Silverman DT, Hsing AW, et al. Cigarette smoking and cancers of the renal pelvis and ureter. Cancer Res. 1992;52:254–7.
6. McLaughlin JK, Blot WJ, Mandel JS, et al. Etiology of cancer of the renal pelvis. J Natl Cancer Inst. 1983;71:287–91.
7. Bringuier PP, McCredie M, Sauter G, et al. Carcinomas of the renal pelvis associated with smoking and Phenacetin abuse: p53 mutations and polymorphism of carcinogen-metabolising enzymes. Int J Cancer. 1998;79:531–6.
8. Delahunt B, Amin MB, Hofstadter F, et al. Tumours of the renal pelvis and ureter. In: Eble JN, Sauter G, Epstein JI, editors. World health organization classification of tumours: tumours of the urinary system and male genital organs. Lyon: IARC Press; 2004. p. 150–3.
9. Jensen OM, Knudsen JB, McLaughlin JK, et al. The Copenhagen case-control study of renal pelvis and ureter cancer: role of smoking and occupational exposures. Int J Cancer. 1988; 41:557–61.
10. Sanderson KM, Roupret M. Upper urinary tract tumour after radical cystectomy for transitional cell carcinoma of the bladder: an update on the risk factors, surveillance regimens and treatments. BJU Int. 2007;100:11–6.
11. Wu F, Wang T. Risk assessment of upper tract urothelial carcinoma related to aristolochic acid. Cancer Epidemiol Biomarkers Prev. 2013;22(5):812–20.
12. Lord GM, Cook T, Arlt VM, et al. Urothelial malignant disease and Chinese herbal nephropathy. Lancet. 2001;358:1515.
13. Hisataki T, Miyao N, Masumori N, et al. Risk factors for the development of bladder cancer after upper tract urothelial cancer. Urology. 2000;55:663–7.
14. Miyake H, Hara I, Arakawa S, et al. A clinicopathological study of bladder cancer associated with upper urinary tract cancer. BJU Int. 2000;85:37–41.
15. Kang CH, Yu TJ, Hsieh HH, et al. The development of bladder tumours after primary transitional cell carcinoma of the upper urinary tract. Cancer. 2003;98:1620–6.
16. Kauffman EC, Raman JD. Bladder cancer following upper tract urothelial carcinoma. Expert Rev Anticancer Ther. 2008;8:75–85.
17. Ruta G, Gladell PP, Mahul BA. Neoplasms of the upper urinary tract. A review with focus on urothelial carcinoma of the pelvicalyceal system and aspects related to its diagnosis and reporting. Adv Anat Pathol. 2008;15(3):127–39.
18. Langner C, Ratschek M, Tsybrovskyy O, Schips L, Zigeuner RJ. P63 immunoreactivity distinguishes upper urinary tract transitional-cell carcinoma and renal-cell carcinoma even in poorly differentiated tumours. Histochem Cytochem. 2003;51(8):1097–9.
19. Renal pelvis and ureter. In: Edge SB, Byrd DR, Compton CC, Fritz AG, Greene FL, Trotti A, editors, AJCC Cancer Staging Manual. 7th ed. New York: Springer; 2010. p. 491–6.

Chapter 10
Diagnosis of UTUC

Kurian George

10.1 Symptoms and Signs

The ominous presenting symptom of upper tract urothelial tumours is haematuria which may be either gross or microscopic. This may be associated with a dull flank pain or an acute clot colic. A minority of patients may be diagnosed as an incidental finding on radiological imaging. Advanced disease may manifest with symptoms from metastasis.

10.2 Imaging

Computed tomographic (CT) urography is the gold standard for imaging of the upper urinary tract and has replaced intravenous excretory urography (Fig. 10.1a, b). It can also detect thickening of the wall of the renal pelvis or ureter as a sign of upper urinary tract urothelial carcinoma. It has been shown that hydronephrosis on preoperative imaging was associated with advanced pathologic disease and poorer oncologic outcomes [1].

The evaluation of the contralateral kidney is important because of the possibility of bilateral lesions and also for determination of the function in that kidney. Unlike renal cell carcinomas that tend to distort the renal outline, even large infiltrating TCCs tend to maintain a normal renal shape and contour (Fig. 10.2) [2, 3].

Magnetic resonance urography imaging is useful in those who cannot be subjected to CT imaging and has a detection rate of 75 % after contrast injection for tumours <2 cm [4].

Despite limited publication, [18F] Fluorodeoxyglucose PET can be used in UTUC for a better definition of LNs and distant metastases when CT-scan and MRI findings are equivocal.

K. George
Senior Consultant, Urology Department, The Royal Hospital, Muscat, Oman
e-mail: kuriangeorge60@gmail.com

S.A. Al-Mamari, S.S. Al-Busaidy (eds.), *Urological Cancer Management*,
DOI 10.1007/978-3-319-16301-7_10

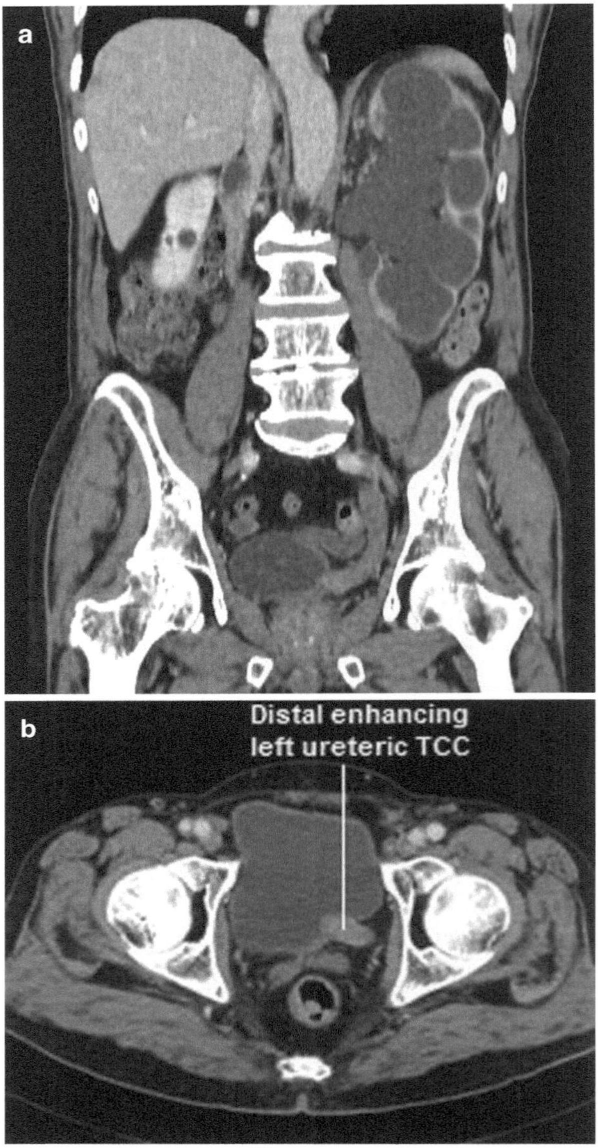

Fig. 10.1 (**a**, **b**) CT images showing hydronephrosis of the left kidney due to a distal left ureteric TCC

10.3 Urine Cytology and Cystoscopy

Positive urine cytology is highly suggestive of upper tract urothelial carcinoma when cystoscopy shows normal findings and if carcinoma in situ (CIS) of the bladder is excluded.

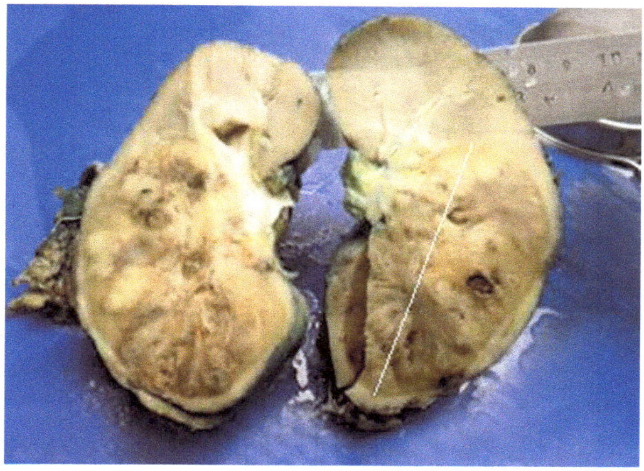

Fig. 10.2 Gross pathology of a large TCC infiltrating the left kidney. The tumour involves the lower 3/4 of the kidney, but the outside contour is maintained

10.4 Diagnostic Ureteroscopy

A rigid or flexible ureteroscopy can be performed to obtain a tumour biopsy and determine tumour grade. When the ureteroscopy is unavailable or not feasible, one can also perform *selective ureteral cytology* and a *retrograde pyelogram*.

Take-Home Message: Diagnosis of UTUC

Disease extent	*Multicentricity is a characteristic of these tumours*, with possible involvement of the bladder
	Recurrences are very common; bilateral presentation is uncommon
Presenting symptom	*Haematuria*
Imaging investigation	*Computed tomography (CT) scan is the gold standard*
	Retrograde pyelogram is also very useful
Final diagnosis	Histopathology. Rigid or flexible ureteroscopy is useful to provide biopsy specimen using the cold cup forceps

References

1. Ng CK, Shariat SF, Lucas SM, et al. Does the presence of hydronephrosis on preoperative axial CT imaging predict worse outcomes for patients undergoing nephroureterectomy for upper-tract urothelial carcinoma? Urol Oncol. 2011;29(1):27–32.
2. Vikram R, Sandler CM, Ng CS. Imaging and staging of transitional cell carcinoma: part 2, upper urinary tract. AJR Am J Roentgenol. 2009;192(6):1488–93.
3. Browne RF, Meehan CP, Colville J, et al. Transitional cell carcinoma of the upper urinary tract: spectrum of imaging findings. Radiographics. 2005;25(6):1609–27.
4. Takahashi N, Kawashima A, Glockner JF, et al. Small (<2-cm) upper-tract urothelial carcinoma: evaluation with gadolinium-enhanced three-dimensional spoiled gradient-recalled echo MR urography. Radiology. 2008;247(2):451–7.

Chapter 11
Treatment of UTUC, Prognosis and Follow-Up

Kurian George

11.1 Primary Treatment

11.1.1 Radical Nephroureterectomy (RNU)

Radical nephroureterectomy (RNU) is the standard management of UTUC, because of the known high rate of recurrence of this disease. The main concern with radical nephrectomy is that it predisposes to chronic kidney disease, which is associated with cardiovascular events and increased mortality rates. The risk of contralateral tumours should also be considered. In a Chinese population-based study, older age, lower preoperative GFR, renal pelvic location of the tumour and multifocality were noted to be predictors of postoperative renal insufficiency [1]. Therefore, an organ-sparing approach may be beneficial in selected patients. During radical nephroureterectomy, care should be taken to prevent tumour seeding by avoiding entry into the urinary tract [2, 3]. The different surgical approaches are as follows.

11.1.1.1 Open Radical Nephroureterectomy

RNU with excision of the bladder cuff is the gold standard treatment for upper urinary tract urothelial carcinomas (Fig. 11.1), regardless of the location of the tumour in the upper urinary tract [2]. There are various surgical approaches for this surgery. Most frequently two *separate incisions* are performed: *a loin incision and a lower abdominal Gibson incision*. The kidney, the perinephric fat and the Gerota fascia are mobilized, and the renal vessels are secured and divided. It is not necessary to remove the adrenals if their gross and imaging appearances are normal. After distal

K. George
Senior Consultant, Urology Department, The Royal Hospital, Muscat, Oman
e-mail: kuriangeorge60@gmail.com

S.A. Al-Mamari, S.S. Al-Busaidy (eds.), *Urological Cancer Management*,
DOI 10.1007/978-3-319-16301-7_11

Fig. 11.1 A nephroureterectomy specimen

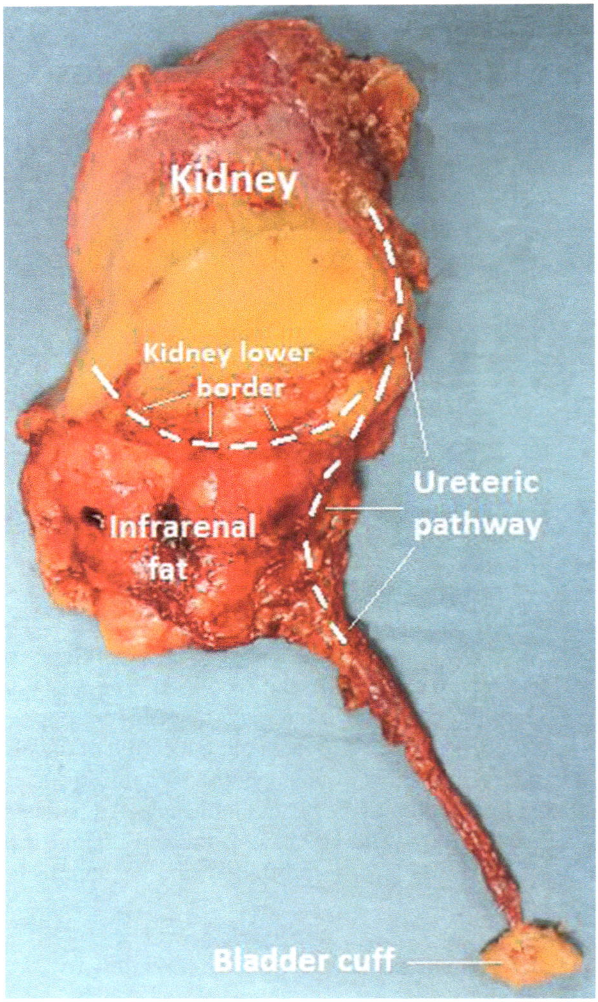

ureterectomy with a cuff of bladder, the whole specimen is removed intact through the lower incision. Lymph node dissection associated with RNU is of therapeutic interest and facilitates optimal staging of the disease [4, 5].

11.1.1.2 Laparoscopic Nephroureterectomy

Laparoscopic nephroureterectomy is now known to have equivalent oncologic results as open surgery and is gaining in popularity among urologists.

Notes: A single-dose mitomycin C intra-vesical instillation (40 mg) can be performed soon after nephroureterectomy as it was shown to prevent bladder recurrence at 1 year by 40 % [6]. *Contrary to bladder cancer, there is no consensus yet about the role of neoadjuvant chemotherapy prior to RNU for high-risk upper tract TCC.* A study has shown a 14 % complete remission and a significant rate of pathological downstaging associated with a neoadjuvant chemotherapy; however, further studies are lacking to corroborate this evidence [7].

11.1.2 Nephron-Sparing Management of Upper Tract Urothelial Carcinoma

This was initially limited to patients with a solitary kidney, bilateral disease, severe renal insufficiency or significant perioperative risk. Many authors still advocate the use of this approach. However improvement in technology and the imaging modalities may result in the expansion of endoscopic treatment to patients with normal contralateral kidneys [8–10].

Low-grade tumours which are unifocal, less than 1.5 cm in size and readily accessible within the kidney are suitable for nephron-sparing surgery by endoscopic resection or partial nephrectomy and segmental ureterectomy.

The different approaches for nephron-sparing surgery are as follows.

11.1.2.1 Endoscopic Management

The tumours in the renal collecting system can be approached either by ureterorenoscopy (retrograde approach) or percutaneously (antegrade approach).

(a) *Retrograde ureterorenoscopy* can be performed either through a rigid or a flexible ureteroscope. *This is usually suitable for tumours less than 1.5 cm in size.* The lesion is biopsied and sent for histopathology. Cold cup forceps or stone baskets can be used for debulking. Deep resection should be avoided in the proximal ureter and renal pelvis due to their thin wall to avoid perforation and spillage of tumour cells. The small calibre of ureteroscopic instruments and working channels and the low irrigant flow are factors which make ureteroscopic resection technically difficult. Complications of ureteroscopic management occur in 8–13 % of cases which include perforation and ureteral stricture [11].
(b) *Percutaneous nephroureteroscopy* allows larger instruments and facilitates better resection of larger tumours (>1.5 cm) of the renal pelvis and proximal ureter. The disadvantage of this approach is the violation of the urinary tract and risk of tumour spillage, although rare. A percutaneous tract is created and a larger sheath used to keep the intrapelvic pressure low. The tumour can be debulked by using forceps to remove its base and can be resected using a standard resectoscope. If the resection is technically difficult, the tumour is biopsied for diagnostic purposes and treated by holmium or neodymium laser sources through a

nephroscope or with a flexible cystoscope. Complications of this method range from 21.4 to 31 % [12–14] which include bleeding, infection, pelviureteric junction obstruction, adjacent organ injury and pleural injury.

11.1.2.2 Partial Nephrectomy

Partial nephrectomy may be considered when the endoscopic approach is not feasible due to a polar location or high tumour grade, stage and size.

11.1.2.3 Segmental Ureterectomy

Segmental ureterectomy is usually considered for distal ureteric tumours which are high grade, invasive or bulky and are not suitable for endoscopic management. It may require a psoas hitch or a Boari bladder flap. Other indications are grade 1 and 2 tumours of the proximal or mid ureter that are too large for endoscopic surgery or grade 3 tumours when nephron-sparing surgery is desirable. After segmental resection, up to 4 cm gap can be managed by performing a direct end-to-end ureteric anastomosis, i.e. ureteroureterostomy.

11.2 Adjuvant Therapy After Organ-Sparing Surgery

The benefits of adjuvant therapy with chemotherapy and radiation are still debated. However, since clinical studies continue to report some improvement in disease-specific survival with both forms of treatment, either therapy may be used in patients undergoing nephron-sparing management of upper tract TCC. Patients' consent and awareness about this is mandatory, and they should be under stringent surveillance [15].

BCG, mitomycin and epirubicin have been used for local instillation therapy. Focal radiation therapy has been tried to decrease the risk of local relapse after radical surgery for locally advanced non-organ-confined disease. The same systemic chemotherapy agents used in bladder TCC are prescribed here for metastatic disease or distant relapses.

11.3 Prognosis

The most significant prognostic factor for patients with upper tract urothelial carcinomas is the TNM stage [16, 17]. The 5-year specific survival is less than 50 % for pT2/pT3 and less than 10 % for pT4 [18, 19]. Histological features of high tumour grade, extensive tumour necrosis and lymphovascular invasion are associated with unfavourable prognosis.

11.4 Follow-Up

All patients should be evaluated at 3-month intervals during the first year by *repeated cystoscopies and urine cytology* following treatment with open or endoscopic methods. *Ureteroscopy* should also be performed after all conservative approaches. *CT urography* is also repeated at 3 and 6 months after a conservative approach or 6 monthly after a radical procedure during the first year. This close follow-up aims at an early detection of metachronous bladder tumours, local recurrences, metachronous tumours in the contralateral side and distant metastases. Subsequently, regular check-ups will be continued 6 monthly during the second year and then annually indefinitely.

Take-Home Message: Treatment of UTUC

Surgical treatment	*Gold standard: radical nephroureterectomy with a bladder cuff.* Traditionally by open surgery through two incisions. Laparoscopic route is also possible
	Nephron-sparing techniques are traditionally indicated in solitary kidney, borderline renal function or bilateral involvement. New indications now include unifocal, low-grade, solitary and less than 1-cm-size tumours: They are performed by endourological procedures (through retrograde ureterorenoscopy or percutaneous nephroureteroscopy), by partial nephrectomy (open or laparoscopic) or by segmental ureterectomy (open or laparoscopic)
Adjuvant therapy	*The same as for bladder TCC* after conservative surgery (instillation of various agents: mitomycin C, epirubicin, BCG), after radical surgery with suspicion of residual disease (EBRT) or in distant relapse or inoperable tumours (G-C or MVAC chemotherapy)
Prognosis	*The TNM stage is the most important factor*
Follow-up after radical treatment	3-monthly check cystoscopy + cytology (+ureteroscopy if conservative approaches)/1 year and CT urography at 3, 6 and 12 months for conservative surgery or at 6 and 12 months for radical approaches
	Continue the follow-up 6 monthly for the 2nd year and then annually indefinitely

References

1. Fang D, Zhang Q, Li X, et al. Nomogram predicting renal insufficiency after nephroureterectomy for upper tract urothelial carcinoma in the Chinese population: exclusion of ineligible candidates for adjuvant chemotherapy. Biomed Res Int. 2014;2014:529186.
2. Margulis V, Shariat SF, Matin SF, et al. Outcomes of radical nephroureterectomy: a series from the upper tract urothelial carcinoma collaboration. Cancer. 2009;115(6):1224–33.
3. Remzi M, Haitel A, Margulis V, et al. Tumour architecture is an independent predictor of outcomes after nephroureterectomy: a multi-institutional analysis of 1363 patients. BJU Int. 2009;103(3):307–11.
4. Lughezzani G, Jeldres C, Isbarn H, et al. A critical appraisal of the value of lymph node dissection at nephroureterectomy for upper tract urothelial carcinoma. Urology. 2010;75(1):118–24.
5. Roscigno M, Shariat SF, Margulis V, et al. Impact of lymph node dissection on cancer specific survival in patients with upper tract urothelial carcinoma treated with radical nephroureterectomy. J Urol. 2009;181(6):2482–9.
6. O'Brien T, Ray E, Singh R, Coker B, Beard R. Prevention of bladder tumours after nephroureterectomy for primary upper urinary tract urothelial carcinoma: a prospective, multicentre, randomised clinical trial of a single postoperative intravesical dose of mitomycin C (the ODMIT-C Trial). Eur Urol. 2011;60(4):703–10.
7. Matin SF, Margulis V, Kamat A, Wood CG, Grossman HB, Brown GA, Dinney CP, Millikan R, Siefker-Radtke AO. Incidence of downstaging and complete remission after neoadjuvant chemotherapy for high-risk upper tract transitional cell carcinoma. Cancer. 2010;116(13):3127–34.
8. Chen GL, Bagley DH. Ureteroscopic management of upper tract transitional cell carcinoma in patients with normal contra lateral kidneys. J Urol. 2000;164:1173–6.
9. Jabbour ME, Smith DA. Primary percutaneous approach to upper urinary tract transitional cell carcinoma. Urol Clin North Am. 2000;27:739–50.
10. Elliott DS, Segura JW, Lightner D, et al. Is nephroureterectomy necessary in all cases of upper tract transitional cell carcinoma? Long-term results of conservative endourologic management of upper tract transitional cell carcinoma in individuals with a normal contra lateral kidney. Urology. 2001;58:174–8.
11. Soderdahl DW, Fabrizio MD, Rahman NU, et al. Endoscopic treatment of upper tract transitional cell carcinoma. Urol Oncol. 2005;23:114–22.
12. Martínez-Piñeiro JA, García Matres MJ, Martínez-Piñeiro L. Endourological treatment of upper tract urothelial carcinomas: analysis of a series of 59 tumours. J Urol. 1996;156(2 Pt 1): 377–85.
13. Goel MC, Mahendra V, Roberts JG. Percutaneous management of renal pelvic urothelial tumours: long term follow-up. J Urol. 2003;169:925–9; discussion 929–30.
14. Jarrett TW, Sweetser PM, Weiss GH, Smith AD. Percutaneous management of transitional cell carcinoma of the renal collecting system: 9-year experience. J Urol. 1995;154:1629–35.
15. Kalyan CL, Christopher RP. Treatment of upper tract urothelial carcinoma: a review of surgical and adjuvant therapy. Rev Urol. 2006;8(2):61–70.
16. Olgac S, Mazumdar M, Dalbagni G, et al. Urothelial carcinoma of the renal pelvis: a clinicopathologic study of 130 cases. Am J Surg Pathol. 2004;28:1545.
17. Chromecki TF, Bensalah K, Remzi M, et al. Prognostic factors for upper urinary tract urothelial carcinoma. Nat Rev Urol. 2011;8:440.
18. Abouassaly R, Alibhai SM, Shah N, et al. Troubling outcomes from population-level analysis of surgery for upper tract urothelial carcinoma. Urology. 2010;76(4):895–901.
19. Jeldres C, Sun M, Isbarn H, et al. A population-based assessment of perioperative mortality after nephroureterectomy for upper-tract urothelial carcinoma. Urology. 2010;75(2):315–20.

Part IV
Renal Cell Carcinomas

Santhosh Narayana Kurukkal and Salim Said Al-Busaidy

Introduction

Renal cell carcinoma (*RCC*) arises from the renal parenchyma and accounts for more than 90 % of kidney cancers. The eponymous term *Grawitz' tumour* was referring to this tumour in the past, but is now seldom used. *In children, Nephroblastoma or Wilms tumour forms the majority of renal cancers* and has not been included in this part.

RCCs have a wide variety of symptoms, but *most of them are asymptomatic and detected incidentally with the liberal use of cross-sectional imaging. The tumour is essentially chemo-resistant and radio-resistant, and surgical extirpation remains the only curative treatment*. Management of RCC has undergone a tremendous change in the last few decades. Advances in diagnostic imaging, minimally invasive techniques such as surgery by laparoscopy and robotics and technical developments in partial nephrectomy have revolutionized the management of RCC. With a better understanding of the less aggressive nature of small renal masses, *management approaches have become more individualized nowadays* and include more options like active surveillance, thermal ablation and nephron-sparing surgery. The advent of targeted therapy has added new drug families in the treatment of metastatic RCC (mRCC); however the *mortality rate remains unchanged in these patients*.

Chapter 12
Epidemiology and Aetiology

Santhosh Narayana Kurukkal and Salim Said Al-Busaidy

12.1 Epidemiology

Kidney cancer is the 13th most common cancer worldwide with approximately 338,000 new cases, including 214,000 men and 124,000 women, and an associated specific mortality of 143,000 in 2012 [1]. Incidence is generally high in Europe and North America and low in Asia and South America [2].

In the USA, the incidence has been rising constantly over time (Fig. 12.1) [3]. There were 358,603 people living with kidney cancer in the USA in 2011. The estimated number of new cases in the USA in 2014 is 63,920, accounting for 3.8 % of all new cancer cases. The overall 5-year survival is 72.4 %.

Kidney cancer affects mostly old age, in the sixth to eighth decade, and the median age at diagnosis is 64 years, and median age of death is 71 years in the USA.

There has been a shift towards smaller tumour sizes and earlier stage at diagnosis (stage I – localized) attributed to the incidental diagnosis following more liberal use of imaging procedures. Nowadays *tumours <2.0 cm outpace tumours of larger sizes.*

The survival rates of patients diagnosed with tumours of all stages have improved over time.

S.N. Kurukkal (✉)
Urology Department, The Royal Hospital, Muscat, Oman
e-mail: drsanthoshnrn@gmail.com

S.S. Al-Busaidy
Senior Consultant and HOD, Urology Department, The Royal Hospital, Muscat, Oman
e-mail: salimalbusaidy@hotmail.com

S.A. Al-Mamari, S.S. Al-Busaidy (eds.), *Urological Cancer Management*,
DOI 10.1007/978-3-319-16301-7_12

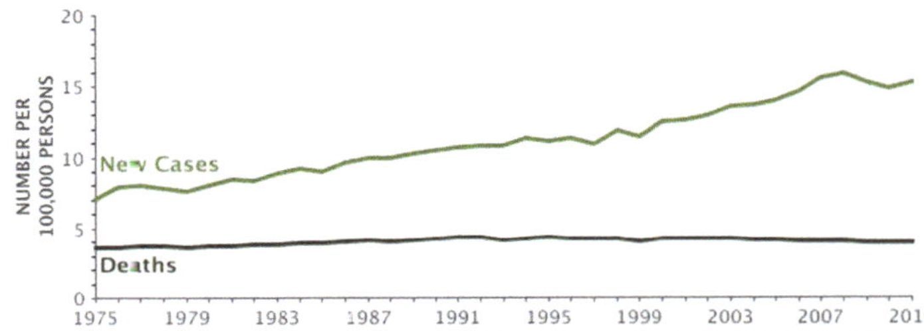

Year	1975	1980	1985	1990	1994	1998	2002	2006
5-Year Relative Survival	52.3%	54.3%	55.2%	59.7%	61.9%	63.2%	67.6%	73.5%

SEER 9 Incidence & U.S. Mortality 1975-2011, All Races, Both Sexes. Rates are Age-Adjusted.

Fig. 12.1 New cases, deaths and 5-year relative survival of RCC patients in the USA (By Howlader et al. [3])

12.2 Aetiology of RCC

1. *Cigarette smoking is an established risk factor for RCC.* There is a strong dose-dependent increase in risk [4]. Heavier smoking is an independent risk factor which increases the likelihood of advanced RCC [5]. The mechanism of action may be chronic tissue hypoxia due to carbon monoxide exposure and damage to DNA caused by tobacco-specific *N*-nitrosamine and benzo[α]pyrene diol epoxide. *Durable smoking cessation of 10 or more years attenuates the risk of advanced disease and is among the few modifiable risk factors* [6].
2. *Metabolic syndrome (MS)* is a cluster of abnormalities including *obesity, hypertension, diabetes and dyslipidaemia*. It forms the pivotal risk factor for cardiovascular diseases. Recent studies have recognized the significant role of MS in carcinogenesis and suggested a strong association with RCC [7]. In addition each component of MS is considered to have a close causal association with RCC:

   (a) *RCC is the third cancer most robustly associated with increased BMI* after endometrial and oesophageal tumours [8–10]. There is a growing knowledge on the impact of obesity and the role of adipose tissue in renal carcinogenesis. Obesity in both men and women increases the risk. The relative risk ranged from 1.04 to 1.08 per unit of increase in BMI (corresponding to 3 kg body weight increase for a subject of average height) [11]. Several mechanisms were hypothesized, but direct evidence is limited. *Abdominal fat is an endocrine organ producing adipose tissue-derived hormones (adipokines)* which play a role in conflicting between growing tumours and the immune system. Other mechanisms include chronic tissue hypoxia, insulin resistance, compensatory hyperinsulinaemia, altered endocrine milieu, obesity-induced inflammatory response, lipid peroxidation and oxidative stress [6, 12, 13].

There is inverse association of physical activity with obesity but little evidence to support the relation with RCC [14]. A recent population-based case control study suggested that physical activity may be inversely associated with RCC risk in whites, but there was no evidence of such an association in blacks [15]. Further investigations are needed to clarify the relationship in this population.

(b) There is sufficient evidence to support that *long-term hypertension* predisposes to RCC [16, 17]. *Users of diuretics and antihypertensive medications were associated with an elevated risk of RCC, but an independent effect of hypertension per se has not been established.* Risk is higher among individual who are both hypertensive and obese than those affected by one of these. The mechanisms attributed are chronic hypoxia and lipid peroxidation with formation of reactive oxygen species [6].

(c) *DM* has been linked to RCC risk, but its independent role from obesity and hypertension was not demonstrated conclusively.

3. *Renal pathologies*: Patients with ARCD [18] (acquired renal cystic disease), end-stage renal disease (ESRD) undergoing long-term hemodialysis and renal transplantation have increased risk of developing RCC [19]. The native kidney is more affected than the transplanted kidney in post-renal transplant patients.
4. *RCC is not an occupational disease.* However, exposure to trichloroethylene (TCE), a metal degreaser and chemical additive as well as an environmental contaminant, has been incriminated as a possible etiological factor in RCC [20]. No link to RCC was shown with other chemical agents like cadmium, uranium, arsenic, nitrate and radon in drinking water. Dietary factors such as diet deficient in fruits and vegetables, antioxidants, vitamins A, C and E and carotenoids and diet rich in fat and protein of animal origin were discussed, but more evidence is needed. Coffee and tea intake also did not show an established role in the risk of RCC [21]. Metachronous cancer in the contralateral kidney has been reported and occurs in younger age. This may be a metastasis; however, occurring after prolonged interval indicates a new lesion [22, 23]. Occurrence of RCCs in the setting of inherited cancer syndromes is also widely described (see special paragraph later).

Alcohol consumption has been reported to lower the risk of renal cell cancer [24].

Take-Home Message: Etiological Factors of RCC

Established risk factors	Putative risk factors
Tobacco smoking	Lack of physical activity
Metabolic syndrome	Second primary in cancer survivors
Obesity	Metachronous bilateral in young age
Hypertension	TCE, trichloroethylene
ARCD	Dietary factors
Post-renal transplant	
Association with hereditary syndromes	

References

1. Ferlay J, Soerjomataram I, Ervik M, Dikshit R, Eser S, Mathers C, Rebelo M, Forman D, Bray F. GLOBOCAN 2012 v1.0, cancer incidence and mortality worldwide: IARC Cancer Base No. 11 [internet]. Lyon: International Agency for Research on Cancer; 2013. Available from: http://globocan.iarc.fr.
2. American Cancer Society. Cancer facts and figures 2014. Atlanta: American Cancer Society; 2014. Available online last revised on 24/2/2014.
3. Howlader N, Noone AM, Krapcho M, et al. SEER cancer statistics review, 1975–2011. Bethesda: National Cancer Institute. http://seer.cancer.gov/csr/1975_2011/
4. Hunt JD, van der Hel OL, McMillan GP, Boffetta P, Brennan P. Renal cell carcinoma in relation to cigarette smoking: meta-analysis of 24 studies. Int J Cancer. 2005;114(1):101–8.
5. Tsivian M, Moreira DM, Caso JR, Mouraviev M, Polascik TJ. Cigarette smoking is associated with advanced renal cell carcinoma. J Clin Oncol. 2011;29(15):2027–31.
6. Chow W-H, Dong LM. Epidemiology and risk factors for kidney cancer. Nat Rev Urol. 2010;7(5):245–57.
7. Zhang GM, Zhu Y, Ye DW. Metabolic syndrome and renal cell carcinoma. World J Surg Oncol. 2014;12:236.
8. Gati A, Kouidhi S, et al. Obesity and renal cancer: role of adipokines in the tumour-immune system conflict. Oncoimmunology. 2014;1:3(1).
9. Ildaphonse G, George PS, et al. Obesity and kidney cancer risk in men: a meta-analysis (1992–2008). Asian Pac J Cancer Prev. 2009;10(2):279–86.
10. Mathew A, George PS, Ildaphonse G. Obesity kidney cancer risk in women a meta-analysis (1992–2008). Asian Pac J Cancer Prev. 2009;10(3):471–8.
11. Bergström A, Hsieh CC, et al. Obesity and renal cell cancer – a quantitative review. Br J Cancer. 2001;85(7):984–90.
12. Drabkin HA, Gemmill RM. Obesity, cholesterol and clear cell carcinoma (RCC). Adv Cancer Res. 2010;107:39–56.
13. Drabkin HA, Gemmil RM. Cholesterol and the development of clear cell renal carcinoma. Curr Opin Pharmacol. 2012;12(6):742–50.
14. Chiu BC, Gapstur SM, et al. Body mass index, physical activity, and risk of renal cell carcinoma. Int J Obes (Lond). 2006;30(6):940–7.
15. Xiao Q, Liao L, Matthews CE, et al. Physical activity and renal cell carcinoma among black and white Americans: a case-control study. BMC Cancer. 2014;14:707.
16. Stojanovic M, Goldner B, et al. Renal cell carcinoma and arterial hypertension. Clin Exp Nephrol. 2009;13(4):295–9.
17. Colt JS, Schwartz K, et al. Hypertension and risk of renal cell carcinoma among white and black Americans. Epidemiology. 2011;22(6):797–804.
18. Kuroda N, Ohe C, et al. Review of acquired cystic disease-associated renal cell carcinoma with focus on pathobiological aspects. Histol Histopathol. 2011;26(9):1215–8.
19. Gigante M, Neuzillet Y, et al. Renal cell carcinoma (RCC) arising in native kidneys of dialyzed and transplant patients: are they different entities? BJU Int. 2012;110(11 Pt B):E570–3.
20. Dubosq F, Linke C, et al. Renal cell carcinoma and trichloroethylene. Prog Urol. 2005;15(3):525–8.
21. Montella M, Tramacere I, et al. Coffee, decaffeinated coffee, tea intake, and risk of renal cell cancer. Nutr Cancer. 2009;61(1):76–80.
22. Klatte T, Patard JJ, et al. Metachronous bilateral renal cell carcinoma: risk assessment, prognosis and relevance of the primary-free interval. J Urol. 2007;177(6):2081–6; discussion 2086–7.
23. Kume H, Teramoto S, Kitamura T. Metachronous bilateral renal cell carcinoma with an interval of more than 10 years. Int Urol Nephrol. 2009;41(4):843–6.
24. Song DY, Song S, Song Y, Lee JE. Alcohol intake and renal cell cancer risk: a meta-analysis. Br J Cancer. 2012;106(11):1881–90.

Chapter 13
Pathology, Genetic Profile and Hereditary Syndromes

Santhosh Narayana Kurukkal and Salim Said Al-Busaidy

13.1 Pathology and Genetic Profile

RCC comprises of a heterogeneous group of tumours with diverse pathological molecular and genetic patterns and variable clinical outcomes. The World Health Organization (WHO 2004) has classified RCCs based primarily on morphology and genetic and molecular features but has also taken into account previous classifications, particularly the Mainz and Heidelberg classifications. The WHO 2004 classification includes *ten subtypes* (Table 13.1) [1], and nearly each RCC type occurs in the sporadic and in the hereditary form.

Recently the International Society of Urological Pathology (ISUP) has reached a consensus to add five new entities as distinct epithelial tumours [2]: tubulocystic renal cell carcinoma (RCC), acquired cystic disease-associated RCC, clear cell (tubulo)papillary RCC, the MiT family translocation RCCs (in particular t(6;11) RCC) and hereditary leiomyomatosis RCC syndrome-associated RCC. In addition three others were proposed for consideration: thyroid-like follicular RCC, succinate dehydrogenase B deficiency-associated RCC and ALK translocation RCC. However, in our present study, we will only consider the 2004 WHO classification as given in the table below.

1. *Clear cell renal cell carcinoma (CCRCC) is the most common histological subtype accounting for 60–70 % and arises from the proximal tubules.* In 2–4 % it is a part of inherited cancer syndrome including von Hippel-Lindau (VHL) and Birt-Hogg-Dubé (BHD) syndromes. *It is usually single*, with only 4 % multi-

S.N. Kurukkal (✉)
Urology Department, The Royal Hospital, Muscat, Oman
e-mail: drsanthoshnrn@gmail.com

S.S. Al-Busaidy
Senior Consultant and HOD, Urology Department, The Royal Hospital, Muscat, Oman
e-mail: salimalbusaidy@hotmail.com

S.A. Al-Mamari, S.S. Al-Busaidy (eds.), *Urological Cancer Management*,
DOI 10.1007/978-3-319-16301-7_13

Table 13.1 WHO histological classification of renal carcinomas (2004) [1]

1. Clear cell renal cell carcinoma (CCRCC)
2. Multilocular clear cell renal cell carcinoma
3. Papillary renal cell carcinoma (PRCC)
4. Chromophobe renal cell carcinoma (ChRCC)
5. Carcinoma of collecting ducts of Bellini
6. Renal medullary carcinoma
7. Xp11 translocation carcinomas
8. Carcinoma associated with neuroblastoma
9. Mucinous tubular and spindle cell carcinoma
10. Renal cell carcinoma unclassified

By Eble et al. With permission from the International Agency for Research on Cancer, 150 Cours Albert Thomas 69372 Lyon cedex 08, France

plicity and 3 % bilaterality. *Section surface is yellow with variable degree of haemorrhage, necrosis, cystic degeneration and calcification* [3] (Fig. 13.1a, b). *The clear cytoplasm of the tumour cells is due to loss of lipid and glycogen during tissue processing* [2] (Fig. 13.2a, b). *Granular eosinophilic cytoplasm indicates high-grade tumour.*

Seventy to ninety percent of CCRCC harbour chromosome 3p alterations. Loss of heterozygosity (LOH) was observed in 78 % of patients with sporadic CCRCC, and almost all the patients showed a likely loss of the whole of the region of 3p examined [3]. Familial VHL cases also exhibited LOH.

VHL protein plays an important role in cellular response to hypoxia through regulation of the hypoxia-inducible factor (HIF), a transcriptional factor. The following sequences are observed [4, 5]:

- Normoxic condition → hydroxylation of HIF → recognition and binding by wild-type VHL protein → degradation of HIF within the proteosomes → HIF levels kept at low level.
- Hypoxic condition → no hydroxylation of HIF → no recognition by VHL → accumulation of HIF → activation of hypoxia-driven genes[1]→activation of intracellular signal transduction pathways (Fig. 13.3).

[1] The genes activated in hypoxic conditions include:

VEGF (vascular endothelial growth factor): promotes angiogenesis

PDGF-β (platelet-derived growth factor): promotes angiogenesis

TGF-α (transforming growth factor): for cell growth and survival

Glut-1: for anaerobic metabolism

CA IX: for acid-base balance

Erythropoietin (EPO): for red cell production

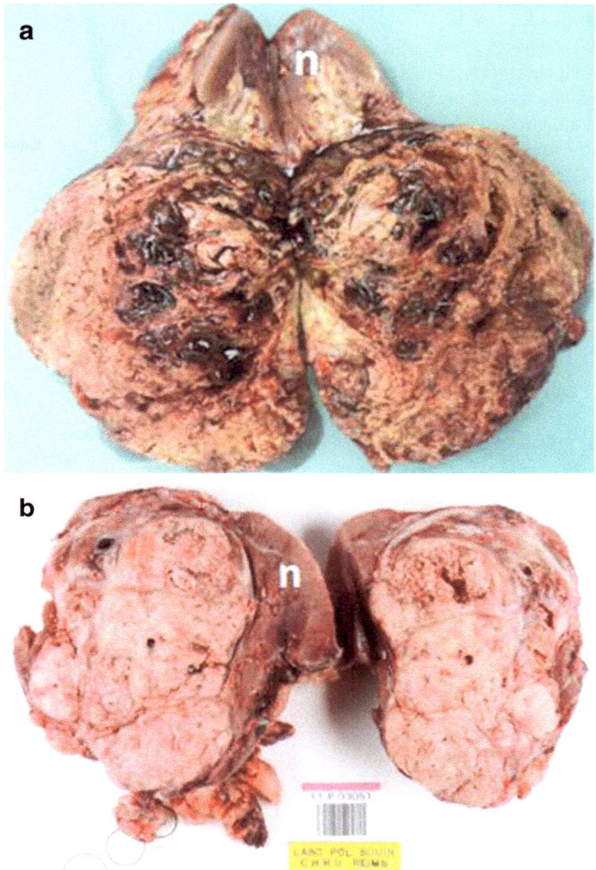

Fig. 13.1 (**a**) A right radical nephrectomy specimen with a huge CCR (*n* normal renal parenchyma) (Courtesy of Kurian George, Urology, The Royal Hospital, Muscat, Oman). (**b**) Section surface of a clear cell RCC with large areas of necrosis (Courtesy of A. Durlach, Pol Bouin Laboratory, University Hospital of Reims, France) (*n* normal renal parenchyma)

These pathways stimulate angiogenesis and compensatory metabolic changes in normal cells when coping with hypoxia [3]. *Therefore, inactivation of VHL gene by mutation or hypermethylation results in uncontrolled cellular proliferation leading to tumorigenesis* [6, 7].

Another signalling pathway important in RCC is *mTOR* [8] (mammalian target of rapamycin[2]). mTOR activation in the presence of phospholipase D enhances the expression of both HIF-1α and HIF-2α in RCC cells [8, 9].

In targeted therapy, critical components of these pathways are targeted as follows:

[2] Rapamycin is the other name of the drug sirolimus.

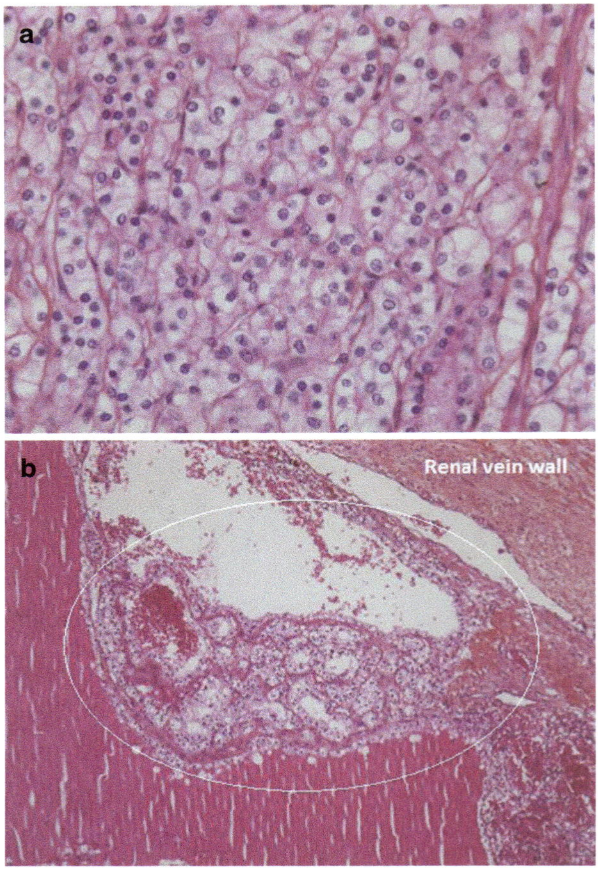

Fig. 13.2 (**a**, **b**) Microphotographs of a clear cell carcinoma showing the characteristic clear cytoplasm and a massive tumour thrombus in the renal vein. The circle does not encompass all the embolus (Courtesy of A. Durlach, Pol Bouin Laboratory, University Hospital of Reims, France)

- VEGFR (R = receptor) using *neutralizing antibody bevacizumab*
- VEGFR and PDGFR using *small molecule inhibitors of tyrosine kinase such as sorafenib and sunitinib*
- EGFR (epidermal growth factor receptor) using *erlotinib*
- mTOR using *temsirolimus*

2. *Papillary Renal Cell Carcinoma (PRCC): Second most common type of RCC accounting for 10–15 %.* PRCC usually present at an early stage and has a *better prognosis* compared to CCRCC of the same stage [10]. The vast majority occurs sporadically; however, there is also a familial variety. They have a well-circumscribed mass enclosed in a pseudocapsule, but some tumours appear necrotic and friable (Fig. 13.4a, b). Bilaterality and multifocality are more frequent than with other RCC varieties [3].
   Two histological types are described [11]:

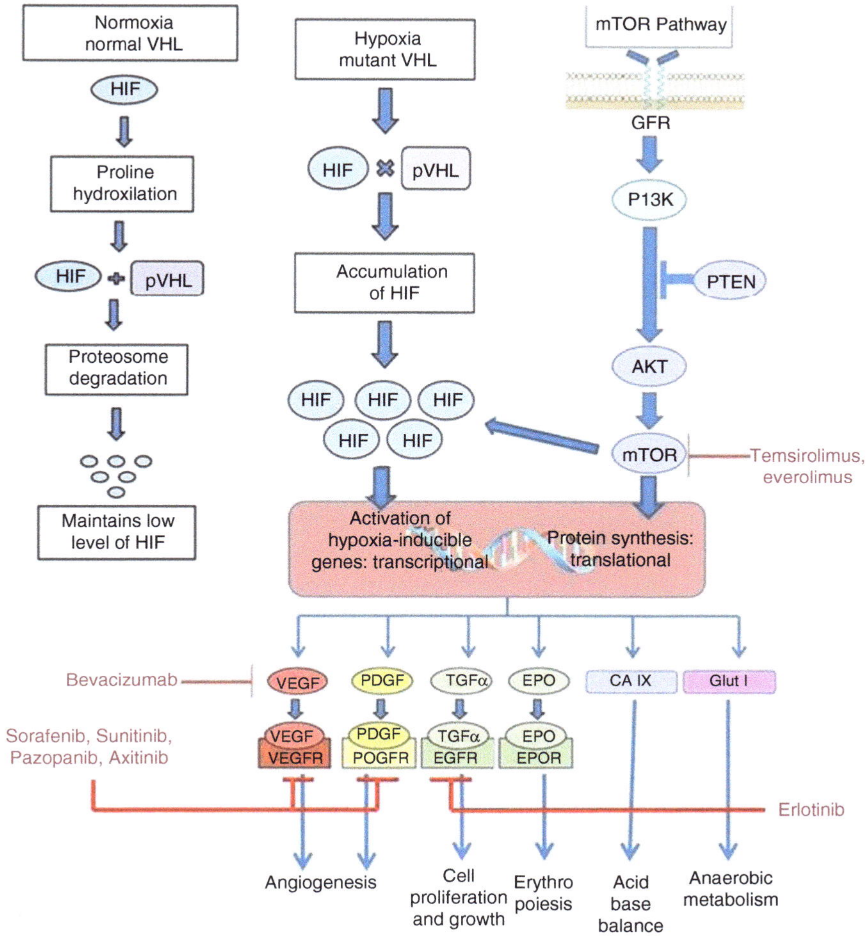

Fig. 13.3 Pathway for VHL and mTOR

- *Type I*: *Cells with scanty pale cytoplasm. Frequent psammoma bodies and foamy macrophages. Cytokeratin +. They have better prognosis.*
- *Type II*: Pseudostratified nuclei, prominent nucleoli, voluminous eosinophilic cytoplasm. *They have worse prognosis.*

3. *Chromophobe renal cell carcinoma* (*ChRCC*): Accounts for 5 % of RCCs. Believed to arise from intercalated cells of collecting ducts. *Prognosis is significantly better than CCRCC. Patients with ChRCC have a low risk of recurrence* (*<5 %*), *tumour progression, metastasis and cancer-specific death* [12].
4. *Multilocular cystic RCC*: 5 % of RCC. Because of their extremely good prognosis after surgery with a 5-year disease-specific survival rate of 100 %, authors

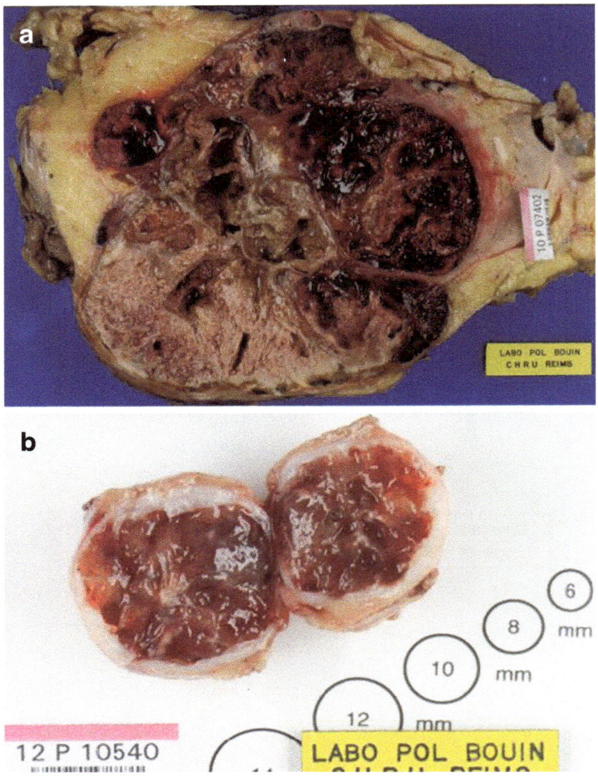

Fig. 13.4 (**a**, **b**) Gross specimens of papillary RCC on radical and partial nephrectomy (Courtesy of A. Durlach, Pol Bouin Laboratory, University Hospital of Reims, France)

have proposed to rename this entity as "multilocular cystic renal cell neoplasm of low malignant potential" [13].

5. *Carcinoma of the collecting ducts of Bellini*: Less than 1 % of all renal tumours. *They are aggressive tumours with 76 and 19 % of patients found respectively to have pT3 and distant metastases at nephrectomy* [14].
6. *Medullary carcinoma*: *Very rare. Occurs in patients with sickle cell haemoglobinopathy or trait, especially African-Americans and Brazilians. Mean age is 22 years*. They are very aggressive with *almost all patients presenting with metastasis and dying within 6 months of diagnosis* (*median survival after nephrectomy*: *15 weeks*) [15, 16]
7. The characteristics of the last classified three subtypes of RCC can be summarized as follows [3]: *Xp11.2 translocation carcinoma* affects children and young adults, accounting for 40 % of RCCs in the latter age group. It is indolent in children but aggressive in adults. The majority of patients with *mucinous tubular and spindle cell carcinoma* remain disease-free after surgical resection. *Post-neuroblastoma renal cell carcinoma* occurs in long-term survivors of neuroblastoma with a mean age of 13.5 years (2–35 years), and its pathological features and prognosis are similar to CCRCC.

Table 13.2 Fuhrman nuclear grading system [17]

Grade	Nuclear size (μm)	Nuclear shape	Chromatin	Nucleoli
1	<10	Round	Dense	Inconspicuous
2	15	Round	Finely granular	Small, not visible at 10×
3	20	Round/oval	Coarsely granular	Prominent, visible at 10×
4	>20	Pleomorphic multilobated	Open, hyperchromatic	Macronucleoli

Table 13.3 Familial renal tumours [3, 18–20]

Syndrome	Chromosome	Gene	Protein	Tumour type
von Hippel-Lindau	3p25	VHL	pVHL	Multiple, bilateral
				Clear cell RCC
				Renal cysts
Tuberous sclerosis	9q34	TSC1	Hamartin and tuberin	Multiple bilateral angiomyolipomas
	16p13	TSC2		Lymphangioleiomyomatosis
				Clear cell RCC
Hereditary papillary RCC	7p31	c-MET	HGF-R	Multiple, bilateral papillary RCC type I
Birt-Hogg-Dubé	17p11	BHD	Folliculin	Multiple chromophobe RCC
				Oncocytoma
				Papillary RCC
Constitutional translocation chromosome 3	3p13–14	–	–	Multiple bilateral clear cell RCC
Hereditary leiomyoma RCC	1q42	FH	FH	Papillary RCC type II

13.1.1 Fuhrman Nuclear Grading

Fuhrman nuclear grading is a histological predictor of prognosis for CCRCC [17]. First described in 1982, it is based on nuclear size, shape, chromatin and nucleolar prominence and is categorized into 4 grades (Table 13.2).

13.2 Hereditary Syndromes

A high number of hereditary syndromes predispose to development of RCC [3, 18–20] (Table 13.3). The predisposing genes identified include von Hippel-Lindau (VHL), met proto-oncogene (MET), fumarate hydratase (FH), folliculin (FLCN;

synonym: BHD) and cell division cycle 73, Paf1/RNA polymerase II complex component and homolog (CDC73; previously known as HRPT2). Less than 5 % of RCC occur in the setting of inherited cancer syndrome.

1. *von Hippel-Lindau* disease is an *autosomal dominant hereditary condition* with stigmata including CCRCCs, central nervous system haemangioblastomas, pheochromocytomas, pancreatic cysts and endolymphatic sac tumours of the inner ear. It is caused by mutations in VHL gene. *CCRCCs in VHL syndrome tend to be bilateral and multifocal, dozens or even hundreds of microscopic tumour foci can be identified in resected kidney specimens. RCC is the leading cause of death in VHL patients* [3].
2. *Tuberous sclerosis*: *First described by Désiré-Magloire Bourneville in 1880, it is also called tuberous sclerosis complex, Bourneville syndrome or EPILOIA* (epilepsy, low intelligence, adenoma sebaceum). It is an autosomal dominant hereditary disease included in the phacomatoses group. But it is also seen in sporadic forms. It is very rare and occurs in 1 in 6,000 live births [21]. It is characterized by hypomelanic skin macules, angiofibromas, retinal hamartomas, infantile epilepsy (West syndrome), renal angiomyolipomas (AML) in teenagers and adults and very rarely renal carcinoma. Very rarely it may present with spontaneous perirenal bleeding known as Wunderlich's syndrome [22].
3. *Hereditary papillary RCC* (*HPRCC*): There are *multiple bilateral type I PRCC. Contrary to the other hereditary syndromes, the kidney is the only organ affected in this group*. This disorder was described in a three generation family with no abnormality of the Xme 3p [23].
4. *Birt-Hogg-Dubé syndrome is an autosomal dominant disorder characterized by benign cutaneous fibrofolliculomas, renal tumours, lung cysts and spontaneous pneumothorax* [24]. The genetic alteration for BHD syndrome is located in chromosome 17p12q11. *The renal tumours are multiple and bilateral* chromophobe RCC and hybrid oncocytomas [25].
5. *Hereditary leiomyomatosis and renal cell cancer* (*HLRCC*) *is an autosomal dominant disease which* predisposes to cutaneous leiomyomas, uterine leiomyomas and papillary RCCs type II. Renal tumours are often solitary, unilateral and more aggressive [3]

Take-Home Message: Pathology, Genetic Profiles and Hereditary Syndromes

Clear cell RCC is the most common histological subtype of RCC accounting for 60–70 %. It arises from the proximal tubules, and 70–90 % of CCRCC harbour *chromosome 3p alterations*.

The 2nd most common subtype is *papillary RCC* which accounts for 10–15 % and has a better prognosis than CCRCC. Among the other variants, *chromophobe and multilocular cystic RCCs* have a good prognosis, while *carcinoma of the collecting ducts of Bellini and medullary carcinoma* have a very bad prognosis.

Medullary carcinoma characteristically occurs in young African-American patients with sickle cell haemoglobinopathy or traits

VHL protein plays an important role in cellular response to hypoxia through regulation of hypoxia-inducible factor (HIF).

In hypoxic conditions, angiogenesis and compensatory metabolic changes occur in normal cells. The involved pathways include activation of the following genes: VEGF, PDGF-β, TGF-α, Glut-1, CA IX and erythropoietin (EPO).

Inactivation of the VHL gene by mutation or hypermethylation results in uncontrolled cellular proliferation leading to tumorigenesis.

mTOR is another signalling pathway, and its activation in the presence of phospholipase D enhances the expression of both HIF-1α and HIF-2α in RCC cells.

The concept of *targeted therapy* is an attempt to selectively block the above-mentioned pathways. Hence, bevacizumab is targeting the receptor of VEGF, while sorafenib and sunitinib are used to block both receptors of VEGF and PDGF. Erlotinib and temsirolimus target the receptors of EGFR and mTOR, respectively.

Fuhrman nuclear grading is a widely used histological predictor of prognosis for CCRCC.

Several hereditary syndromes are known to be associated with renal carcinomas:

von Hippel-Lindau disease: Characteristically associated with bilateral and numerous microscopic foci of CCRCC. It is caused by mutations in VHL gene located on chromosome 3p. Other components of this syndrome are central nervous system haemangioblastomas, pheochromocytomas, pancreatic cysts and endolymphatic sac tumours of the inner ear.

Tuberous sclerosis: This syndrome is defined by the abbreviation EPILOIA (epilepsy, low intelligence, adenoma sebaceum) and is associated with renal angiomyolipoma and very rarely renal carcinoma.

Others: Hereditary papillary RCC, Birt-Hogg-Dubé syndrome and the combination hereditary leiomyomatosis and renal cell cancer.

References

1. Eble JN, Sauter G, Epstein JI, Sesterhenn IA. World Health Organization classification of tumours: pathology and genetics of tumours of the urinary system and male genital organs. Lyon: IARC; 2004. p. 10.
2. Srigley JR, Delahunt B, Eble JN, et al., ISUP Renal Tumour Panel. The International Society of Urological Pathology (ISUP) Vancouver classification of renal neoplasia. Am J Surg Pathol. 2013;37(10):1469–89.

3. Ming Z, Huiying H. Pathology of renal cell carcinoma. In: Campbell SC, Rini BI, editors. Renal cell carcinoma: clinical management, Current clinical urology. New York: Springer; 2013. p. 23–41.
4. Banks RE, Tirukonda P, Taylor C, Hornigold N, Astuti D, Cohen D, Maher ER, Stanley AJ, Harnden P, Joyce A, Knowles M, Selby PJ. Genetic and epigenetic analysis of von Hippel-Lindau (VHL) gene alterations and relationship with clinical variables in sporadic renal cancer. Cancer Res. 2006;66(4):2000–11.
5. Kaelin Jr WG. Molecular basis of the VHL hereditary cancer syndrome. Nat Rev Cancer. 2002;2(9):673–82.
6. Hudson CC, Liu M, Chiang GG, et al. Regulation of hypoxia-inducible factor 1alpha expression and function by the mammalian target of rapamycin. Mol Cell Biol. 2002;22(20):7004–14.
7. Wykoff CC, Pugh CW, Harris AL, Maxwell PH, Ratcliffe PJ. The HIF pathway: implications for patterns of gene expression in cancer. Novartis Found Symp. 2001;240:212–25.
8. Battelli C, Cho DC. mTOR inhibitors in renal cell carcinoma. Therapy. 2011;8(4):359–67.
9. Toschi A, Edelstein J, Rockwell P, Ohh M, Foster DA. HIFα expression in VHL-deficient renal cancer cells is dependent on phospholipase D. Oncogene. 2008;27(19):2746–53.
10. Amin MB, Corless CL, et al. Papillary (chromophil) renal cell carcinoma: histomorphologic characteristics and evaluation of conventional pathologic prognostic parameters in 62 cases. Am J Surg Pathol. 1997;21(6):621–35.
11. Delahunt B, Eble JN McCredie MR, Bethwaite PB, Stewart JH, Bilous AM. Morphologic typing of papillary renal cell carcinoma: comparison of growth kinetics and patient survival in 66 cases. Hum Pathol 2001;32(6):590–5.
12. Volpe A, Novara G, Antonelli A, et al. Chromophobe renal cell carcinoma (RCC): oncological outcomes and prognostic factors in a large multicentre series. BJU Int. 2012;110(1):76–83.
13. Suzigan S, López-Beltrán A, Montironi R, et al. Multilocular cystic renal cell carcinoma: a report of 45 cases of a kidney tumour of low malignant potential. Am J Clin Pathol. 2006;125(2):217–22.
14. Karakiewicz PI, Trinh QD, Rioux-Leclercq N, et al. Collecting duct renal cell carcinoma: a matched analysis of 4 cases. Eur Urol. 2007;52(4):1140–5.
15. Davis Jr CJ, Mostofi FK, Sesterhenn IA. Renal medullary carcinoma. The seventh sickle cell nephropathy. Am J Surg Pathol. 1995;19(1):1–11.
16. Watanabe IC, Billis A, Guimarães MS, et al. Renal medullary carcinoma: report of seven cases from Brazil. Mod Pathol. 2007;20(9):914–20.
17. Fuhrman SA, Lasky LC, et al. Prognostic significance of morphologic parameters in renal cell carcinoma. Am J Surg Pathol. 1982;6(7):655–63.
18. Algaba F, Akaza H, Lopez-Beltrán A, Martignoni G, Moch H, Montironi R, Reuter V. Current pathology keys of renal cell carcinoma. Eur Urol. 2011;60(4):634–43.
19. Lopez-Beltran A, Montironi R, Egevad L, Caballero-Vargas MT, Scarpelli M, Kirkali Z, Cheng L. Genetic profiles in renal tumours. Int J Urol. 2010;17:6–19.
20. Lopez-Beltran A, Cheng L, Vidal A, Scarpelli M, Kirkali Z, Blanca A, Montironi R. Pathology of renal cell carcinoma, an update. Anal Quant Cytopathol Histpathol. 2013;35(2):61–75.
21. Osborne JP, Freyer A, Webb D. Epidemiology of tuberous sclerosis. Ann N Y Acad Sci. 1991;615:125–7.
22. Sparks D, Chase D, Thomas D, Arnott J. The Wunderlich's syndrome secondary to massive bilateral angiomyolipomas associated with advanced tuberous sclerosis. Saudi J Kidney Dis Transpl. 2011;22(3):534–7.
23. Zbar B, Tory K, Merino M, et al. Hereditary papillary renal cell carcinoma. J Urol. 1994;151(3):561–6.
24. Toro JR, Wei MH, Glenn GM, et al. BHD mutations, clinical and molecular genetic investigations of Birt-Hogg-Dube syndrome: a new series of 50 families and a review of published reports. J Med Genet. 2008;45:321.
25. Adley BP, Smith ND, Nayar R, Yang XJ. Birt-Hogg-Dubé syndrome: clinicopathologic findings and genetic alterations. Arch Pathol Lab Med. 2006;130(12):1865–70.

Chapter 14
Clinical Features

Santhosh Narayana Kurukkal and Salim Said Al-Busaidy

As the kidneys are retroperitoneal in location, renal tumours remain asymptomatic until advanced stages. Local symptoms arise only after reaching enough size to displace or invade other organs. The manifestations are diverse, signs and symptoms are often latent. In the past, RCC used to be called '*Internist's tumour*'. *Now due to the liberal use of imaging modalities, about 60 % of RCCs are detected incidentally at early stage,* Hence Novick and Campbell renamed it '*Radiologist's tumour*' [1, 2]. The incidental tumours are clinically and histologically less aggressive and leads to better patient survivals and decreased recurrences [3, 4].

14.1 Classic Triad

Nowadays the 'classic triad' combining flank pain, haematuria and palpable abdominal mass is seen in fewer than 10 % of cases and is considered as 'too late a triad'. Most of the patients presenting with all the three symptoms already suffer from metastatic disease. When present, symptoms are most frequently isolated [5]:

- *Haematuria is the most common, and is seen in 40–60 % of cases.*
- *Flank pain is seen in 40 %, caused by bleeding within the tumour or invasion into adjacent tissue.*
- *Palpable mass* is present in fewer than a third of patients (Fig. 14.1a, b).
- *Constitutional symptoms* like fatigue, loss of weight, fever and nausea occur in advanced disease.

S.N. Kurukkal (✉)
Urology Department, The Royal Hospital, Muscat, Oman
e-mail: drsanthoshnrn@gmail.com

S.S. Al-Busaidy
Senior Consultant and HOD, Urology Department, The Royal Hospital, Muscat, Oman
e-mail: salimalbusaidy@hotmail.com

S.A. Al-Mamari, S.S. Al-Busaidy (eds.), *Urological Cancer Management*,
DOI 10.1007/978-3-319-16301-7_14

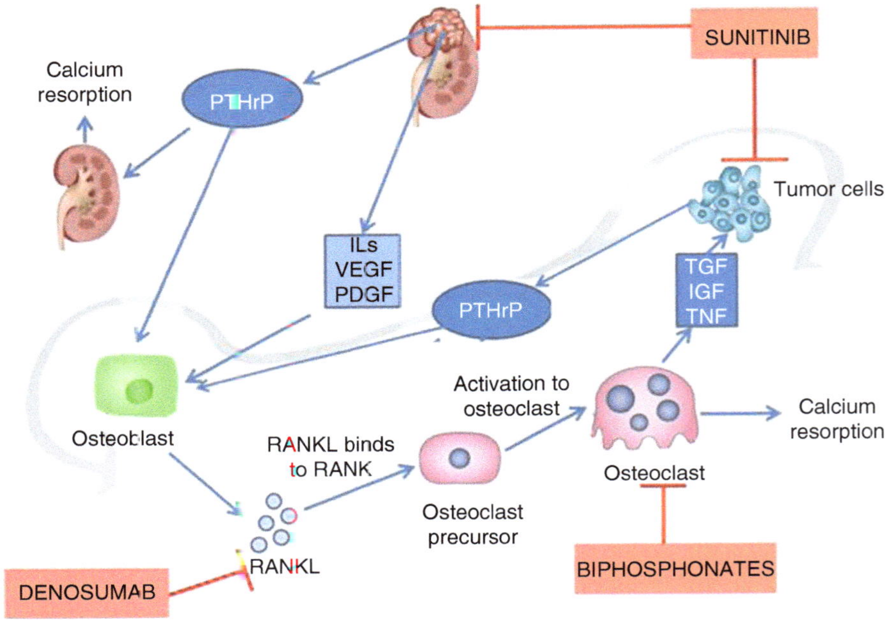

Fig. 14.3 Mechanism of hypercalcaemia in RCC. Vicious cycle of hypercalcaemia. Renal cell carcinoma secreting PTHrP causes renal reabsorption of calcium and stimulates osteoblasts. Osteoblasts produce RANKL which in turn binds to RANK receptor on the surface of osteoclast precursor, resulting in activation to osteoclasts. Osteoclasts cause bone resorption and produce tumour growth factors which enhance metastatic tumour growth. Denosumab is a monoclonal antibody that binds to RANK inhibiting the formation of osteoclasts

PTH-rP binds to PTH receptors in renal tubules and bone. This increases bone resorption of calcium, decreases renal clearance of calcium and increases phosphorus excretion. Also PTH-rP inhibits 1.25 hydroxylase in kidneys lowering the level of active vitamin D3. The net result is hypercalcaemia, reduced levels of PTH and Vit D3 and renal phosphate wasting. Other mediators are also known to potentiate this cascade, like TGF α and β, IL-1, IL-6 and TNF [20, 21].

Note: *Hypercalcaemia secondary to bone metastasis accounts for 50 % of hypercalcaemia in RCC and is not a true PNS*. Metastatic tumour in the bone liberates substances that activate osteoclasts causing the release of calcium from bone. Local secretion of prostaglandins and IL-6 were attributed to this reaction. Patients may have bone pain, which can be alleviated by radiotherapy. Medical therapy is beneficial in managing systemic effects. Agents such as biphosphonates and osteoprotegerin were proven effective in the treatment of lytic bone disease mediated by osteoclast activation [22].

Symptoms and signs of hypercalcaemia are systemic such as fatigue, lethargy, nausea, weakness, confusion, constipation, reduced deep tendon reflexes (DTRs) and impaired level of consciousness. Other signs include dehydration, ECG changes such as prolonged PR and QT interval, bradyarrhythmias and asystole. Patients presenting in hypercalcemic coma have also been reported [23]. Management includes initial hydration by intravenous infusion of normal saline and loop diuretics (furosemide), and avoidance of thiazide diuretics. Biphosphonates are effective in long-term management. Indomethacin (NSAID drug) has been reported as effective in patients with high serum prostaglandins. Nephrectomy was reported to be effective in relieving the associated hypercalcaemia [24, 25].

Treatment with sunitinib, tyrosine kinase inhibitor has been reported to successfully control paraneoplastic hypercalcaemia which was resistant to conventional therapy. Sunitinib also helps in alleviating symptoms [26].

14.2.2 Hypertension

Long-standing hypertension is a risk factor for RCC and evidence also suggests that RCC causes hypertension [27]. Hypertension is experienced in 40 % of patients with RCC as a PNS, whereas the incidence in age-matched control is 20 %. Cause is attributed to various peptides released from RCC, increased renin secretion (by the tumour itself or by the adjacent renal parenchyma due to tumour compression and hypoxia), presence of arteriovenous fistula, tumour compression of the renal artery or its branches and polycythaemia. Nephrectomy has been reported to reduce the hypertension in these patients. Renin elevation was found in up to 37 % of patients. It was correlated with high grade and stage of RCC with mixed histological subtypes and indicated poor prognosis. The role of renin as the cause of hypertension in RCC is controversial [28, 29]. Many renal epithelial neoplasms like oncocytoma and chromophobe carcinoma express renin in the cytoplasm of tumour cells. However, the role of this renin in hypertension is not clear, being structurally abnormal and biologically inactive, and its secretion into circulation is doubtful. Most of the RCC tumours are hypervascular and may harbour small arteriovenous fistulas (AVF) [30, 31]. Rarely tumour AVF produces sufficient left to right shunting to cause decompensation of the cardiovascular system, leading to intractable hypertension and congestive cardiac failure. Nephrectomy offers a dramatic improvement in hypertension and resolution of clinical cardiovascular symptoms.

14.2.3 Polycythaemia

Erythropoietin (EPO) is a glycoprotein normally produced by the peritubular interstitial cells of the kidney and functions to promote red cell production from bone marrow. *RCC behaves as an ectopic site of EPO synthesis and raised EPO has been observed in 63 % of cases* [32, 33]. *Level of EPO in RCC was not shown to correlate directly with tumour grade, stage, histological type, prognosis or haematocrit and haemoglobin levels*. Even though most of patients with RCC produce EPO, erythrocytosis and polycythaemia has been noted only in about 5 % of RCCs. Tumour cells may be producing inactive forms of EPO. *In patients with organ-confined disease, EPO falls to normal after nephrectomy, but in mRCC, it tends to remain elevated.* EPO can have a role as a marker during therapy. It has been reported recently that targeted presurgical sunitinib therapy in mRCC successfully controlled polycythaemia caused by EPO production in tumour cells [34].

14.2.4 Anaemia

Anaemia is more common in RCC than polycythaemia. *Tumour cachexia* is an important cause of the anaemia. *Lactoferrin*, a glycoprotein produced by RCC cells is another suggested cause [35]. Lower serum iron levels correlate with the RCC stage, the effects of surgery and the advent of recurrence [36].

Ferritin is produced by kidney tumour cells [37]. Intraoperative renal vein ferritin has positive correlation to tumour size and volume. The practical clinical role of peripheral serum ferritin as an indicator of disease status, and as a prognosticator of survival has not been established [38].

14.2.5 Stauffer's Syndrome

Maurice H. Stauffer, a gastroenterologist in Mayo clinic, first characterized the syndrome in 1961, with the original name '*nephrogenic hepatomegaly*' [39]. This unique paraneoplastic syndrome associated with RCC, is *a nonmetastatic hepatic dysfunction* and comprises a constellation of signs and symptoms. It is characterized by an elevation of liver enzymes and abnormal levels of hepatic synthetic products and has been reported in *3–20 % of RCC patients. Clinically patients present with hepatosplenomegaly, fever and weight loss*. There is *a raised serum alkaline phosphate in all patients, an elevated prothrombin time or hypoalbumineamia in 66 %, an elevated serum bilirubin or transaminase levels in 20 % and an elevated gammaglobulin in 54 %*.

Diagnosis requires at least three of these serum abnormalities. Thrombocytopenia and neutropenia are other findings.

The exact mechanism of hepatic injury is not completely understood. *Liver biopsy reveals generalized hepatitis with lymphocyte infiltration and hepatocellular degeneration and shows discrete regions of hepatic necrosis in many patients.* Hepatic function normalizes in 66 % of patients after nephrectomy, and persistence of hepatic dysfunction is consistent with persistence of a viable tumour and poor prognosis [40–43].

Take-Home Message: RCC – Clinical Manifestations

Incidental detection	Nowadays about 60 % of RCCs are detected serendipitously at early stage due to the liberal use of imaging modalities. *The Internist's tumour has become a Radiologist's tumour*
Local tumour effect	The classic triad is seen in <10 % cases. The symptoms are mostly isolated including haematuria, flank pain, palpable mass, retroperitoneal bleeding
Metastatic manifestations	Cough and chest pain, bone pain, neurological symptoms
IVC thrombus	Bilateral lower limb oedema, nonreducing and right-sided varicocoele
Paraneoplastic syndromes	Constitutional symptoms, fever, hypercalcaemia, hypertension, polycythaemia, anaemia, Stauffer's syndrome, amyloidosis, neuromyopathy, Cushing syndrome, galactorrhoea, vasculopathy, coagulopathy

References

1. Jayson M, Sanders H. Increased incidence of serendipitously discovered renal cell carcinoma. Urology. 1998;51(2):203–5.
2. Campbell SC, Lane BR. Chapter 49. Malignant renal tumours. In: Campbell-Walsh urology. 10th ed. Philadelphia: Saunders Elsevier; 2012. p. 1437.
3. Patard JJ, Rodriguez A, Rioux-Leclercq N, Guillé F, Lobel B. Prognostic significance of the mode of detection in renal tumours. BJU Int. 2002;90(4):358–63.
4. Tsui KH, Shvarts O, Smith RB, Figlin R, de Kernion JB, Belldegrun A. Renal cell carcinoma: prognostic significance of incidentally detected tumours. J Urol. 2000;163(2):426–30.
5. Pantuck AJ, Zisman A, Belldegrun AS. The changing natural history of renal cell carcinoma. J Urol. 2001;166(5):1611–23.
6. Brown ET, Perlmutter AE, Oliverio B, Williams HJ, Zaslau S. Chromophobe renal cell carcinoma presenting as hemorrhagic shock: case report. Can J Urol. 2008;15(5):4276–8.
7. Mikami K, Takei K, Naito H. A case of spontaneous rupture of renal cell carcinoma. Hinyokika Kiyo. 1997;43(12):867–70.
8. Seseke S, Schreiber M, Rebmann U, Seseke F. Spontaneous perirenal hematomas in patients taking anticoagulation medication or having a bleeding diathesis. Aktuelle Urol. 2008;39(3): 215–8.
9. Nakai M, Nakamura N. A case report of spontaneous rupture of renal cell carcinoma difficult to be distinguished from angiomyolipoma. Hinyokika Kiyo. 2003;49(2):99–101.
10. Yang Y, Mao QZ, Li HZ, et al. Clinical features of urological malignancies with paraneoplastic syndromes. Zhonghua Yi Xue Za Zhi. 2010;90(48):3411–4.
11. Feng CC, Ding GX, Song NH, Li X, Wu Z, Jiang HW, Ding Q. Paraneoplastic hormones: parathyroid hormone-related protein (PTHrP) and erythropoietin (EPO) are related to vascular endothelial growth factor (VEGF) expression in clear cell renal cell carcinoma. Tumour Biol. 2013;34(6):3471–6.
12. Alsirafy SA, El Mesidy SM, Abou-Elela EN, Elfaramawy YI. Naproxen test for neoplastic fever may reduce suffering. J Palliat Med. 2011;14(5):665–7.

13. Tsukamoto T, Kumamoto Y, Miyao N, Masumori N, Takahashi A, Yanase M. Interleukin-6 in renal cell carcinoma. J Urol. 1992;148(6):1778–81; discussion 1781–2.
14. Palapattu GS, Kristo B, Rajfer J. Paraneoplastic syndromes in urologic malignancy: the many faces of renal cell carcinoma. Rev Urol. 2002;4(4):163–70.
15. Albright F. Case records of the Massachusetts General Hospital: case 39061. N Engl J Med. 1941;225:789–96.
16. Goldberg MF, Tashjian Jr AH, Order SE, Dammin GJ. Renal adenocarcinoma containing a parathyroid hormone-like substance and associated with marked hypercalcemia. Am J Med. 1964;36:805–14.
17. Sourbier C, Massfelder T. Parathyroid hormone-related protein in human renal cell carcinoma. Cancer Lett. 2006;240(2):170–82.
18. Mangin M, Webb AC, Dreyer BE, et al. Identification of a cDNA encoding a parathyroid hormone-like peptide from a human tumour associated with humoral hypercalcemia of malignancy. Proc Natl Acad Sci U S A. 1988;85(2):597–601.
19. Wysolmerski JJ. Parathyroid hormone-related protein: an update. J Clin Endocrinol Metab. 2012;97(9):2947–56.
20. Mundy GR, Edwards JR. PTH-related peptide (PTHrP) in hypercalcemia. J Am Soc Nephrol. 2008;19(4):672–5.
21. Ueno M, Ban S, Nakanoma T, Tsukamoto T, Nonaka S, Hirata R, Iida M, Deguchi N. Hypercalcemia in a patient with renal cell carcinoma producing parathyroid hormone-related protein and interleukin-6. Int J Urol. 2000;7:239–42.
22. Paule B. Interleukin-6 and bone metastasis of renal cancer: molecular bases and therapeutic implications. Prog Urol. 2001;11(2):368–75.
23. Pepper K, Jaowattana U, Starsiak MD, et al. Renal cell carcinoma presenting with paraneoplastic hypercalcemic coma: a case report and review of the literature. J Gen Intern Med. 2007;22(7):1042–6.
24. Walther MM, Patel B, et al. Hypercalcemia in patients with metastatic renal cell carcinoma: effect of nephrectomy and metabolic evaluation. J Urol. 1997;158(3):733–9.
25. Clines GA. Mechanisms and treatment of hypercalcemia of malignancy. Curr Opin Endocrinol Diabetes Obes. 2011;18(6):339–46.
26. Karaca H, Lale A, Dikilitas M, Ozkan M, Er O. Recovery of paraneoplastic *hypercalcemia* by sunitinib *treatment* for renal cell carcinoma: a case report and review of the literature. Med Oncol. 2010;27(3):1023–6.
27. Stojanovic M, Goldner B, Ivkovic D. Renal cell carcinoma and arterial hypertension. Clin Exp Nephrol. 2009;13(4):295–9.
28. Arias LF, Bruneval P, Blanco J. Renin expression in adult renal epithelial tumours with granular cells. Pathol Res Pract. 2010;206:731–4.
29. Lindop GB, Fleming S. Renin in renal cell carcinoma – an immunocytochemical study using an antibody to pure human rennin. J Clin Pathol. 1984;37(1):27–31.
30. Crawford ED, Skinner DG, Mallamo JT. Renal arteriovenous fistulas secondary to bilateral renal cell carcinoma. Urology. 1979;13(5):525–8.
31. Esquerre C, Delahaye RP, Carle S, Metges PJ, Moine D, Maydat L, Bon JF, Duriez R. Arteriovenous fistulas in renal carcinoma. Diagnosis in one case. J Radiol Electrol Med Nucl. 1973;54(5):389–94.
32. Da Silva J-L, Lacombe C, Bruneval P, et al. Tumour cells are the site of erythropoietin synthesis in human renal cancers associated with polycythemia. Blood. 1990;75(3):577–82.
33. Sherwood JB, Burns ER, Shouval D. Stimulation by cAMP of erythropoietin secretion by an established human renal carcinoma cell line. Blood. 1987;69(4):1053–7.
34. Ueda K, Suekane S, Chikui K, Nakiri M, Moriya F, Hayashi T, Miyajima J, Matsuoka K. Successful treatment of erythropoietin-producing advanced renal cell carcinoma after targeted therapy using sunitinib: case report and review of the literature. Mol Clin Oncol. 2013;1:112–6.
35. Loughlin KR, Gittes RF, Partridge D, Stelos P. The relationship of lactoferrin to the anemia of renal cell carcinoma. Cancer. 1987;59(3):566–71.

36. Yu CC, Chen KK, Chen MT, Huang JK, Lin AT, Lee YH, Chang LS. Serum iron as a tumour marker in renal cell carcinoma. Eur Urol. 1991;19(1):54–8.
37. Kirkali Z, Güzelsoy M, Mungan MU, Kirkali G, Yörükoglu K. Serum ferritin as a clinical marker for renal cell carcinoma: influence of tumour size and volume. Urol Int. 1999; 62(1):21–5.
38. Partin AW, Criley SR, Steiner MS, Hsieh K, Simons JW, Lumadue J, Carter HB, Marshall FF. Serum ferritin as a clinical marker for renal cell carcinoma: influence of tumour volume. Urology. 1995;45(2):211–7.
39. Stauffer MH. Nephrogenic hepatomegaly. Gastroenterology. 1961;40:694.
40. Hanash KA. The nonmetastatic hepatic dysfunction syndrome associated with renal cell carcinoma (hypernephroma): Stauffer's syndrome. Prog Clin Biol Res. 1982;100:310–6.
41. Boxer RJ, Waisman J, Lieber MM, Mampaso FM, Skinner DG. Non-metastatic hepatic dysfunction associated with renal carcinoma. J Urol. 1978;119(4):468–71.
42. Kranidiotis GP, Voidonikola PT, Dimopoulos MK, Anastasiou-Nana MI. Stauffer's syndrome as a prominent manifestation of renal cancer: a case report. Cases J. 2009;2:49.
43. Tomadoni A, García C, Márquez M, Ayala JC, Prado F. Stauffer's syndrome with jaundice, a paraneoplastic manifestation of renal cell carcinoma: a case report. Arch Esp Urol. 2010; 63(2):154–6.

Chapter 15
Physical Examination, Laboratory and Radiological Investigations

Santhosh Narayana Kurukkal and Salim Said Al-Busaidy

15.1 Physical Examination

Physical examination should be as complete as possible from the head to the feet. This is needed to detect an eventual left supraclavicular lymph node (Troisier's sign or Virchow's node), elicit an abdominal mass and find a non-reducing varicocoele or pedal oedema.

15.2 Laboratory Parameters

Routine tests include complete blood cells count, serum creatinine and glomerular filtration rate, liver function tests, alkaline phosphate, lactate dehydrogenase, serum calcium, coagulation profile and urinalysis.

15.3 Radiological Investigations

15.3.1 Ultrasound (US)

Ultrasound (US) is the initial imaging modality for assessment of suspected renal masses. It is easy and quick to perform with the added advantages of less cost and no radiation exposure. *It is accurate in detecting a renal cyst.* Ultrasound differentiates mass lesion into cystic, solid and indeterminate group with mixed elements.

S.N. Kurukkal (✉)
Urology Department, The Royal Hospital, Muscat, Oman
e-mail: drsanthoshnrn@gmail.com

S.S. Al-Busaidy
Senior Consultant and HOD, Urology Department, The Royal Hospital, Muscat, Oman
e-mail: salimalbusaidy@hotmail.com

S.A. Al-Mamari, S.S. Al-Busaidy (eds.), *Urological Cancer Management*,
DOI 10.1007/978-3-319-16301-7_15

Difficult differential diagnoses often exist between small homogenous solid renal masses and renal pseudotumours. There are some tools which assist the sonologist in difficult situations: colour Doppler US (CDUS), power Doppler US (PDUS), spectral US (SDUS) and contrast-enhanced US (CEUS) [1, 2]. *Pseudotumour is just a prominent column of Bertin* but can sometimes be confused with a renal tumoural mass. *One important feature to remember is that dominant vessels are displaced around a true renal tumour while they go through the pseudotumour.*

RCC should be considered in all solid masses unless there is a strong evidence to suggest other diagnoses.

Tumour thrombus is well demonstrated by US. Sliding between organs demonstrates the direct invasion into liver or spleen. US is also useful in biopsy guidance and intraoperative tumour assessment.

15.3.2 CT Scan

CT scan is considered the gold standard in the radiological diagnosis of renal masses [3]. Multidetector CT (MDCT) scan allows rapid acquisition and multiplanar reconstruction of the acquired data. A noncontrast CT followed by contrast-enhanced CT in the corticomedullary phase and nephrographic phase is best for detection of renal mass (Fig. 15.1a–e). When a centrally located tumour or tumour of urothelial origin is considered, an excretory phase study (urogram) is added. The following are important features to remember when interpreting CT findings during renal investigation:

(a) *Solid mass:* This lesion contains little or no fluid component; hence, the fluid attenuation is <20 HU. It consists of predominantly enhancing tissue. *A change in attenuation of ≥15 HU is considered as enhancement and is characteristic of RCC.* One should bear in mind that *renal tumour do not enhance as much as the normal renal parenchyma*, especially in the nephrographic phase [3]. Avid enhancement (140 HU), presence of necrosis and heterogeneity are more in favour of clear cell pathology than of chromophobe and papillary variants which are less vascular and homogenously enhancing.

(b) *Tumour size*: Many small renal masses are benign, and CT cannot accurately differentiate them. *Here the size is used as "an indicator" of the likelihood of malignancy. Among renal masses <1 cm, 46 % are benign. In 1–2 cm tumours, 20–22 % are benign. When size is more than 4 cm, only <10 % turn out to be benign. There is an increase in likelihood of malignancy by 16 % per cm of diameter* [4, 5]. *Obviously ruling out or confirming a renal tumour cannot be based solely on the initial lesion size.* Therefore, when surveillance criteria apply (see later), a regular follow-up of such small lesions is necessary to detect if they are rapidly growing, i.e. more likely to be malignant and high-grade tumours, or very slowly or non-growing and mostly consistent with benign or low-grade tumours

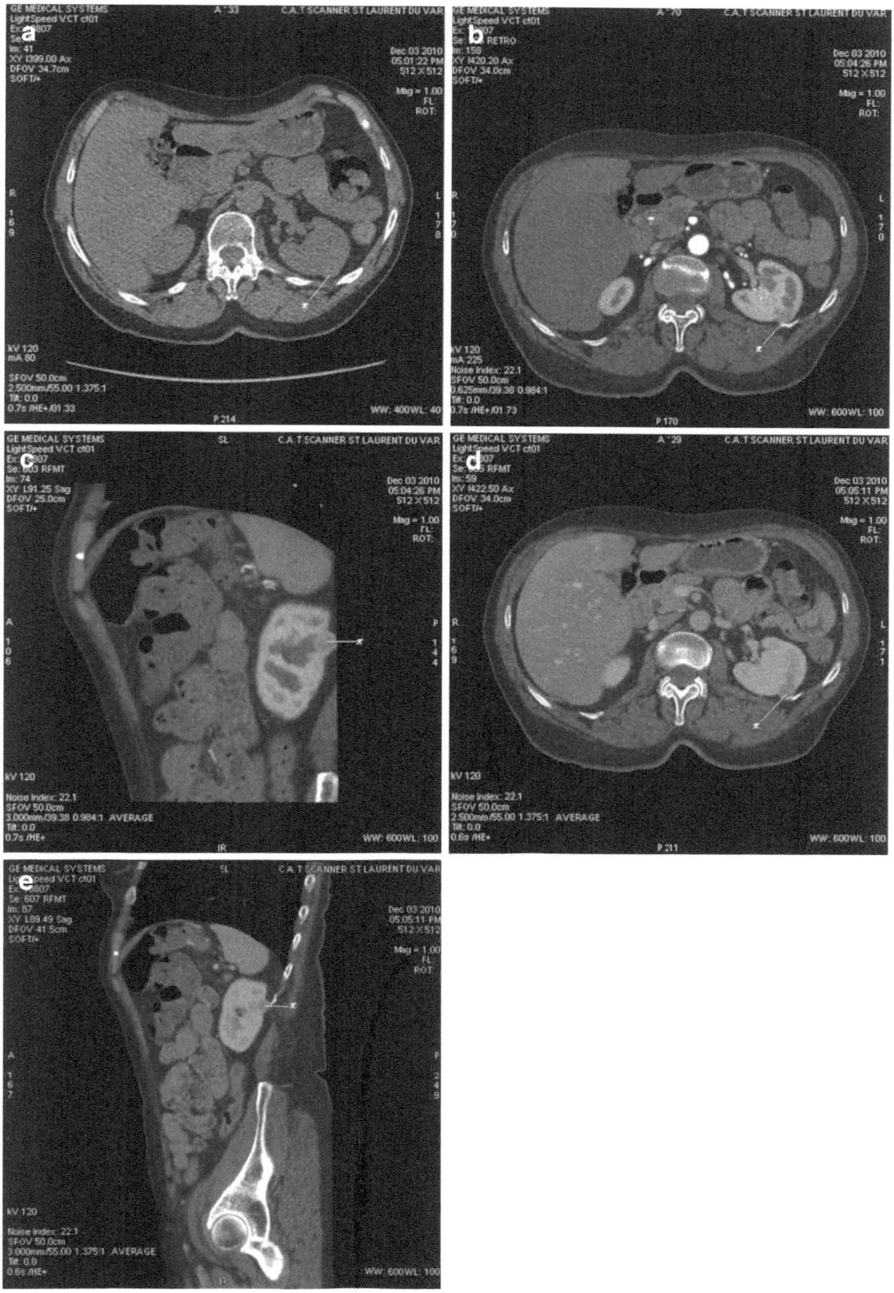

Fig. 15.1 (**a**–**e**) CT scan pre- and post-contrast showing a small tumour (**x**) before injection (**a**), in arterial time (**b**, **c**) and venous time (**d**, **e**) (Courtesy of S. Novellas, Radiology, Arnault-Tzanck Institute, Saint-Laurent-du-Var and CHU Nice, Nice, France)

(c) *Evidence of fat in the mass suggests angiomyolipoma (AML). An area within the tumour of more than 20 pixels with an attenuation of* <-20 *HU or* >5 *pixels with attenuation* <-30 *HU is indicative of fat and consistent with the diagnosis of AML.*

(d) *Oncocytoma is another benign renal tumour. It shows a characteristic central stellate scar in one third of cases* (Fig. 15.2). Segmental enhancement inversion in the corticomedullary phase and early excretory phase may help to distinguish RCC from oncocytoma with 80 % sensitivity and 99 % specificity.

(e) *Metanephric adenoma is a benign tumour indistinguishable by CT scan from RCC*. It is a solitary lesion with poor vascularity similar to PRCC and may contain fine calcific foci. These lesions are treated by surgery and only histopathological studies will allow their diagnosis.

(f) *Calcifications within a solid tumour* are also frequently encountered.

(g) *Perirenal fat invasion* (IIIa) detected in CT scan has 98 % positive predictive value. However, the sensitivity of CT is low here since it predicts only 46 % of cases. MDCT is superior in the detection of *renal vein and IVC thrombus* (IIIb and IIIc).

(h) *CT scan can predict the need for adrenalectomy during nephrectomy when there is direct invasion into the adrenal gland, tumours larger than 7 cm in the upper pole, multifocal tumours or IVC tumours.*

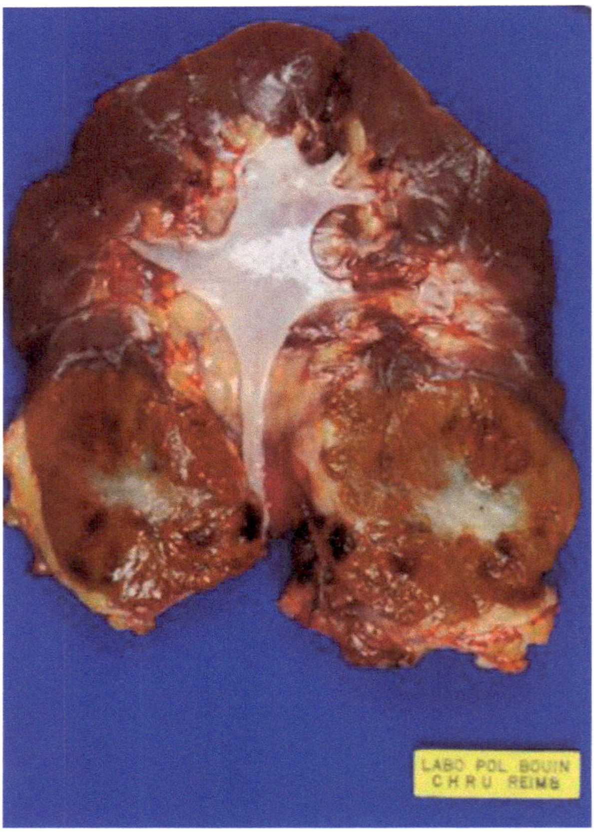

Fig. 15.2 Features of an oncocytoma. See the characteristic central stellate whitish scar (Courtesy of A. Durlach, Pol Bouin Laboratory, University Hospital of Reims, France)

(i) Number and size of loco-regional lymph nodes and the need for lymphadenectomy are also evaluated in preoperative CT [6].

(j) Angiographic CT and 3D reconstruction are helpful in *planning for nephron-sparing* surgery by evaluating the tumour and vascular anatomy.

15.3.3 MRI

MRI is indicated when CT scan is inconclusive, in patients in whom iodinated contrast medium is contraindicated, or when more evaluation of a tumour thrombus is needed. It also avoids the hazard of ionising radiation (Fig. 15.3a–d).

It is important to note that gadolinium is not always safe. It is known to cause *nephrogenic systemic fibrosis in patients with GFR below 30 ml/min, particularly*

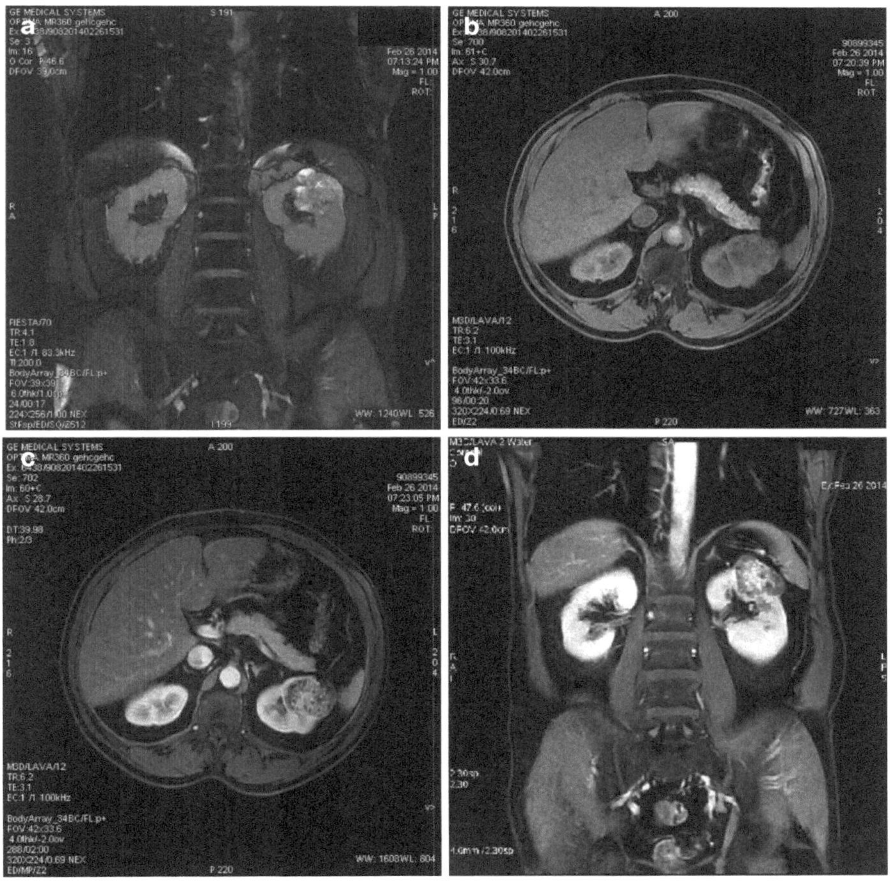

Fig. 15.3 (**a–d**) MRI showing a cystic renal carcinoma: (**a**) T2-weighted, (**b**) T1-weighted without gadolinium, (**c, d**) T1-weighted with gadolinium (Courtesy of S. Novellas, Radiology, Arnault-Tzanck Institute, Saint-Laurent-du-Var and CHU Nice, Nice, France)

those on dialysis, post renal transplant and with acute renal failure. The nephrogenic systemic fibrosis is consistent with abnormal proliferation of fibroblasts in skin, muscles, liver, lungs and heart leading to organ dysfunctions, immobility and contractures. Strategies to overcome these complications include using low dosage, early post-MRI dialysis and avoidance of the agent during acute renal failure [7].

(a) *Solid renal masses are isointense or moderately hypointense in T1-weighted images and hyperintense in T2-weighted images.* Papillary RCC is hypointense in T2-weighted image. Gadolinium is used to study the degree of enhancement which is less than 5 % in renal cysts and at least 97 % in solid masses. *The degree of enhancement is often useful in subtyping*, as the percentage of signal intensity change in clear cell carcinoma is significantly higher than in papillary carcinoma with chromophobe carcinoma falling intermediate [8, 9].
(b) *Macroscopic fat is well detected by MRI which suggests AML.* The presence of microscopic fat is also seen in both clear cell RCC and papillary RCC.
(c) *MRI* is a useful tool in diagnosing perirenal fat invasion (IIIa), tumour invasion into the renal vein IVC and cephalad extent of tumour thrombus. Distinction of blood and thrombus without contrast is possible. *In this regard MRI is superior to spiral CT, but MDCT is considered comparable* [10, 11].

The urologist should be aware of the MRI protocol sequences used for evaluating the renal tumour [12].

- T2HASTE (*h*alf-Fourier *a*cquisition *s*ingle-shot *t*urbo-spin *e*cho): It is done in coronal and axial planes and rapidly acquired. It provides good anatomy and overview. Fluid-containing structures appear bright.
- T1-gradient echo: Fat is bright and AML and myelolipomas are conspicuous. Complex fluid (e.g. haemorrhage) is also bright. Adenopathy is easily visualised.
- T1-gradient echo with fat saturation: Fat-containing structures become dark; complex fluid remains bright.
- T1-gradient echo 3D dynamic sequence after IV gadolinium: Enhancement within any portions of a mass or cyst is consistent with a neoplasm. Vessels also enhance.
- MR angiography and MR venography: Vessels enhance allowing for detection of renal vein and IVC involvement. Vascular anatomy can be mapped.
- CT/MRI angiography is useful in selected cases to obtain information about renal vascular anatomy especially when planning for selective vessel clamping in partial nephrectomy. CTA is more accurate than MRA in detecting supernumerary vessels.

15.3.4 PET Scan

PET scan is not recommended as a standard investigation either in initial diagnosis, initial staging or follow-up of RCC. *There is no advantage of PET scan over CT scan in the characterisation and initial staging*. The reported sensitivity of PET in detecting primary RCC is far less (47–60 %) compared to CT (92–97 %) with comparable specificity (100 % for both) and accuracy [13, 14].

PET scan can have a role in restaging of metastatic RCC (mRCC) and is useful in characterising an anatomical lesion of unknown significance [15]. PET scan is helpful for clarifying findings on other imaging modalities suggestive of metastatic disease, bilateral disease or recurrence, particularly in settings where a positive PET will avoid an invasive biopsy. PET may be appropriate if there is suspicion of a metastatic lesion and biopsy of that lesion is considered potentially less invasive than biopsy of the kidney or performing nephrectomy. The overall PET scan sensitivity for detection of metastatic RCC lesions is inferior being 75 % in lung metastasis, 78 % in bone lesions, 64 % in soft tissue lesions and 75 % in retroperitoneal lymph nodes. In no case has PET scan detected a metastasis that had not been visualised in CT or MRI. However, the overall specificity is higher than any other tests [16, 17].

15.3.5 Categorisation of Renal Cysts

Classically ultrasound is the diagnostic tool for a simple renal cyst. Rounded, well-demarcated lesion with regular sharp borders, imperceptible wall, anechoic content and strong posterior sonic/acoustic enhancement are the features of a simple renal cyst and do not need further studies, namely, CT or MRI.

The presence of varying degrees of complexity in a cystic lesion, like *internal echoes, septa, thickness of wall, calcification and mural nodularity*, requires further evaluation with CT scan (Fig. 15.4a, b). Based on the CT findings, Morton Bosniak classified cystic lesions into four classes in 1986 [18] and added class 2 F later on (Table 15.1).

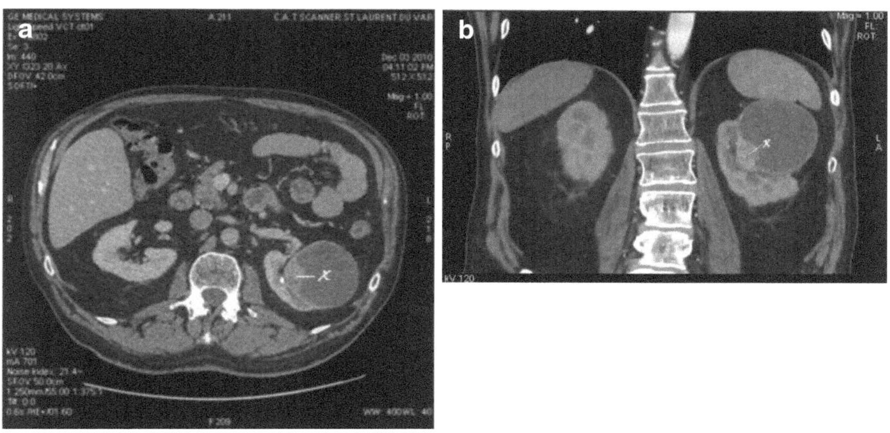

Fig. 15.4 (**a**, **b**) A Bosniak IV left renal cyst seen on CT scan (horizontal and sagittal plans). It was proven to be a clear cell carcinoma (Courtesy of S. Novellas, Radiology, Arnault-Tzanck Institute, Saint-Laurent-du-Var and CHU Nice, Nice, France)

Table 15.1 The Bosniak classification of renal cystic disease

Category		Features	Malignant risk	Management
Category I	Simple renal cyst	Round or oval shape, anechoic posterior enhancement (through transmission), thin, smooth wall Homogeneous water content, sharp delineation with the renal parenchyma, no calcification, no enhancement or wall thickening	Less than 1 %	No follow-up needed
Category II	Minimally complicated cyst	Cystic lesion with some abnormal radiological features <1 mm septations (hairline thin) Fine calcifications within the septum or wall <3 cm in diameter Hyperdense cysts (>20 Hounsfield units)	Less than 3 %	No follow-up needed
Category IIF	Complicated cyst for follow-up	Cystic lesion with increased abnormal findings, multiple thin septum *Septa thicker than hairline or slightly thick wall calcification, which may be thick intrarenal, >3 cm* *No contrast enhancement*	5–10 %	Follow-up recommended
Category III	Indeterminate	More complicated uniform wall thickening/nodularity Thick/irregular calcification Thick septa *Enhances with contrast*	50 %	Surgery recommended
Category IV	Malignant	Large cystic components Irregular margins/prominent nodules Solid enhancing elements, independent of septa	75–90 %	Surgery recommended

Bosniak category I and II renal cysts do not require further imaging or follow-up as the malignancy risk is low. Patients in category IIF, because of the approximate 5 % malignant risk, do require periodic imaging. For category III (50 % malignant risk) and category IV (75–90 % malignant risk), surgical excision is recommended. Although MRI may add further information, it should be used as an adjunct to CT scans in difficult cases [19, 20].

15.3.6 Renal Tumour Biopsy

Percutaneous needle biopsy of the renal mass was traditionally limited by concerns about its safety, accuracy and sampling errors. Biopsy was reserved for patients suspected of having unresectable or disseminated RCC, renal metastasis, renal abscess or lymphoma [21] (Fig. 15.5). With improvement in diagnostic accuracy of biopsy, refinements in image guiding and better understanding of small renal masses, the indications for tumour biopsy have changed. The increasing incidence in the diagnosis of incidental small renal masses (SRMs), the development of conservative and minimally invasive treatments for low-risk RCCs and the discovery of novel targeted treatments for metastatic disease are now leading to wider indications for renal tumour biopsy [22].

According to the EAU guidelines [3], renal tumour biopsies are presently used for:

- Histological diagnosis of radiologically indeterminate renal masses
- Selecting patients with small renal masses for surveillance approaches
- Obtaining histology before ablative treatments
- Selecting the most suitable form of targeted therapy in the setting of metastatic disease

It is not indicated, however, for healthy patients who are unwilling to accept the uncertainty associated with the procedure or for older patients who will only be considered for conservative management option regardless of the biopsy result [23].

Updated indications have been proposed for renal mass sampling aiming at tailoring the treatment for each individual patient and optimising the oncological efficacy (Table 15.2, Fig. 15.6a–c) [24].

15.3.7 Staging of RCC

This is done according to the 2010 AJCC cancer staging manual (identical to the TNM UICC classification system) [25] (Table 15.3).

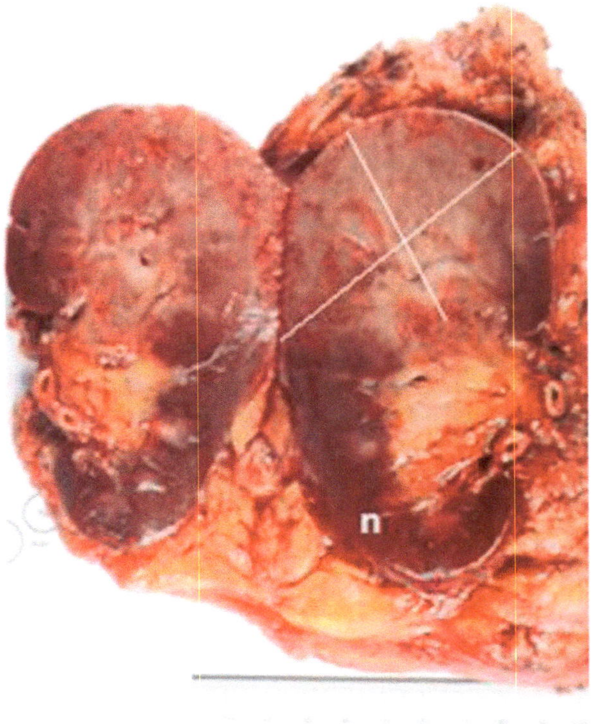

Fig. 15.5 B-cell lymphoma with a diffuse infiltration of the upper half of the right kidney in a 83-year-old man (n = grossly normal parenchyma) (*Caution: lymphoma is not an indication for nephrectomy. This was decided solely on the basis of CT scan findings suggestive of tumour and could have been avoided if a biopsy was performed, especially in an elderly patient*)

Table 15.2 Indications for renal mass sampling [22]

Absolute indications
Renal tumour with known extrarenal primary
Suspicion of renal abscess
Suspected lymphoma
Prior to thermal ablation
Relative indications
Tumour in solitary kidney (Fig. 15.5)
Bilateral renal tumour
Unresectable tumour
Medically unfit
Emerging indications
Small renal enhancing mass
Complex cystic lesions – indeterminate
In metastatic RCC to determine the subtype

15.3.8 Nephrometry Scoring Systems

The number of nephron-sparing surgeries over radical nephrectomies is increasing since the beginning of the twenty-first century because more small-size tumours are diagnosed [26]. Recently nephrometry scoring systems were developed to better

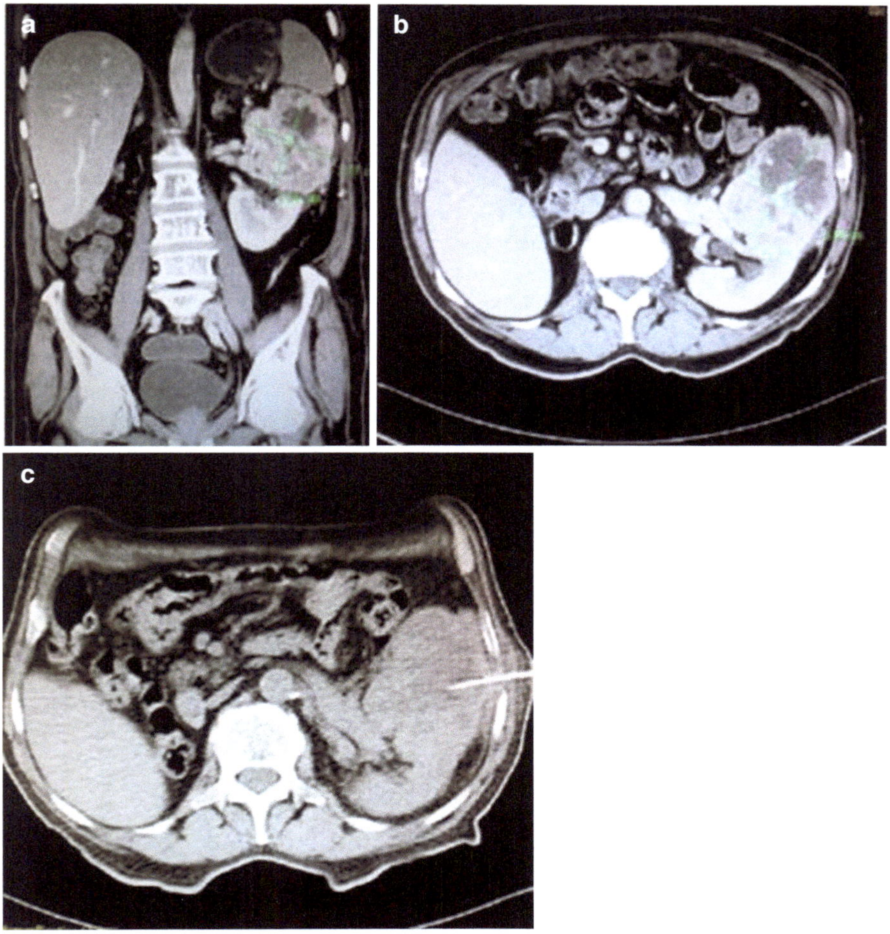

Fig. 15.6 (**a**–**c**) A case of expanding indications for renal tumour biopsy: a 51-year-old male patient with tumour in a solitary left kidney. A clear cell RCC was proven after CT-guided biopsy (Courtesy of Kurian George, Urology, The Royal Hospital, Muscat, Oman)

characterise the anatomy of these small renal masses. The score is an objective and useful tool which defines the character of a renal mass, aids clinical decision-making and enhances communication between professionals. Three nephrometry scoring systems were proposed:

- RENAL nephrometry (*R*adius, *E*xophytic/endophytic, *N*earness to collecting system, *A*nterior or posterior, *L*ocation relative to polar lines) [27]
- PADUA (Preoperative Aspects and Dimensions for an Anatomical Classification) [28]
- C-index method [29]

The RENAL nephrometry is the most studied and discussed. It includes the assessment of tumour radius (the maximal diameter), its exophytic or endophytic

Table 15.3 The 2010 AJCC staging for renal cancer [25]

Primary tumour (T)			
TX	Primary tumour cannot be assessed		
T0	No evidence of primary tumour		
T1	*Tumour ≤7 cm in greatest dimension, limited to the kidney*		
T1a	Tumour ≤4 cm in greatest dimension, limited to the kidney		
T1b	Tumour >4 cm but ≤7 cm in greatest dimension, limited to the kidney		
T2	*Tumour >7 cm in greatest dimension, limited to the kidney*		
T2a	Tumour >7 cm but ≤10 cm, limited to the kidney		
T2b	Tumours >10 cm limited to the kidney		
T3	*Tumour extends into major veins or perinephric tissue but not into the ipsilateral adrenal gland and not beyond the Gerota's fascia*		
T3a	Tumour grossly extends into the renal vein or its segmental (muscle-containing) branches, or tumour invades perirenal and/or renal sinus fat but not beyond Gerota's fascia		
T3b	Tumour grossly extends into the vena cava below the diaphragm		
T3c	Tumour grossly extends into the vena cava above the diaphragm or involves the wall of the vena cava		
T4	*Tumour invades beyond the Gerota's fascia (including contiguous extension into the ipsilateral adrenal gland)*		
Regional lymph nodes (N)			
NX	Regional lymph nodes cannot be assessed		
N0	No regional lymph node metastasis		
N1	Metastasis in regional lymph node(s) (*N1 disease is defined as a single or multiple regional lymph nodes involvement*)		
Distant metastasis (M)			
M0	No distant metastasis		
M1	Distant metastasis		
Anatomic stage/prognostic groups			
Stage I	T1	N0	M0
Stage II	T2	N0	M0
Stage III	T1–T2	N1	M0
	T3	N0–N1	M0
Stage IV	T4	Any N	M0
	Any T	Any N	M1

Used with the permission of the American Joint Committee on Cancer (AJCC), Chicago, Illinois. The original source for this material is the *AJCC Cancer Staging Manual*, Seventh Edition (2010), published by Springer Science and Business Media LLC, www.springer.com

properties, the nearness to the collecting system or sinus, the anterior/posterior position and the location relative to polar lines. In the original description by Kutikov and Uzzo, standardised points (1–3 points per descriptor) are assigned onto each parameter, except the anterior or posterior component [27] (Table 15.4 and Fig. 15.7).

Table 15.4 The RENAL nephrometry scoring system [27]

	1 point	2 points	3 points
R – radius (maximal diameter) (cm)	<4	4–7	>7
E – exophytic or endophytic	>50 % exophytic	<50 % exophytic	Entirely endophytic
N – nearness to collecting system (mm)	>7	4–7	<4
A – anterior or posterior	a – anterior, p – posterior or x		
L – location relative to polar lines	Entirely above the upper or below the lower polar lines	Lesion crosses the polar lines	>50 % crosses the polar line, or entirely between the polar lines or crosses the axial midline

Fig. 15.7 Nephrometry landmarks

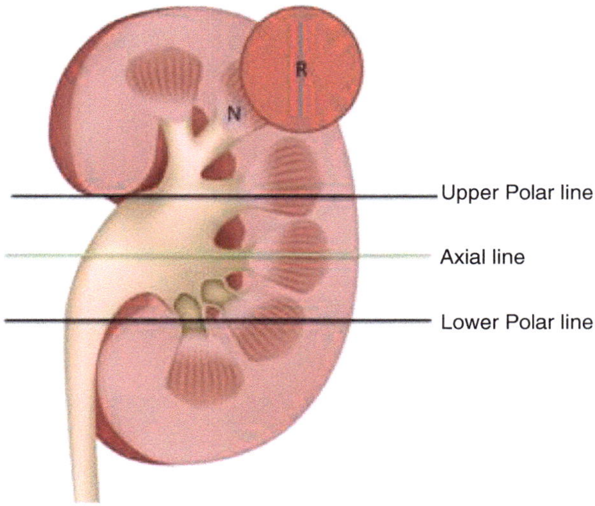

The score is calculated by totalling the points of each parameter. Scores of 4–6 are considered low complexity for resection, 7–9 moderate complexity and 10–12 high complexity.

This nephrometry scoring system was proven useful in many instances:

- Preoperative planning: Choice of surgical modality (partial or radical nephrectomy) and approach (open or minimally invasive).
- Deciding for alternative treatment modalities (thermal ablation) [30–32].

- Predicting intraoperative ischemia, perioperative urine leak and functional outcome in partial nephrectomy, in standard laparoscopic and robotic-assisted procedure [30]. The significant correlation of the score with warm ischaemia time, blood loss, complications like urinary leak and length of hospital stay helps an enhanced preoperative counselling of patients undergoing partial nephrectomy [33].

Available data so far have provided more evidence in support of the use of this scoring system when making more objective therapeutic choices for renal masses.

Take-Home Message: Imaging Investigations of a Renal Mass

Ultrasound (US) is the initial imaging modality for assessment of suspected renal masses. It is accurate in detecting a renal cyst and is considered satisfactory in the presence of a simple cyst where there is none of internal echoes, septa, thickness of wall, calcification and mural nodularity

CT scan is the gold standard in the radiological diagnosis of renal masses. Its important features are:

- For solid tumours, a change in attenuation of ≥15 HU after IV contrast is considered as enhancement and is characteristic of RCC
- The bigger the tumour, the more likely malignant. At >4 cm, only <10 % of tumour masses turn out to be benign
- An area within the tumour of more than 20 pixels with an attenuation of <–20 HU or >5 pixels with attenuation <–30 HU is indicative of fat and consistent with the diagnosis of AML
- Oncocytoma is a benign renal tumour showing a characteristic central stellate scar in one third of cases
- Metanephric adenoma is a benign tumour indistinguishable by CT scan from RCC
- CT scan can predict the need for adrenalectomy when there is direct invasion into the adrenal gland, tumours larger than 7 cm in the upper pole, multifocal tumours or IVC tumours
- MDCT is superior to spiral CT in the detection of renal vein and IVC thrombus
- Angiographic CT and 3D reconstruction are helpful in planning for nephron-sparing surgery by evaluating the tumour and vascular anatomy

MRI is indicated when CT scan is inconclusive, in patients in whom iodinated contrast medium is contraindicated, or when more evaluation of a tumour thrombus is needed. It also avoids the hazard of ionising radiation. However, gadolinium is not always safe and may cause nephrogenic systemic fibrosis in patients with GFR below 30 ml/min, particularly those on dialysis, post renal transplant and with acute renal failure

There is no advantage of PET scan over CT scan in the characterisation and initial staging. PET may be appropriate if there is suspicion of a metastatic lesion and biopsy of that lesion is considered potentially less invasive than biopsy of the kidney or performing nephrectomy

If initial US detects the presence of varying degrees of complexity in a cystic lesion such as internal echoes, septa, thickness of wall, calcification and mural nodularity, the lesion has to be further characterised by CT. The lesion will then be defined as per *Bosniak classification* where categories I and II do not require further imaging or follow-up, category IIF requires periodic imaging, and categories III and IV require surgical excision

References

1. Kim SH, Cho JY, Kim SY, et al. Ultrasound evaluation of renal masses: grey scale, Doppler and more. Ultrasound Clin. 2013;8(4):565–79.
2. Houtzager S, Wijkstra H, de la Rosette JJ, Laguna MP. Evaluation of renal masses with contrast-enhanced ultrasound. Curr Urol Rep. 2013;14(2):116–23.
3. Ljungberg B, Bensalah K, Bex A, et al. Guidelines on renal cell carcinoma. EAU update. Apr 2014. http://uroweb.org/wp-content/uploads/10-Renal-Cell-Carcinoma_LR.pdf.
4. Israel GM, Bosniak MA. How i do it: evaluating renal masses. Radiology. 2005;236:441–50.
5. Sohaib A. Incidental solid cystic renal lesion. Cancer Imaging. 2012;12(2):385–6.
6. Türkvatan A, Akdur PO, Altinel M, Olçer T, Turhan N, Cumhur T, Akinci S, Ozkul F. Preoperative staging of renal cell carcinoma with multidetector CT. Diagn Interv Radiol. 2009;15:22–30.
7. Perazella MA. Gadolinium-contrast toxicity in patients with kidney disease: nephrotoxicity and nephrogenic systemic fibrosis. Curr Drug Saf. 2008;3(1):67–75.
8. Ergen FB, Hussain HK, Caoili EM. MRI for preoperative staging of renal cell carcinoma using the 1997 TNM classification: comparison with surgical and pathologic staging. Am J Roentgenol. 2004;182:217–25.
9. Shirkhoda A. Imaging of cystic and solid renal mass and the role of MRI. Iran. J. Radiol. 2005;3(1):1–6.
10. Lawrentschuk N, Gani J, Riordan R, Esler S, Bolton DM. Multidetector computed tomography vs magnetic resonance imaging for defining the upper limit of tumour thrombus in renal cell carcinoma: a study and review. BJU Int. 2005;96(3):291–5.
11. Hallscheidt PJ, Fink C, Haferkamp A, et al. Preoperative staging of renal cell carcinoma with inferior vena cava thrombus using multidetector CT and MRI: prospective study with histopathological correlation. J Comput Assist Tomogr. 2005;29(1):64–8.
12. Bassignani MJ. Understanding and interpreting MRI of the GU tract. Urol Clin North Am. 2006;33:135–51.
13. De Jong IJ, Breeuwsma AJ, Pruim J. Positron emission tomography in urology. EAU-EBU Upd Ser. 2007;5:93–104.
14. Kang DE, White Jr RL, Zuger JH, Sasser HC, Teigland CM. Clinical use of fluorodeoxyglucose F 18 positron emission tomography for detection of renal cell carcinoma. J Urol. 2004;171(5):1806–9.
15. Rioja J, Rodríguez-Fraile M, Lima-Favaretto R, Rincón-Mayans A, Peñuelas-Sánchez I, Zudaire-Bergera JJ, Parra RO. Role of positron emission tomography in urological oncology. BJU Int. 2010;106(11):1578–93.
16. Dilhuydy MS, Durieux A, Pariente A, de Clermont H, Pasticier G, Monteil J, Ravaud A. PET scans for decision-making in metastatic renal cell carcinoma: a single-institution evaluation. Oncology. 2006;70(5):339–44.
17. Wang HY, Ding HJ, Chen JH, Chao CH, Lu YY, Lin WY, Kao CH. Meta-analysis of the diagnostic performance of [^{18}F]FDG-PET and PET/CT in renal cell carcinoma. Cancer Imaging. 2012;12(3):464–74.
18. Bosniak MA. The current radiological approach to renal cysts. Radiology. 1986;158(1):1–10.
19. O'Malley RL, Godoy G, Hecht EM, Stifelman MD, Taneja SS, Bosniak Category IIF. Designation and surgery for complex renal cysts. J Urol. 2009;182(3):1091–5.
20. Whelan TF. Guidelines on the management of renal cyst disease. Can Urol Assoc J. 2010;4(2):98–9.
21. Herts BR, Baker ME. The current role of percutaneous biopsy in the evaluation of renal masses. Semin Urol Oncol. 1995;13(4):254–61.
22. Volpe A, Terrone C, Scarpa RM. The current role of percutaneous needle biopsies of renal tumours. Arch Ital Urol Androl. 2009;81(2):107–12.
23. Campbell SC, Novick AC, Belldengrun A, et al. Guidelines for the management of the Clinical stage 1 Renal Mass. J Urol. 2009;182(4):1271–9.
24. Samplaski MK, Zhou M, Lane BR, Herts B, Campbell SC. Renal mass sampling: an enlightened perspective. Int J Urol. 2011;18:5–19.

25. Kidney. In: Edge SB, Byrd DR, Compton CC, Fritz AG, Greene FL, Trotti A, editors. AJCC cancer staging manual. 7th ed. New York: Springer; 2010. p. 479–89.
26. Dall'Oglio MF, Crippa A, Camara C, et al. The beginning of the 21st century: a paradigm shift in the surgical management of renal cell carcinoma in South America. Clin Urol. 2010;36(6):670–7.
27. Kutikov A, Uzzo RG. The R.E.N.A.L. nephrometry score: a comprehensive standardized system for quantitating renal tumour size, location and depth. J Urol. 2009;182:844–53.
28. Ficarra V, Novara G, Secco S, et al. Preoperative aspects and dimensions used for an anatomical (PADUA) classification of renal tumours in patients who are candidates for nephron-sparing surgery. Eur Urol. 2009;56:786–93.
29. Simmons MN, Ching CB, Samplaski MK, Park CH, Gill IS. Kidney tumour location measurement using the C index method. J Urol. 2010;183:1708–13.
30. Yeon JS, Son SJ, Lee YL, et al. The nephrometry score: is it effective for predicting perioperative outcome during robot-assisted partial nephrectomy? Korean J Urol. 2014;55(4):254–9.
31. Canter D, Kutikov A, Manley B, et al. Utility of the R.E.N.A.L. nephrometry scoring system in objectifying treatment decision-making of the enhancing renal mass. Urology. 2011;78(5):1089–94.
32. Wong MH, Cho KY, Ho KL, Wong KW, Lai CT, Man CM, Yiu MK. How can the R.E.N.A.L. nephrometry scoring system aid management of a solid renal mass? Hong Kong Med J. 2014;20(1):37–44.
33. Ellison JS, Montgomery JS, Hafez KS, et al. Association of RENAL nephrometry score with outcomes of minimally invasive partial nephrectomy. Int J Urol. 2013;20:564–70.

Chapter 16
Treatment of Renal Cell Carcinomas

Santhosh Narayana Kurukkal and Salim Said Al-Busaidy

16.1 Management of Incidental Small Renal Mass

Small renal masses (SRMs) are defined as *lesions ≤4 cm in dimension, i.e. T1a.* They are an increasingly common clinical scenario for practising urologists and physicians, and contemporary epidemiological studies indicate that *SRMs account for nearly one half of all diagnosed renal masses diagnosed.* SRMs are biologically heterogeneous with 20 % being benign lesions, while 20–30 % others are potentially aggressive at the time of diagnosis [1] (Fig. 16.1).

SRMs are slow growing, and the average growth rate of RCC is *0.28 cm/year.* They seldom progress to metastasize, which was reported in only 1 % of patients [3]. However, the growth rate of a renal mass does not predict malignancy with certainty as even tumours with zero growth rate have a malignant potential [4]. Neither clinical nor radiographic features can reliably categorize SRMs as benign or malignant and differentiate between indolent and potentially aggressive tumours.

So far, there is no established protocol for active surveillance of renal tumours. The tumour size may be an indicator of biological aggressiveness. In clinical T1b lesions (4–7 cm), the rate of tumour growth is *1.43 cm/year*, and one out of nine patients develops metastasis. The risk of synchronous metastases increases to 22 % with each 1 cm rise in tumour size [5].

Renal mass biopsy with molecular analysis can assess the aggressive potential and guide in decision-making between active surveillance and active treatment.

S.N. Kurukkal (✉)
Urology Department, The Royal Hospital, Muscat, Oman
e-mail: drsanthoshnrn@gmail.com

S.S. Al-Busaidy
Senior Consultant and HOD, Urology Department, The Royal Hospital, Muscat, Oman
e-mail: salimalbusaidy@hotmail.com

S.A. Al-Mamari, S.S. Al-Busaidy (eds.), *Urological Cancer Management*,
DOI 10.1007/978-3-319-16301-7_16

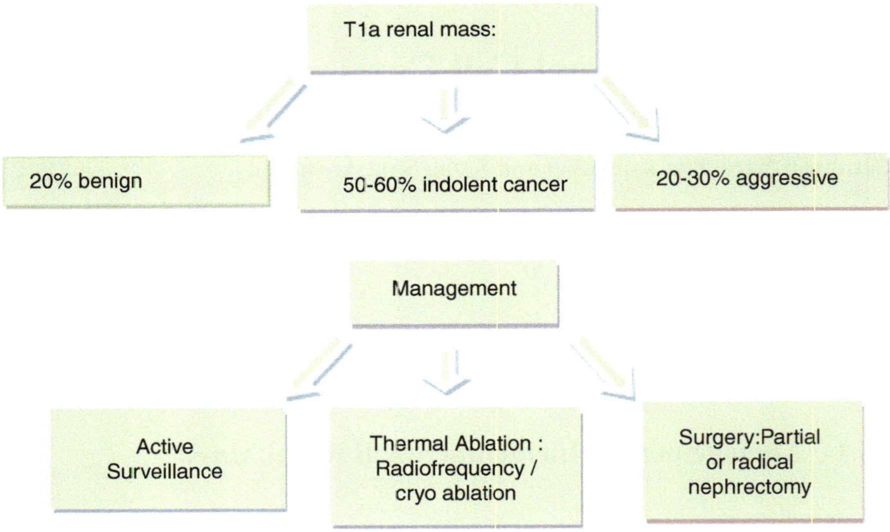

Fig. 16.1 Clinical behaviour and management of a T1a renal mass [1, 2]

16.2 Active Surveillance (AS)

Elderly patients and patients with co-morbidities with an incidentally detected SRM have a relatively low RCC-specific mortality. They can be considered for active surveillance. Active surveillance is defined as the initial monitoring of tumour size by serial abdominal imaging (ultrasound, CT, or MRI) with delayed intervention reserved for those tumours that show clinical progression during follow-up [6].

AS is a reasonable option in [2]:

1. Patients with limited life expectancy
2. Patients unfit for intervention
3. Patients who do not desire immediate intervention

All the patients should be counselled about the small but real risk of cancer progression, the possibility to lose an opportunity for nephron-sparing surgery, the lack of curative therapies if metastases develop during the surveillance period and the limitations of renal mass biopsy in assisting the decision for active surveillance or active treatment.

16.3 Ablation Therapies

Many novel treatment modalities have evolved in the treatment of renal tumours: high intensity-focused ultrasound (HIFU), radiosurgery (CyberKnife), microwave thermal therapy (MWT), laser interstitial thermal therapy (LITT) and pulsed cavitational ultrasound (PCU). However, only two ablation therapies are recommended by expert panels for the treatment of renal tumours: cryoablation and radiofrequency ablation.

Ablative therapies are indicated in elderly patients (>70 years), small renal tumours (T1a), solitary kidneys, impaired renal function, post-surgical locally recurrent low-grade cancers and hereditary RCC (VHL, hereditary papillary RCC and tuberous sclerosis). Ideally, tumours treated with these techniques should be exophytic and distant from the hilum.

16.3.1 Radiofrequency Ablation (RFA)

It is a minimally invasive treatment option for localized renal masses in patients with high surgical risk. RFA is produced by an alternating electrical current of a frequency between 350 and 500 kHz through an electrode inserted in the tumour. The following sequence is observed [7]:

> Ionic agitation → frictional tumour heating beyond 55 °C → coagulative necrosis.

It is important that the heat doesn't exceed 100 °C, because that would produce an immediate local vaporization and carbonization limiting the electrical conductivity.

The resulting ablation zone generally encompasses the initial tumour with a 5–10 mm excess (Fig. 16.2a–d).

Relative contraindications: Large contact between the tumour and the renal excretory system (renal pelvis, upper ureter), the vessels or the bowels (anteriorly located tumours).

Absolute contraindications: Impaired coagulation, sepsis and severe mental retardation (non-compliance for regular follow-up).

16.3.2 Cryoablation (CA)

In the past, liquid nitrogen was used to perform CA. It has been replaced now by liquid argon, and the cooling can reach up to −185°. Cryotherapy causes tissue destruction using repeated freeze/thaw cycles. *The use of multi-probes technique*

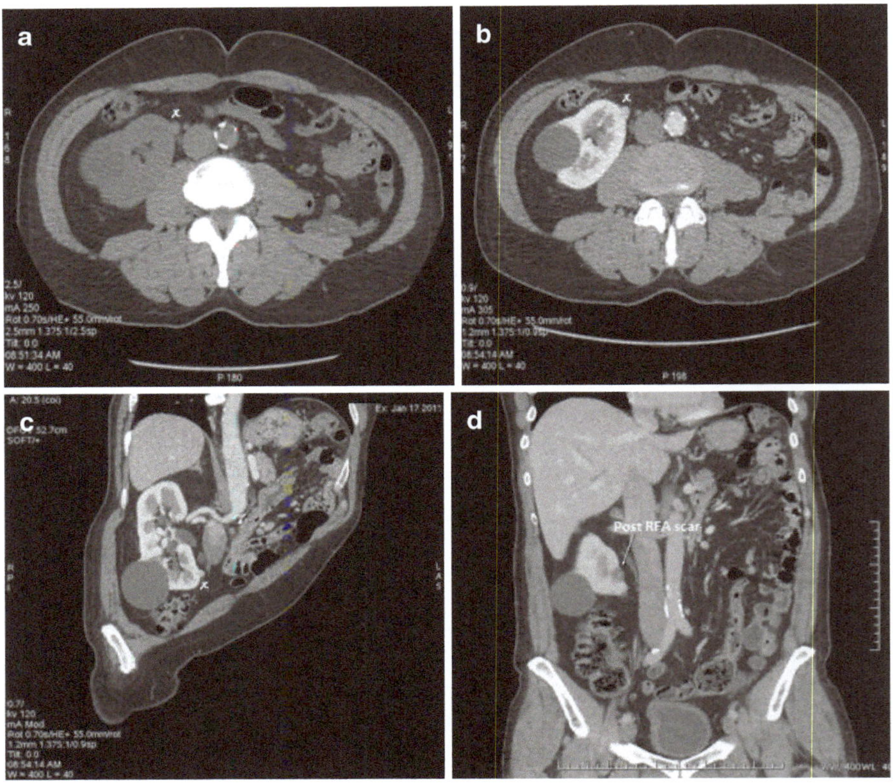

Fig. 16.2 (**a–d**) CT scan showing a small (1 cm) exophytic tumour (**x**) in a solitary right kidney in a 66 years man. This is a typical indication for ablative therapies. There is also a benign cyst. The tumour is very close to the upper ureter and the IVC (**c**). The patient had a laparoscopy-guided RFA. (**d**) Shows a post-treatment scar which is larger than the treated tumour

has the advantage of treating larger renal lesions than RFA. Unlike RFA, cryotherapy is also MRI compatible. MRI-guided ablation has the advantage of real-time guidance for probe placement, multiplanar imaging, exquisite soft tissue contrast and lack of ionizing radiation [8]. Also, there seems to be less damage to the urothelium, and the treated zone will be well defined by CT in the follow-up. Authors have also reported less pain associated with CA than RFA [9]. Cryoablation may be a treatment option for patients with high surgical risk and who are not candidates for observation. When cryoablation has failed, salvage surgery can be difficult due to fibrotic reaction within the perinephric space.

Both RFA and CA can be performed either by percutaneous approach with ultrasound or CT guidance or laparoscopically and are treatment options for patients with high surgical risk who want active treatment and accept the need for long-term radiographic surveillance after treatment. Renal biopsies are strongly recommended prior to ablation therapies to confirm and document the histopathology of the tumour. There is an increased risk of local recurrence, and a repeat renal tumour biopsy may sometimes be considered with the potential need for a second therapeutic intervention. Larger tumours, tumours with irregular shape or with an infiltrative appearance have an increased risk of recurrence when treated with thermal ablation.

16.4 Surgical Resection

RCC is resistant to radiotherapy and chemotherapy. Surgical extirpation remains the only curative therapy for RCC even in the era of targeted therapy. Various systemic treatment modalities such as immunotherapy were developed for advanced RCC, but targeted therapy has been accepted widely despite being costly. As for all malignant tumours, the treatment strategy is based on the stage of the disease. For operable tumours, there is a net demarcation between localized (stages I and II) and locally advanced tumours (stages III and IV).

1. *Stage I: (T1 N0 M0; ≤7 cm tumours):*

   The standard of care is partial nephrectomy [2, 10]. This can be performed by open-, laparoscopic- or robotic-assisted technique. Radical nephrectomy is recommended if partial nephrectomy is not technically feasible due to unfavourable tumour localization and characteristics (mid-polar endophytic tumour near the hilum). Other alternative modalities are *thermal ablations: radiofrequency ablation and cryoablation*. These are suitable for small cortical tumours, multiple, hereditary and bilateral tumours or in solitary kidneys.

   Active surveillance is an alternative in patients who are at high risk for surgery and for those with a short life expectancy and tumour size smaller than 4 cm.

> As stated by the American Expert Panel, there is no statistically significant difference in overall survival and cancer-specific survival observed between radical nephrectomy, partial nephrectomy and active surveillance for clinically T1a renal mass [2].

2. *Stage II: (T2 N0 M0; >7 cm tumours):*

   Primary treatment is radical nephrectomy, preferably by laparoscopy.

3. *Stage III: (T3 N0 M0; perinephric tissue invasion and venous thrombus):*

   Open radical nephrectomy is the standard of care. Laparoscopy can be considered. *Tumour thrombectomy from renal vein or venal cava is indicated if involved.*

4. *Stage IV: (T4, any T with N1 ± M1):*

   Locally invasive RCC may require aggressive surgical management with resection of adjacent organs. 40–60 % of patients may be cured by such aggressive surgical management [11].

   When there is a solitary resectable metastasis, nephrectomy can be combined with metastasectomy. In patients with multiple metastases, a cytoreductive nephrectomy may be recommended prior to systemic therapy.

   Systemic targeted therapy is recommended in patients unfit for surgery or unresectable tumour or mRCC [10].

16.4.1 Surgical Modalities and Approaches

16.4.1.1 Open Radical Nephrectomy (RN)

RN includes ligating the renal artery and vein, removing the kidney without opening the Gerota's fascia, removing the ipsilateral adrenal gland and complete regional lymphadenectomy from ipsilateral crus of the diaphragm to aortic bifurcation [12] (Fig. 16.3).

Thoracoabdominal, anterior subcostal and flank incisions are the most commonly used. Transperitoneal or extraperitoneal approaches are used depending on the size and location of tumour and patient habitus. Transperitoneal approach has the advantage of an excellent initial exposure of renal pedicle. Thoracoabdominal route is best for a large upper pole tumour. Extraperitoneal flank approach is preferable when the kidney is chronically infected, in obese patients, when there are multiple prior abdominal surgeries and if partial nephrectomy is considered. Details of the technique are beyond the scope of this book.

The oncological outcomes of open versus *laparoscopic radical nephrectomy were found to be similar* [13]. Laparoscopic radical nephrectomy (LRN) allows a shorter hospital stay and lower analgesic requirement. There is longer operative time in LRN, but less peri-operative blood loss and shorter convalescence time. There is no difference in complications rate and in post-operative quality of life (QoL) between the two techniques. No differences were also noted between retroperitoneal and trans-peritoneal approaches of LRN in oncological outcomes and QoL [14].

Adrenalectomy is not always necessary and is not routinely recommended. The tumour size is predictive of adrenal involvement but not its sole upper pole localization. Nephrectomies with and without adrenalectomy did not show any difference in overall survival at 5 and 10 years. *Adrenalectomy is justified only if there is evidence of radiological invasion or intra-operative findings of involvement* [15].

Lymph node dissection: Only 20 % of clinically detected lymph nodes by CT/MRI and intra-operative assessment are confirmed to be metastatic on histology.

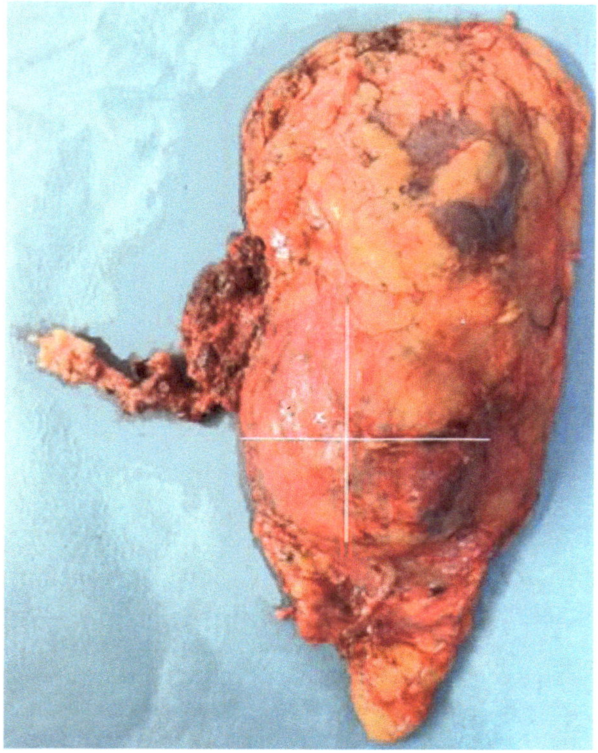

Fig. 16.3 Gross specimen of a radical laparoscopic left nephrectomy: there was a large tumour (**x**) involving all the lower half of the left kidney as well as few hilar LN

Furthermore, an EORTC study has shown that only 4 % of clinically N0 patients were found to have a positive lymph node in the final pathology [16]. *These findings suggest that routine LND is clearly an over-treatment in the majority of N0 patients. Therefore, LND is not recommended in localized tumour without clinical evidence of lymph node invasion* [10]. When there are clinically enlarged lymph nodes, LND can be performed for staging purposes or for local control.

16.4.1.2 Open Partial Nephrectomy (PN) or Nephron-Sparing Surgery (NSS)

This can be approached through a flank retroperitoneal approach or an anterior subcostal incision *according to the surgeon's preference*. Whatever the approach, the kidney must be dissected free from the perirenal fat to leave only the fat overlying the site of tumour. Here again, details of the technique are beyond the scope of this book.

There is no difference in survival between laparoscopic PN (LPN) and open PN. The mean blood loss is generally lower, but operative time is longer in laparoscopic PN [17]. A study has noted a deeper decline in GFR in the immediate postoperative period in LPN but no difference in 3.6-year follow-up [18].

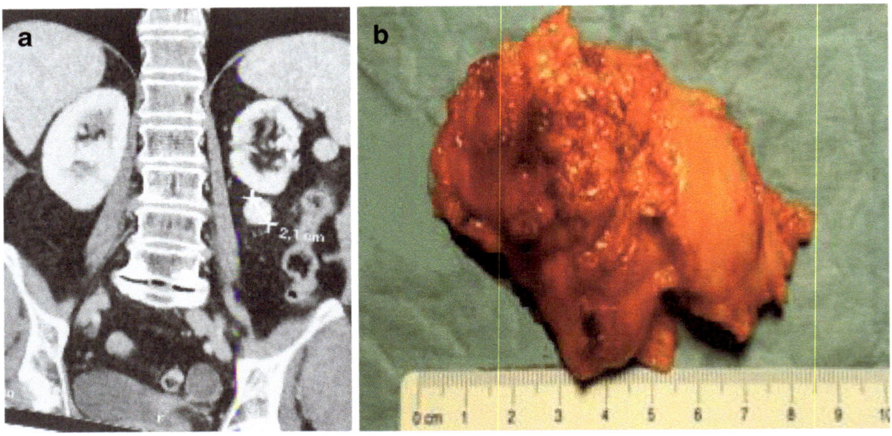

Fig. 16.4 (**a**, **b**) Local recurrence in the Gerota's fascia 2 years after a laparoscopic left partial nephrectomy for a lower pole tumour. The recurrent lesion was estimated to be 2–3 cm diameter and was safely removed laparoscopically with enough peri-renal fat to ensure negative margins

There are similar outcomes when comparing retroperitoneal versus transperitoneal LPN [19].

The cancer-specific survival of radical nephrectomy versus partial nephrectomy at 5 years is comparable for tumours less than 5 cm in size and a normal contralateral kidney. Although local recurrence rate is potentially higher in the partial nephrectomy group (Fig. 16.4a, b), a recent meta-analysis has shown that NSS had a significantly lower cancer-specific death rate compared with RN, but there was no significant difference in the rate of tumour recurrence and complications between the two techniques [20].

In T1a RCC, radical nephrectomy, partial nephrectomy and radiofrequency ablation all showed a 5-year cancer-specific survival of 100 %.

The oncological outcome of partial nephrectomy supports that localized RCCs are best managed by nephron-sparing surgeries than by radical nephrectomy. However, in some patients with localized RCC, nephron-sparing surgery is not suitable because of locally advanced tumour growth, unfavourable location of tumour and a poor general condition. In these situations, radical nephrectomy is the rule [21].

16.4.1.3 Laparoscopic Radical Nephrectomy

Laparoscopic nephrectomy has become one of the commonest laparoscopic urologic procedures. Laparoscopy is the preferred approach in experienced centres for all indications of radical nephrectomy, and the larger tumour size is not considered a contraindication. *The only limiting factor is the expertise of the urologist.* Certain situations may be challenging such as large venous thrombus, adjacent organ infiltration and widespread metastases.

A transperitoneal approach has the advantage of a large working space with presence of familiar anatomical landmarks. Difficulties should be anticipated when there is history of multiple previous abdominal surgeries. On the other hand, a retroperitoneal approach performed over the triangle of Jean Louis Petit avoids the intra-abdominal viscera in the field and allows a rapid access to the renal artery, but the working space is limited, and the surrounding anatomy is less familiar.

Hand-assisted laparoscopic nephrectomy utilizes a 7–8 cm incision for the hand to retract, dissect and guide the laparoscopic tools. It is reported to have a shorter operative time.

16.4.1.4 Laparoscopic Partial Nephrectomy

This has emerged as an attractive minimally invasive alternative to open partial nephrectomy and is considered as the standard of care when facilities and expertise are available. It is a technically challenging procedure because of its intra-operative complexities and potential complications. It should be reserved for urologists with adequate prior laparoscopic experience.

> *Absolute indications* of partial nephrectomy (open or laparoscopic) are tumour in a solitary kidney, patients with compromised renal function and bilateral renal tumours.

Relative indications are current or future threat to renal function such as diabetes, hypertension, contralateral kidney affected by renovascular disease, recurrent stone disease, cysts, ureteropelvic junction obstruction or other anatomical or functional abnormalities.

The elective indications include small renal tumours in the presence of a contralateral functioning kidney. Initially, elective partial nephrectomy was performed for exophytic tumours less than 4 cm size, but with the increasing experience nowadays, highly specialized centres regularly record partial nephrectomy for bigger size tumours, larger infiltrating tumours requiring heminephrectomy, centrally located and para-hilar tumours.

A pre-operative CT angiogram evaluates the tumour as well as the vascular anatomy. Intra-operative laparoscopic ultrasonography can also be useful to delineate the contour of an endophytic tumour during the resection.

Specific complications of nephron-sparing surgery include delayed haemorrhage and urinary leak, as well as the risk of renal function deterioration in longer warm ischemia time, especially if >30 min [22].

In Western Europe and North America, many centres routinely now perform robotic-assisted partial nephrectomy aiming at facilitating the endocorporeal dissection and stitching. Among other positive results, this technique helps to significantly reduce the warm ischaemia time [23].

Non-clamping techniques or selective arterial occlusion can be used for smaller exophytic lesions, with the purpose of avoiding warm ischemia insult to the remaining renal parenchyma.

16.4.1.5 Positive Surgical Margin After Nephron-Sparing Surgery

Positive surgical margins (PSM) were reported in 0–7 % of patients after open PN, in 0.7–4 % after laparoscopic PN and in 3.9–5.7 % after robot-assisted PN [24]. *The thickness of healthy parenchyma surrounding the tumour is irrelevant as long as complete tumour removal is achieved. PSM is mostly associated with small and endophytic tumours. Gross evaluation of the resection margins by the surgeon is reliable, and routine frozen section is unnecessary* [25]. A PSM raises the risk of local recurrence, especially in high-grade tumours. Large-scale data with nephrometry scores and long-term follow-up are lacking in this subject. *Available data indicate that majority of patients with PSMs after partial nephrectomy will not experience disease recurrence. Moreover, prophylactic secondary nephrectomy of the renal remnant has shown residual tumour in only a minority (0–39 %) of patients with PSM* [26]. Development of metastasis and cancer-specific survival was comparable to those in patients with negative surgical margins. *Therefore, a surveillance strategy with adherence to vigilant follow-up is the best management option over surgical re-intervention* [26, 27].

16.4.2 Management of Vena Caval Thrombus

Venous thrombus formation is a unique feature of RCC. It has been reported in 4–10 % of patients and was even found to involve the infrarenal vena cava [28, 29].

Although involvement of the IVC in renal cancer is generally not a vascular invasion by the neoplastic process but mostly an intraluminal extension of the tumour mass, such intravascular growth implies a heightened biologic behaviour of the tumour. Previous reports have shown that total resection of tumour, i.e. including any eventual venous thrombus, affords the best chance of cure and long-term survival when distant metastases are not present [29, 30].

Caval thrombus is one of the most technically challenging surgeries, but it is also rewarding for the urologist, because the 5-year survival rates, even in the face of intra-atrial tumour thrombus (Fig. 16.5a, b), *are comparable to lesions confined to the kidney* [29].

A number of patients with caval thrombus are asymptomatic. But depending on the extent of occlusion, certain signs and symptoms may develop: lower extremity oedema, isolated right-sided varicocoele (irreducible), dilated superficial abdominal

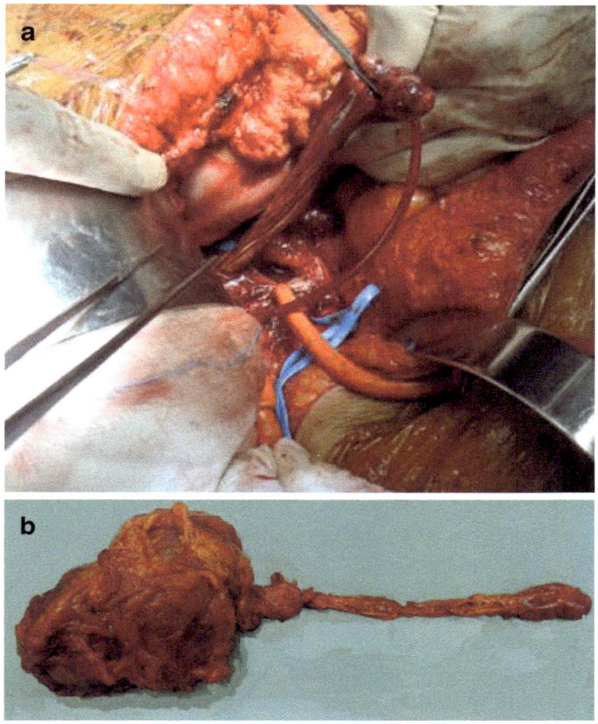

Fig. 16.5 (**a**, **b**) Cardiothoracic team removing a right atrial tumour thrombus from an RCC under extracorporeal circulation

veins (caput medusae), proteinuria and even pulmonary embolism. Careful perioperative planning is essential to optimize the outcome. Traditionally, venocavography was used as gold standard for the diagnosis of venacaval thrombus, but it is now rarely used as it does not show caval wall invasion and does not add any further information compared to US. MRI is considered the gold standard imaging for delineating the upper limit for tumour thrombosis as well as the extent of the caval wall invasion [30] (Fig. 16.6a, b). Alternatively, multidetector CT can be used with nearly equal performance [31].

A multidisciplinary surgical team approach involving vascular, hepatobiliary and cardiothoracic surgical teams is needed in addition to the urologist.

In the presence of a large renal tumour with venacaval thrombus, the following surgical principles apply [30, 32]:

1. Complete resection of the tumour and caval thrombus
2. Mobilization of inferior vena cava (IVC) and the contralateral renal vein (RV)
3. Vascular control of the contralateral RV and IVC proximal and distal to the thrombus
4. Restoration of hemodynamic stability by vascular bypass
5. Reconstruction of IVC if more than 50 % of the wall is involved by tumour

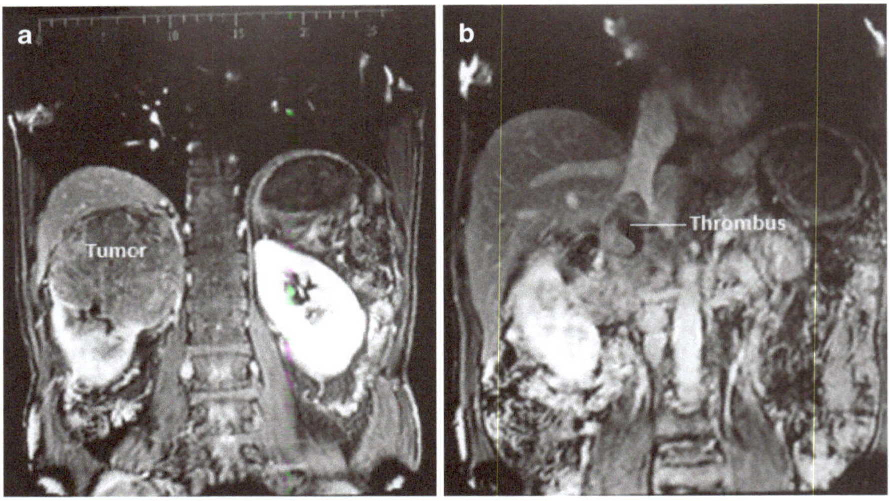

Fig. 16.6 (**a**, **b**) MRI showing a large right upper pole tumour (**a**) with venacaval thrombus (**b**) (Courtesy of Kurian George, Urology, The Royal Hospital, Muscat, Oman)

Various classification systems were developed to characterize the venacaval thrombi on the basis of their cranial extent (Neves, Novick, Hinman and Mayo classification systems). The most commonly used system and the appropriate corresponding management are given in Table 16.1.

16.4.3 Cytoreductive Nephrectomy (CN)

Cytoreductive nephrectomy (CN) was considered as an integral part of multimodality treatment of advanced RCC in the cytokine era. Patients who underwent CN had an improved overall survival when treated with interferon-alpha immunotherapy. This was independent of the performance status and site of metastasis. However, the overall survival advantage was only 5.8 months [33].

Presently, drugs targeting angiogenesis and cellular growth pathways have transformed the treatment of mRCC, and the new place of non-palliative CN needs to be established with ongoing randomized trials. Meanwhile, 90 % of patients entering target therapy trial had prior nephrectomy. CN is recommended for patients with potentially resectable primary and resectable solitary or oligometastasis and continues to play a role in VEGF-targeted treatment. CN is not recommended in patients with poor performance status [34].

The concept of CN which is performed to optimize the effect of a subsequent systemic therapy should not be confused with *palliative nephrectomy* which may be indicated in some surgically fit mRCC patients to relieve intractable haematuria and local symptoms.

Table 16.1 Classification and management of IVC tumour thrombus in RCC

Levels	TNM stage	Cranial extend of tumour	Surgical planning	Incision	Thrombectomy technique
Level I	T3a	Renal vein extending <2 cm within IVC	Experienced urologist alone	Flank	Nephrectomy + RV thrombectomy, Satinsky parallel to wall of IVC to include only the ipsilateral RV ostium
Level II	T3b	Infrahepatic	Vascular	Flank vs. Chevron[a]	Mobilization of entire IVC
					Ligation of lumbar veins
					Infrarenal, suprarenal and opposite renal vein control
Level III	T3b	Intrahepatic	Hepatobiliary ± cardiovascular	Thoracoabdominal	Mobilization of entire IVC
				Or Chevron	Piggyback liver mobilization
				Or midline	Pringle manoeuvre[b]
					Control of suprahepatic IVC
					Venovenous bypass
Level IV (Fig. 16.4a, b)	T3c	Supradiaphragmatic and atrial thrombus	Cardiovascular	Combined Chevron + median sternotomy	Cardiopulmonary bypass
					Hypothermic circulatory arrest

[a]A Chevron incision is a double Kocher or rooftop incision. It crosses the abdominal wall below the ribcage from one midaxillary line to another

[b]Pringle manoeuvre (named after *James Hogarth Pringle*) describes the technique of applying a clamp or other compressive device to the hepatoduodenal ligament at the foramen of Winslow. This is an effective means to control the portal vein and the hepatic artery during liver surgery

Table 16.2 Further post-nephrectomy follow-up (a first review at 4–6 weeks post-operatively applies for all)

	pT1	pT2	pT3
History, physical examination and labs	Every 6 months for 3 years and then annually	Every 6 months for 3 years and then annually	Every 6 months for 3 years and then annually
Chest X-ray	Every 6 months for 3 years and then annually	Every 6 months for 3 years and then annually	Every 6 months for 3 years and then annually
Abdominal CT	Not mandatory	CT/US every 2 years	Every 6 months for 2 years, then every 2 years

Role of Metastasectomy

Metastasectomy can be performed after multidisciplinary review in selected patients with solitary or easily accessible pulmonary metastases and solitary resectable intra-abdominal metastasis (e.g. liver, pancreas, contralateral ureter). Apart from the brain and bone, metastasectomy remains an appropriate local treatment for most sites [35–38].

16.4.4 Follow-up After Surgery

Follow-up allows monitoring for surgical complications and possible impairment of renal function as well as early detection of local recurrence, recurrence in the contralateral kidney and distant metastasis. At 4–6 weeks post-operatively, the first follow-up assesses the patient's history, physical examination, serum creatinine and haemoglobin. Further schedules are given in Table 16.2 [39]. *Thirty % of the patients with RCC develop relapse after surgery and need long-term follow-up* (Fig. 16.7a, b).

16.4.5 Best Supportive Care

About one third of patients with mRCC develop bone involvement with osteolytic lesions [40] (Figs. 16.8a, b and 16.9a, b). For metastases in the brain and bone, *radiotherapy* can induce significant relief of local symptoms. Surgery and radiotherapy are often needed in spinal cord compression, pathological fractures and pain management. Bone modifying agents like bisphosphonates (zoledronic acid) and monoclonal antibody RANKL (receptor activator of nuclear factor kappa-B ligand) inhibitor (denosumab) help in delaying skeletal-related events [41]. When the disease is well controlled extracranially, surgery can be considered for solitary brain metastasis. *Stereotactic radiotherapy* for limited volume brain metastasis and whole brain irradiation for multiple brain metastases are recommended [42].

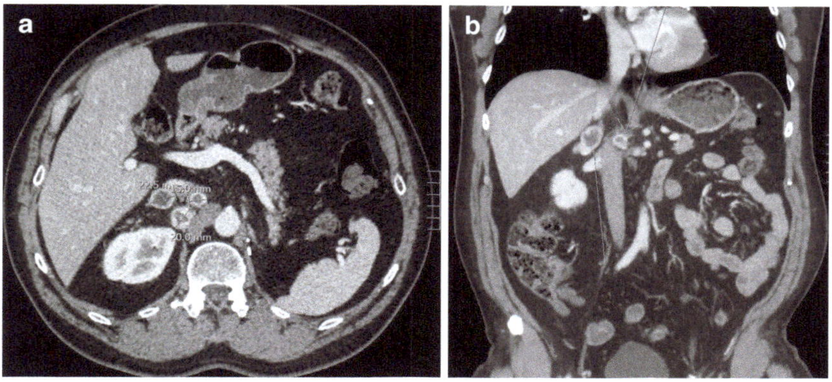

Fig. 16.7 (**a**, **b**) CT scan showing peri-caval LNs recurrence after left laparoscopic nephrectomy done 15 months back in a 62-year-old man (all the LNs were removed laparoscopically)

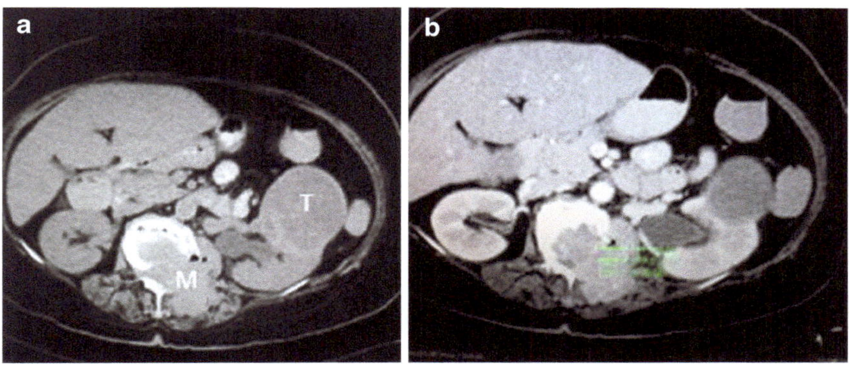

Fig. 16.8 (**a**, **b**) Plain and contrast CT showing a left renal tumour (*T*) with vertebral metastasis (*M*) (Courtesy of Sadiq Lala, Urology, the Royal hospital, Muscat, Oman)

16.5 Systemic Therapy

RCCs express high levels of P-glycoprotein, the multiple drug resistance protein which is responsible for their chemoresistance. In the last few decades, several trials were conducted to find effective systemic therapy for mRCC. These included immunotherapy with interferon-alpha (IFN α), interleukin-2 (IL-2), vaccine therapy with tumour antigen MVA-5 T4 and, most recently, targeted therapy. Vaccines and monotherapy with cytokines are no longer recommended by any guideline, but *the cure horizon is still not in sight even with the current systemic therapy*.

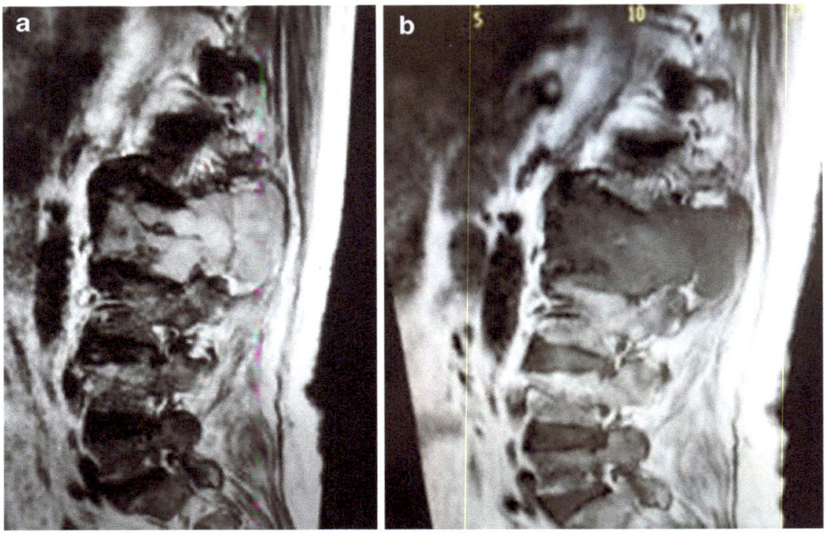

Fig. 16.9 (**a**, **b**) T2- and T1-weighted MRI showing vertebral metastasis (same patient in Fig. 16.8) (Courtesy of Sadiq Lala, Urology, the Royal hospital, Muscat, Oman)

Risk Stratification for mRCC

When immunotherapy was the standard treatment, various risk models were developed for prognostic risk stratification and treatment planning [43]. The most popular and standard one was the Memorial Sloan-Kettering Cancer Center (MSKCC) model. More recently, the International Metastatic RCC Database Consortium (IMDC) model was introduced to suit the targeted therapy. This model is based on six risk factors. The number of the risk factors present is added up and stratified into three risk categories: favourable, intermediate and poor-risk groups [44] (Table 16.3).

IMDC has now been validated and compared with other risk models, the Cleveland Clinic Foundation (CCF) model, the International Kidney Cancer Working Group (IKCWG) model, the French model and the Memorial Sloan-Kettering Cancer Center (MSKCC) model [45, 46].

16.5.1 Immunotherapy

(a) *High-Dose Interleukin-2 (HDIL-2):* The American National Comprehensive Cancer Network (NCCN) recommends *HDIL-2 as an option in first-line and second-line treatment* [47] in selected patients with good performance status and normal organ function. In the experience of National Cancer Institute, out of the 906 patients included in the kidney cancer database during 2004–2011, 91 patients with mRCC were treated with HDIL-2. Four patients (4.5 %) had a

Table 16.3 International Metastatic RCC Database Consortium model (IMDC/DCM) [44]

Risk factors	Risk group	Number of risk factors	Median overall survival (months)	2-year overall survival (%)
Karnofsky performance status <80 %[a] Haemoglobin < lower limit of normal Time from diagnosis to treatment <1 year Corrected calcium above upper limit of normal Platelets greater than upper limit of normal Neutrophils greater than upper limit of normal	Favourable	0	43	75
	Intermediate	1–2	27	53
	Poor risk	3–6	8.8	7

[a]80 % in the Karnofsky criteria is defined as normal activity with effort with some signs or symptoms of disease. It corresponds to the grade 1 of the ECOG performance status (see Table 7.3)

complete response, 10 (11.4 %) had a partial response and 28 (31.8 %) had stable disease. Median progression-free survival and overall survival (OS) were 8.6 and 35.5 months, respectively. The estimated 2-year OS rate was 60.6 % [48].

(b) *IFN-α monotherapy* has been reported to have a modest impact on survival with 15 % objective response rate in appropriately selected cases. Average improvement in survival was only 2.6 months. *Both EAU and NCCN*[1] *are not recommending IFN-α monotherapy* [49],*but they do recommend the combination of IFN-α and bevacizumab as first-line option for clear cell mRCC* [10, 47].

16.5.2 Targeted Therapy

The US FDA has approved seven targeted agents in the treatment of advanced RCC. Agents that target the VEGF pathway, namely, *sunitinib* and *pazopanib,* are first-line drugs. The monoclonal antibody *bevacizumab* (in combination with IFN-α) is also listed as first-line agent, while *sorafenib* and *axitinib* are approved as second-line options. The approved agents that inhibit mTOR are *temsirolimus* and *everolimus.*

- *Sunitinib or SU 11248 (Sutent®)* is an oral multitargeted tyrosine-kinase inhibitor (TKI). It has shown high activity in patients with mRCC. *Sunitinib inhibits the vascular endothelial growth factor (VEGF) receptor and other tyrosine kinases, including the platelet-derived growth factor (PDGF) and c-kit receptor at nanomolar concentrations. It has antitumour and antiangiogenic activity.* It was shown to have an objective response rate of 31 % which was far higher than that of IFN-α (6 %) and also a longer median progression-free survival (11 months) [50]. Patients treated with sunitinib were also reported to have a significantly better quality of life compared with IFN-α.

[1] National Comprehensive Cancer Network.

- *Pazopanib (Votrient®)* is an oral angiogenesis inhibitor targeting VEGFR, PDGFR and c-kit. It has a similar efficacy to sunitinib but better safety and quality of life profiles [51].
- *Bevacizumab (Avastin®)* is a humanized monoclonal antibody that binds to the circulating isoforms of VEGF-A. In the double blind phase III trial (AVOREN), the median overall survival time was 23.3 months for patients treated with bevacizumab + IFN-α compared to 21.3 months in the group treated with IFN-α monotherapy [52]. There is an increased toxicity profile in the combination therapy which includes generalized fatigue, proteinuria, hypertension, haemorrhage, venous thromboembolism, gastrointestinal perforation and arterial ischaemia [53].
- *Sorafenib ou BAY 43–9006 (Nexavar®)* is an oral multikinase inhibitor of VEGF and related receptors. It has been recommended as the second-line option after failure of immunotherapy, and as third-line option after failure of mTOR inhibitors.
- *Axitinib (Inlyta®)* is an oral selective inhibitor of VEGFR 1, 2 and 3. It is recommended as second-line option. A comparison of axitinib and sorafenib has shown an overall survival of 20.1 and 19.2 months, respectively, and a clearly better progression-free rate with respective values of 8.3 months and 5.7 months [54]. Axitinib has been licensed as a second-line drug in the USA and Europe.
- *Temsirolimus (Torisel®)* is a specific inhibitor of the mammalian target of rapamycin (mTOR). mTOR is an integral molecule in the signalling pathway, an enzyme that regulates cell growth and proliferation. Temsirolimus monotherapy has been recommended as first-line treatment of clear cell mRCC in the poor prognosis group [10, 43]. The reported median overall survival is 10.9 months compared with 7.3 months in a similar group treated with interferon [55]. Reported adverse effects are rash, peripheral oedema, hyperglycaemia and hyperlipidaemia.
- *Everolimus (Afinitor®)* is an oral mTOR inhibitor and established as second line in VEGF refractory disease. In patients with failed anti-VEGFR therapy, treatment with everolimus + best supportive care (BSC) has been credited with a median progression-free survival of 4.0 months as compared to 1.9 months in placebo + BSC [56].

Systemic Therapy Should Be Based on Targeted Agents

- For advanced/metastatic clear cell RCC patients *with favourable and intermediate prognostic risk criteria*, the first-line options are sunitinib, pazopanib or bevacizumab + IFN-α. Pazopanib has a similar efficacy to sunitinib, with a different toxicity profile. Following progression with VEGF-targeted therapy, recommended second-line agents are everolimus and axitinib. Pazopanib and sorafenib are recommended in patients failing prior cytokine therapy.
- In patients with clear cell mRCC *with poor prognostic risk criteria* (patients with ≥3 risk factors), the only recommended agent in both NCCN and EAU guidelines is anti-mTOR agent *temsirolimus*.
- No standard treatment is available for non-clear cell histology. A recent trial with sunitinib reported median progression-free survival (PFS) of 6.4 months [57].

Erlotinib, an oral EGFR inhibitor, was studied in papillary RCC and produced a median overall survival of 27 months [58].

- Sarcomatoid RCC (sRCC) is an aggressive form of RCC. May be a terminally dedifferentiated clone arising from any of the other subtypes of RCC or may arise from a completely separate clone. A combination chemotherapy similar to treatment of sarcoma, immunotherapy and targeted therapy were used in the treatment of this variety which led to median survival times of 6–12 months [59, 60].
- Medullary carcinoma and collecting duct carcinoma are rare subtypes and carry poor prognosis. Chemotherapy is the modality of treatment.

In conclusion, *the treatment of mRCC is still disappointing despite the years of research and the multiplicity of trials and marketed drugs.* VGEF and tyrosine-kinase inhibitors have not revolutionized this treatment. They merely improved the PFS, but not the overall survival compared to IFN-α. Combination of bevacizumab and mTOR inhibitors does not perform better, and everolimus for second-line treatment only allows stabilization of the patients' condition, but there is no benefit in the overall survival compared to placebo.

Take-Home Message: Systemic Therapy for mRCC – Summary of the Recommendations

RCC type	First line	Second line
Clear cell mRCC, favourable and intermediate risk	Sunitinib or pazopanib	Everolimus or axitinib in failed VGEF inhibitors
	Bevacizumab + IFN-α	Pazopanib or sorafenib in failed cytokine
Clear cell mRCC, poor risk	Temsirolimus	Any targeted agent
Non-clear cell mRCC	Sunitinib or everolimus or temsirolimus	
Predominant sarcomatoid	Gemcitabine, doxorubicin/capecitabine, immunotherapy	
Collecting duct or medullary subtype	Carboplatin, gemcitabine and paclitaxel	

References

1. Rao K, Royce PL. Incidentally detected small renal masses – investigation and management. Aust Fam Physician. 2011;40(10):776–82.
2. Campbell SC, Novick AC, Belldengrun A, et al. Guidelines for the management of the Clinical stage 1 Renal Mass. J Urol. 2009;182(4):1271–9.
3. Chawla SN, Crispen PL, Hanlon AL, Greenberg RE, Chen DY, Uzzo RG. The natural history of observed enhancing renal masses: meta-analysis and review of the world literature. J Urol. 2006;175(2):425–31.

4. Kunkle DA, Crispen PL, Chen DY, Greenberg RE, Uzzo RG. Enhancing renal masses with zero net growth during active surveillance. J Urol. 2007;177(3):849–53; discussion 853–4.
5. Kunkle DA, Crispen PL, Li T, Uzzo RG. Tumour size predicts synchronous metastatic renal cell carcinoma: implications for surveillance of small renal masses. J Urol. 2007;177(5):1692–6; discussion 1697.
6. Pierorazio PM, Hyams ES, Mullins JK, Allaf ME. Active surveillance for small renal masses. Rev Urol. 2012;14(1–2):13–9.
7. McGahan JP, Browning PD, Brock JM, Tesluk H. Hepatic ablation using radiofrequency electrocautery. Invest Radiol. 1990;25:267–70.
8. Ahrar K, Ahrar JU, Javadi S, Pan L, Milton DR, Wood CG, Matin SF, Stafford RJ. Real-time magnetic resonance imaging-guided cryoablation of small renal tumours at 1.5 T. Invest Radiol. 2013;48(6):437–44.
9. Truesdale CM, Soulen MC, Clark TW, Mondschein JI, Wehrenberg-Klee E, Malkowicz SB, Wein AJ, Guzzo TJ, Stavropoulos SW. Percutaneous computed tomography-guided renal mass radiofrequency ablation versus cryoablation: doses of sedation medication used. J Vasc Interv Radiol. 2013;24(3):347–50.
10. Ljungberg B, Bensalah K, Bex A, et al. Guidelines on renal cell carcinoma. EAU update. Apr 2014. http://uroweb.org/wp-content/uploads/10-Renal-Cell-Carcinoma_LR.pdf.
11. Margulis V, Sánchez-Ortiz RF, Tamboli P, Cohen DD, Swanson DA, Wood CG. Renal cell carcinoma clinically involving adjacent organs: experience with aggressive surgical management. Cancer. 2007;109(10):2025–30.
12. Robson CJ. Radical nephrectomy for renal cell carcinoma. J Urol. 1963;89:37–42.
13. Colombo Jr JR, Haber GP, Aron M, Cocuzza M, Colombo R, Kaouk J, Gill IS. Oncological outcomes of laparoscopic radical nephrectomy for renal cancer. Clinics (Sao Paulo). 2007;62(3):251–6.
14. Fan X, Xu K, Lin T, Liu H, Yin Z, Dong W, Huang H, Huang J. Comparison of transperitoneal and retroperitoneal laparoscopic nephrectomy for renal cell carcinoma: a systematic review and meta-analysis. BJU Int. 2013;111(4):611–2.
15. Lane BR, Tiong HY, Campbell SC, Fergany AF, Weight CJ, Larson BT, Novick AC, Flechner SM. Management of the adrenal gland during partial nephrectomy. J Urol. 2009;181(6):2430–6.
16. Blom JH, van Poppel H, Maréchal JM, Jacqmin D, Schröder FH, de Prijck L, Sylvester R, EORTC Genitourinary Tract Cancer Group. Radical nephrectomy with and without lymph-node dissection: final results of European Organization for Research and Treatment of Cancer (EORTC) randomized phase 3 trial 30881. Eur Urol. 2009;55(1):28–34.
17. Gill IS, Kavoussi LR, Lane BR, Blute ML, Babineau D, Colombo Jr JR, Frank I, Permpongkosol S, Weight CJ, Kaouk JH, Kattan MW, Novick AC. Comparison of 1,800 laparoscopic and open partial nephrectomies for single renal tumours. J Urol. 2007;178(1):41–6.
18. Marszalek M, Meixl H, Polajnar M, Rauchenwald M, Jeschke K, Madersbacher S. Laparoscopic and open partial nephrectomy: a matched-pair comparison of 200 patients. Eur Urol. 2009;55(5):1171–8.
19. Tugcu V, Bitkin A, Sonmezay E, Polat H, Ilbey YO, Taşçi AI. Transperitoneal versus retroperitoneal laparoscopic partial nephrectomy: initial experience. Arch Ital Urol Androl. 2011;83(4):175–80.
20. Li W, Cheng Y, Cheng Y, Ren H, Han N. Clinical efficacy of radical nephrectomy versus nephron-sparing surgery on localized renal cell carcinoma. Eur J Med Res. 2014;19(1):58. doi:10.1186/s40001-014-0058-4. Published online Nov 6, 2014.
21. Badalato GM, Kates M, Wisnivesky JP, Choudhury AR, McKiernan JM. Survival after partial and radical nephrectomy for the treatment of stage T1bN0M0 renal cell carcinoma (RCC) in the USA: a propensity scoring approach. BJU Int. 2012;109(10):1457–62.
22. Thompson RH, Lane BR, Campbell SC, et al. Every minute counts when the renal hilum is clamped during partial nephrectomy. Eur Urol. 2010;58(3):340–5.
23. Aboumarzouk OM, Stein RJ, Eyraud R, Haber GP, Chlosta PL, Somani BK, Kaouk JH. Robotic versus laparoscopic partial nephrectomy: a systematic review and meta-analysis. Eur Urol. 2012;62(6):1023–33.

24. Marszalek M, Carini M, Chlosta P, et al. Positive surgical margins after nephron-sparing surgery. Eur Urol. 2012;61:757–63.
25. Yilmaz H, Ciftci S, Ozkan L, Saribacak A, Yildiz K, Dillioglugil O. Gross intraoperative evaluation (GIE): a reliable method for the evaluation of surgical margins at partial nephrectomy. Int J Clin Exp Med. 2014;7(3):792–8.
26. Steinestel J, Steffens S, Steinestel K, Schrader AJ. Positive surgical margins in nephron-sparing surgery: risk factors and therapeutic consequences. World J Surg Oncol. 2014;12:252.
27. Borghesi M, Brunocilla E, Schiavina R, Martorana G. Positive surgical margins after nephron-sparing surgery for renal cell carcinoma: incidence, clinical impact, and management. Clin Genitourin Cancer. 2013;11(1):5–9.
28. Mootha RK, Butler R, Laucirica R, Scardino PT, Lerner SP. Renal cell carcinoma with infra-renal vena caval tumour thrombus. Urology. 1999;54:561–5.
29. Wotkowicz C, Wszolek MF, Libertino JA. Resection of renal tumours invading Vena cava. Urol Clin North Am. 2008;35:657–71.
30. Nouh MA, Inui M, Kakehi Y. Renal cell carcinoma with IVC thrombi; current concepts and future perspectives. Clin Med Oncol. 2008;2:247–56.
31. Lawrentschuk N, Gani J, Riordan R, Esler S, Bolton DM. Multidetector computed tomography vs magnetic resonance imaging for defining the upper limit of tumour thrombus in renal cell carcinoma: a study and review. BJU Int. 2005;96:291–5.
32. Lawindy SM, Kurian T, Kim T, Mangar D, Armstrong PA, Alsina AE, Sheffield C, Sexton WJ, Spiess PE. Important surgical considerations in the management of renal cell carcinoma (RCC) with inferior vena cava (IVC) tumour thrombus. BJU Int. 2012;110(7):926–39.
33. Flanigan RC, Mickisch G, Sylvester R, Tangen C, Van Poppel H, Crawford ED. Cytoreductive nephrectomy in patients with metastatic renal cancer: a combined analysis. J Urol. 2004;171(3):1071–6.
34. Choueiri TK, Xie W, Kollmannsberger C, North S, Knox JJ, Lampard JG, McDermott DF, Rini BI, Heng DY. The impact of cytoreductive nephrectomy on survival of patients with metastatic renal cell carcinoma receiving vascular endothelial growth factor targeted therapy. J Urol. 2011;185(1):60–6.
35. Amiraliev A, Pikin O, Alekseev B, Kalpinksiy A. Treatment strategy in patients with pulmonary metastases of renal cell cancer. Interact CardioVasc Thorac Surg. 2012;15 suppl 1:SXIII–F068.
36. Staehler MD, Kruse J, Haseke N, Stadler T, Roosen A, Karl A, Stief CG, Jauch KW, Bruns CJ. Liver resection for metastatic disease prolongs survival in renal cell carcinoma: 12-year results from a retrospective comparative analysis. World J Urol. 2010;28(4):543–7.
37. Ballarin R, Spaggiari M, Cautero N. Pancreatic metastases from renal cell carcinoma: the state of the art. World J Gastroenterol. 2011;17(43):4747–56.
38. Al-Busaidy SA, George K, Kamona A, Samarasinghe DS. Renal cell carcinoma: synchronous contralateral ureteric metastasis. Br J Med Surg Urol. 2011;4:86–8.
39. Skolarikos A, Alivizatos G, Laguna P, de la Rosette J. A review of follow up strategies for renal cell carcinoma after nephrectomy. Eur Urol. 2007;51(6):1490–500.
40. Sahi C, Knox JJ, Clemons M, Joshua AM, Broom R. Renal cell carcinoma bone metastases: clinical advances. Ther Adv Med Oncol. 2010;2(2):75–83.
41. Henry DH, Costa L, Goldwasser F, et al. Randomized, double-blind study of denosumab versus zoledronic acid in the treatment of bone metastases in patients with advanced cancer (excluding breast and prostate cancer) or multiple myeloma. J Clin Oncol. 2011;29(9):1125–32.
42. Fokas E, Henzel M, Hamm K, Surber G, Kleinert G, Engenhart-Cabillic R. Radiotherapy for brain metastases from renal cell cancer: should whole-brain radiotherapy be added to stereotactic radiosurgery?: analysis of 88 patients. Strahlenther Onkol. 2010;186(4):210–7.
43. Motzer RJ, Bacik J, Murphy BA, et al. Interferon-alfa as a comparative treatment for clinical trials of new therapies against advanced renal cell carcinoma. J Clin Oncol. 2002;20:289–96.
44. Heng DY, Xie W, Regan MM, et al. Prognostic factors for overall survival in patients with metastatic renal cell carcinoma treated with vascular endothelial growth factor-targeted agents: results from a large, multicenter study. J Clin Oncol. 2009;27(34):5794–9.

45. Kwon WA, Cho IC, Yu A, et al. Validation of the MSKCC and Heng risk criteria models for predicting survival in patients with metastatic renal cell carcinoma treated with sunitinib. Ann Surg Oncol. 2013;20(13):4397–404.
46. Heng DY, Xie W, Regan MM, et al. External validation and comparison with other models of the International Metastatic Renal-Cell Carcinoma Database Consortium prognostic model: a population-based study. Lancet Oncol. 2013;14(2):141–8.
47. NCCN (National Comprehensive Cancer Network, Inc. 2014) Clinical Practice Guidelines in Oncology. Kidney Cancer. Version I. 2015.
48. Hanzly M, Aboumohamed A, Yarlagadda N. High-dose interleukin-2 therapy for metastatic renal cell carcinoma: a contemporary experience. Urology. 2014;83(5):1129–34.
49. Coppin C, Porzsolt F, Awa A, Kumpf J, Coldman A, Wilt T. Immunotherapy for advanced renal cell cancer. Cochrane Database Syst Rev. 2005;(1):CD001425.
50. Motzer RJ, Hutson TE, Tomczak P, et al. Sunitinib versus interferon alfa in metastatic renal-cell carcinoma. N Engl J Med. 2007;356:115–24.
51. Motzer RJ, Hutson TE, Cella D, et al. Pazopanib versus sunitinib in metastatic renal-cell carcinoma. N Engl J Med. 2013;369:722–31.
52. Escudier B, Bellmunt J, Négrier S, et al. Phase III trial of bevacizumab plus interferon alfa-2a in patients with metastatic renal cell carcinoma (AVOREN): final analysis of overall survival. J Clin Oncol. 2010;28(13):2144–50.
53. Rini BI, Halabi S, Rosenberg JE, Stadler WM, Vaena DA, Archer L, Atkins JN, Picus J, Czaykowski P, Dutcher J, Small EJ. Phase III trial of bevacizumab plus interferon alfa versus interferon alfa monotherapy in patients with metastatic renal cell carcinoma: final results of CALGB 90206. J Clin Oncol. 2010;28(13):2137–43.
54. Motzer RJ, Escudier B, Tomczak P, et al. Axitinib versus sorafenib as second-line treatment for advanced renal cell carcinoma: overall survival analysis and updated results from a randomised phase 3 trial. Lancet Oncol. 2013;14(6):552–62.
55. Hudes G, Carducci M, Tomczak P, et al. Temsirolimus, interferon alfa, or both for advanced renal-cell carcinoma. N Engl J Med. 2007;356(22):2271–81.
56. Motzer RJ, Escudier B, Oudard S, et al. Efficacy of everolimus in advanced renal cell carcinoma: a double-blind, randomised, placebo-controlled phase III trial. Lancet. 2008;372(9637):449–56.
57. Lee JL, Ahn JH, Lim HY, Park SH, et al. Multicenter phase II study of sunitinib in patients with non-clear cell renal cell carcinoma. Ann Oncol. 2012;23(8):2108–14.
58. Gordon MS, Hussey M, Nagle RB, et al. Phase II study of erlotinib in patients with locally advanced or metastatic papillary histology renal cell cancer: SWOG S0317. J Clin Oncol. 2009;27(34):5788–93.
59. Shuch B, Bratslavsky G, Linehan WM, Srinivasan R, et al. Sarcomatoid renal cell carcinoma: a comprehensive review of the biology and current treatment strategies. Oncologist. 2012; 17(1):46–54.
60. Molina AM, Tickoo SK, Ishill N, et al. Sarcomatoid-variant renal cell carcinoma: treatment outcome and survival in advanced disease. Am J Clin Oncol. 2011;34(5):454–9.

Part V
Male Genital Cancers

Qais Mohamed Al Hooti and Said Abdallah Al-Mamari

Male genital cancers comprise malignancies of the testicles, the penis, the urethra, the scrotal skin, the spermatic cord and the epididymis. Testicular cancers will be mostly addressed in this part which will include a short account of primary extra-gonadal germ cell tumours and penile neoplasms.

Chapter 17
Epidemiology and Aetiology of Testicular Cancers

Qais Mohamed Al-Hooti and Said Abdallah Al-Mamari

17.1 Epidemiology

Testicular cancer is the most common malignancy encountered among males aged 20–40 years and accounts for 1–1.5 % of cancers in men and 5 % of all urological tumours [1]. There is a significant geographic variation in the incidence of this malignancy especially germ cell tumours (GCTs): Scandinavian countries, Germany and Switzerland record the highest incidence, while the lowest is reported in African and Asian countries [1]. The estimated incidence of testicular tumours in Western countries is 3–10 new cases per 100,000 males per year [2]. In the last 30–40 years, a trend towards an increased testicular cancer incidence has been documented in the majority of industrialized countries, especially in Northern European countries, North America and Oceania [3–6]. It has been suggested that the birth cohort hypothesis plays a major role towards this trend, as Nordic men born around 1943 and 1968 showed lower incidences than men born just before or just after these dates [4, 7, 8].

Data from 1973 to 1998 have shown that this increase was mostly due to seminomas in American Caucasian men [1]. Nonetheless, the incidence of both seminoma and non-seminomatous tumours also began to increase among black men in the 1990s [5, 9].

The increased awareness has resulted in earlier diagnosis and an increased incidence of early-stage disease. Localized cancers were reported in 72.7 % of testicular cancers of white Americans since the year 2000 [9].

Q.M. Al-Hooti • S.A. Al-Mamari (✉)
Urology Department, The Royal Hospital, Muscat, Oman
e-mail: sabdal67@yahoo.com

S.A. Al-Mamari, S.S. Al-Busaidy (eds.), *Urological Cancer Management*,
DOI 10.1007/978-3-319-16301-7_17

17.2 Aetiology

Multiple factors are associated with an increased risk of testicular cancer; however, *four are well established*, including *cryptorchidism*, presence of *intratubular germ cells neoplasia* (*ITGCN*), a history of *contralateral testicular cancer* and a *family history of testicular cancer* [10].

1. *Cryptorchidism* (Fig. 17.1): Suspected mechanisms in undescended testis include abnormal germ cell morphology, elevated temperature, endocrine dysfunction and gonadal dysgenesis [11]. Nowadays, the incidence of GCT in patients with cryptorchidism is estimated to be about seven times higher than that of the general population, and biopsy of the undescended testis during orchidopexy has been reported to be a greater risk factor for subsequent development of malignancy [12]. Some studies have revealed that the risk of developing tumour declines if the orchidopexy is performed before puberty [13], but controversy remains. A meta-analysis reported that in patients with unilateral cryptorchidism, the contralateral well-descended testis is also at a slightly increased risk of cancer [14]. It has been estimated that the rate of cancer involvement of the undescended gonad and the well-descended contralateral one were respectively 79 and 21 % [15].
2. *ITGCN or carcinoma in situ of the testis or testicular intraepithelial neoplasia* (*TIN*): This is a noninvasive premalignant precursor of germ cell tumours. It is commonly found in patients with pre-existing ipsilateral testicular GCT (80 % of patients), but may even be encountered in the contralateral "normal" one (5–10 %) [15]. ITGCN has also been found in association with cryptorchidism, atrophic testis, infertility and hermaphroditism. The progression risk into

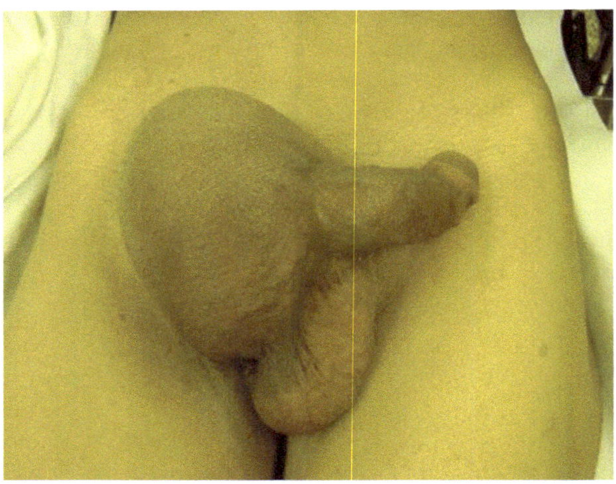

Fig 17.1 Tumour of an undescended right testis (Courtesy of Kurian George, Urology, Royal Hospital, Muscat, Oman)

invasive GCTs increases with time and has been evaluated to be 50 % within 5 years and 70 % within 7 years [16–18].

3. *Past history of a testicular cancer*: This exposes the patient to an increased risk of developing a synchronous or metachronous GCT in the contralateral testis. This risk is reported to be higher in patients who are younger at the time of the diagnosis and in those with seminoma [19, 20].
4. *Family history of testicular tumour*: Having a first-degree relative with testicular cancer increases the risk of developing this tumour. The median age at diagnosis in such patients with a positive family history is 2–3 years younger than in the general population [21]. Family-linked testicular cancers have been extensively studied by Scandinavian authors who found the individual's risks for testicular cancer increased by 8- and 4-folds with an affected brother and father [22–24]. A recessive mode of inheritance was proposed as an explanation for the higher correlation between brothers than between a father and his son [25]. The combination of shared childhood environment and heritable causes were suggested as an explanation of this high familial risk. There are few genetic changes described in association with testicular cancer. The most commonly encountered is an *isochromosome of the short arm of chromosome 12-i(12p)* which was reported in almost all histological types of germ cell tumours [26, 27]. However, a study has shown that the overrepresentation of 12p is more related to invasive growth and is not an early event in the development of testicular GCTs [28]. *Alterations in the p53 locus* have been described in 66 % of cases of ITGCN.
5. *Other possible risk factors*: These include Klinefelter's syndrome, HIV infection [29], testicular atrophy, infertility, testicular feminization, trauma and hormones. Testicular regression syndrome or *vanishing testis syndrome* is believed to carry a potential for malignant degeneration in the long term, and it is a common practice to remove such remnants as a preventive measure. However, a recent literature review failed to identify any report of a GCT arising from this condition [30]. This phenomenon should not be confused with the so-called *burnt-out germ cell tumour*, a yet unexplained regression of the primary testicular lesion in metastatic germ cell tumour which could be due to immunological reactions.

Note: *Testicular tumour has also been described as a causative factor for other pathologies*:

- A small population study in Mayo Clinic has shown that sarcoidosis has a 100-fold increased association with testicular cancer patients compared with the general population of young white men [31]. The onset of sarcoidosis was shown to occur after an average of 5 years following the diagnosis of testicular cancer. This appears to be the strongest association between any solid tumours and sarcoidosis.
- *Testicular sarcoma* with fatal outcome was reported to arise in association with spermatocytic seminomas [32].

Take-Home Message: Epidemiology and Aetiology

Testicular cancer is the most common malignancy encountered in younger men aged 20–40 years.
Higher incidence is observed in Western countries with an estimated incidence of 3–10 new cases/100,000 males.
There are 4 established aetiological factors: cryptorchidism, presence of ITGCN, personal history and family history of testicular cancer.
Associated genetic findings are consistent with an isochromosome of the short arm of chromosome 12-i(12p) and alterations in the p53 locus.

References

1. Horner MJ, Ries LA, et al. SEER cancer statistics review, 1975–2006. Bethesda: National Cancer Institute; 2009.
2. Jemal A, Siegel R, Ward E, Hao Y, Xu J, Thun MJ. Cancer statistics, 2009. CA Cancer J Clin. 2009;59(4):225–49.
3. Huyghe E, Matsuda T, Thonneau P. Increasing incidence of testicular cancer worldwide: a review. J Urol. 2003;170:5–11.
4. Jacobsen R, Moller H, Thoresen SO, Pukkala E, Kjaer SK, Johansen C. Trends in testicular cancer incidence in the Nordic countries, focusing on the recent decrease in Denmark. Int J Androl. 2006;29:199–204.
5. Shah MN, Devesa SS, Zhu K, McGlynn KA. Trends in testicular germ cell tumours by ethnic group in the United States. Int J Androl. 2007;30:206–13; discussion 13–4.
6. Baade P, Carriere P, Fritschi L. Trends in testicular germ cell cancer incidence in Australia. Cancer Causes Control. 2008;19:1043–9.
7. Ekbom A, Akre O. Increasing incidence of testicular cancer – birth cohort effects. APMIS. 1998;106(1):225–9; discussion 229–31.
8. Bergström R, Adami HO, Möhner M, et al. Increase in testicular cancer incidence in six European countries: a birth cohort phenomenon. J Natl Cancer Inst. 1996;88(11):727–33.
9. McGlynn KA, Devesa SS, Graubard BI, Castle PE. Increasing incidence of testicular germ cell tumours among black men in the United States. J Clin Oncol. 2005;23(24):5757–61.
10. Stephenson AJ, Gilligan TD. Neoplasms of the testis. In: Wein AJ, Kavoussi LR, Novick AC, Partin AW, Peters CA, editors. Campbell-Walsh urology. Chapter 31, vol. 1. 10th ed. Philadelphia: Elsevier Saunders; 2012. p. 837–70.
11. Mostofi FK. Proceedings: testicular tumours. Epidemiologic, etiologic, and pathologic features. Cancer. 1973;32(5):1186–201.
12. Swerdlow AJ, Higgins CD, Pike MC. Risk of testicular cancer in cohort of boys with cryptorchidism. BMJ. 1997;314:1507–11.
13. Dieckmann KP, Pichlmeier U. Clinical epidemiology of testicular germ cell tumours. World J Urol. 2004;22:2–14.
14. Akre O, Pettersson A, Richiardi L. Risk of contralateral testicular cancer among men with unilaterally undescended testis: a meta-analysis. Int J Cancer. 2009;124(3):687–9.
15. Berthelsen JG, Skakkebaek NE, von der Maase H, Sørensen BL, Mogensen P. Screening for carcinoma in situ of the contralateral testis in patients with germinal testicular cancer. Br Med J (Clin Res Ed). 1982;285(6356):1683–6.
16. Skakkebaek NE, Berthelsen JG, Müller J. Carcinoma-in-situ of the undescended testis. Urol Clin North Am. 1982;9(3):377–85.
17. Dieckmann KP, Skakkebaek NE. Carcinoma in situ of the testis: review of biological and clinical features. Int J Cancer. 1999;83(6):815–22.

18. Montironi R. Intratubular germ cell neoplasia of the testis: testicular intraepithelial neoplasia. Eur Urol. 2002;41(6):651–4.
19. Theodore C, Terrier-Lacombe MJ, Laplanche A, Benoit G, Fizazi K, Stamerra O, Wibault P. Bilateral germ-cell tumours: 22-year experience at the Institut Gustave Roussy. Br J Cancer. 2004;90(1):55–9.
20. Fosså SD, Chen J, Schonfeld SJ, McGlynn KA, McMaster ML, Gail MH, Travis LB. Risk of contralateral testicular cancer: a population-based study of 29,515 U.S. men. J Natl Cancer Inst. 2005;97(14):1056–66.
21. Mai PL, Chen BE, Tucker K, et al. Younger age at diagnosis for familial malignant testicular germ cell tumour. Fam Cancer. 2009;8(4):451–6.
22. Hemminki K, Chen B. Familial risks in testicular cancer as aetiological clues. Int J Androl. 2006;29:205–10.
23. Hemminki K, Li X. Familial risk in testicular cancer as a clue to a heritable and environmental aetiology. Br J Cancer. 2004;90:1765–70.
24. Dieckmann KP, Pichlmeier U. The prevalence of familial testicular cancer: an analysis of two patient populations and a review of the literature. Cancer. 1997;80:1954–60.
25. Heimdal K, Olsson H, Tretli S, Fossa SD, Borresen AL, Bishop DT. A segregation analysis of testicular cancer based on Norwegian and Swedish families. Br J Cancer. 1997;75:1084–7.
26. Ilson DH, Bosl GJ, Motzer R, Dmitrovsky E, Chaganti RS. Genetic analysis of germ cell tumours: current progress and future prospects. Hematol Oncol Clin North Am. 1991;5(6):1271–83.
27. Bosl GJ, Dmitrovsky E, Reuter VE, Samaniego F, Rodriguez E, Geller NL, Chaganti RS. Isochromosome of the short arm of chromosome 12: clinically useful markers for male germ cell tumours. J Natl Cancer Inst. 1989;81(24):1874–8.
28. Rosenberg C, Van Gurp RJ, Geelen E, Oosterhuis JW, Looijenga LH. Overrepresentation of the short arm of chromosome 12 is related to invasive growth of human testicular seminomas and nonseminomas. Oncogene. 2000;19(51):5858–62.
29. Goedert JJ, Purdue MP, McNeel TS, et al. Risk of germ cell tumours among men with HIV/acquired immunodeficiency syndrome. Cancer Epidemiol Biomarkers Prev. 2007;16(6):1266–9.
30. Pirgon O, Dündar BN. Vanishing testes: a literature review. J Clin Res Pediatr Endocrinol. 2012;4(3):116–20.
31. Rayson D, Burch PA, Richardson RL. Sarcoidosis and testicular carcinoma. Cancer. 1998;83(2):337–43.
32. Eble JN. Spermatocytic seminoma. Hum Pathol. 1994;25(10):1035–42.

Chapter 18
Histological Classification of Testicular Cancer

Qais Mohamed Al-Hooti and Said Abdallah Al-Mamari

Testicular neoplasms are divided morphologically into different types.

- *Germ cell tumours (GCTs) are the most common type of testicular neoplasm comprising approximately 95 % of these malignancies* [1]. *Most of the GCTs are unilateral, predominant in the right testicle owing to a higher incidence of cryptorchidism* (Fig. 17.1). Metachronous or synchronous bilateral testicular tumours are seen in 1–2 % [2]. Of all GCTs, 5 % are extragonadal and most commonly involve the mediastinum and retroperitoneum. *GCTs* are classified as seminoma and non-seminomatous germ cell tumours (NSGCT), and the relative distribution of each is 55 and 45 %, respectively [3, 4]. Pure seminomas are further divided into classic or typical (95 %) and spermatocytic (5 %). The expression NSGCTs includes all other types of GCTs (see below). Either seminomas or NSGCTs can occur in a *pure form or in a mixed fashion* where more than one histological type is found.
- *Non-GCTs* of the testis are uncommon and include sex cord/stromal tumours, lymphoid and haematopoietic tumours, tumours of the collecting duct and rete testis and tumours of the testicular adnexa [2].

The 2004 World Health Organization [WHO] pathological classification of testicular cancers is shown in Table 18.1 [5].

Q.M. Al-Hooti • S.A. Al-Mamari (✉)
Urology Department, The Royal Hospital, Muscat, Oman
e-mail: sabdal67@yahoo.com

S.A. Al-Mamari, S.S. Al-Busaidy (eds.), *Urological Cancer Management*,
DOI 10.1007/978-3-319-16301-7_18

Table 18.1 The 2004 pathological classification of testicular tumours [5]

1. Germ cell tumours
Intratubular germ cell neoplasia, unclassified type (IGCNU)
Seminoma (including cases with syncytiotrophoblastic cells)
Spermatocytic seminoma (mention if there is sarcomatous component)
Embryonal carcinoma
Yolk sac tumour
Choriocarcinoma
Teratoma (mature, immature, with malignant component)
Tumours with more than one histological type (specify percentage of individual components)
2. Sex cord/gonadal stromal tumours
Leydig cell tumour
Malignant Leydig cell tumour
Sertoli cell tumour: lipid-rich variant, sclerosing and large cell calcifying
Malignant Sertoli cell tumour
Granulosa cell tumour: adult type and juvenile type
Thecoma/fibroma group of tumours
Other sex cord/gonadal stromal tumours: incompletely differentiated and mixed
Tumours containing germ cell and sex cord/gonadal stromal (gonadoblastoma)
3. Miscellaneous non-specific stromal tumours
Ovarian epithelial tumours
Tumours of the collecting ducts and rete testis
Tumours (benign and malignant) of non-specific stroma

By Eble et al. With permission from the International Agency for Research on Cancer, 150 cours Albert Thomas 69372 Lyon cedex 08, France

18.1 GCTs

18.1.1 Intratubular Germ Cell Neoplasia (ITGCN)

ITGCN or carcinoma in situ of the testis (CIS) is a non-invasive pre-malignant lesion. *It is the precursor of all testicular germ cell tumours with the exception of spermatocytic seminoma.* It is thought to derive from primordial germ cells. When discovered in an adult testis, it is believed to have been present since birth. *CIS is found in testicular tissue adjacent to testicular GCTs in about 90 % of cases, and it is also observed in the contralateral "normal" testis of 5–10 % of patients with testicular cancer* [6, 7]. It may also occur in patients with cryptorchidism, infertility, atrophic testis (36 %) and intersex. Conversely, CIS is found in less than 1 % of the normal male population. If left untreated, this condition is associated with a *50 % risk of developing GCT within 5 years and a 70 % risk within 7 years* [6, 8, 9]. Although it is not a routine practice in many centres, expert panels advocate contralateral testicular biopsy to rule out ITGCN *in high risk patients*: *age <40 years, history of undescended testis, testicular volume <12 ml, presence of grade 3 microlithiasis* (see details later in radiological procedures) [10]. *The trans-scrotal approach is prohibited* and *an open inguinal biopsy in unanimously recommended* [10, 11].

18.1.2 Seminoma

Seminoma is the most common type of GCT and occurs at an older average age than NSGCTs. Indeed most cases are diagnosed in the fourth or fifth decade of life. *The majority of GCT found in the undescended testis is seminomas* [2]. It has been suggested that seminomas are the common precursor for other NSGCT subtypes [12].

Two types of seminomas are described: *the typical (classic) and spermatocytic seminoma*. The expression "anaplastic seminoma" is now considered obsolete. It was used in the past to refer to a seminoma with high mitotic activity but was not found to influence the treatment since there are no poor prognostic groups for seminomas (see later).

- *Classic seminoma*: *This forms 40 % of GCTs* (Fig. 18.1). Histologically, it is made of clear cells resembling primitive germ cells. Its incidence has doubled during the last 30 years. It mostly affects young men aged 20–55 years. *At presentation, 75 % of classic seminomas are limited to the testes*, 20 % have retroperitoneal extension and the remaining 5 % have supradiaphragmatic and/or visceral metastases. There is an increased serum placental alkaline phosphatase (PLAP) in 33–91 % and an increased beta-human chorionic gonadotropin (βHCG) in 5 % of cases.
- *Spermatocytic seminoma* is rare and accounts for 1–4 % of GCTs. The expression spermatocytic seminoma appears to be a misnomer since this clinicopathological entity is completely distinct from other GCTs. Spermatocytic seminoma has several specific characteristics which differ from other GCTs: It lacks ITGCN and is not associated with a history of cryptorchidism nor bilaterality. Furthermore,

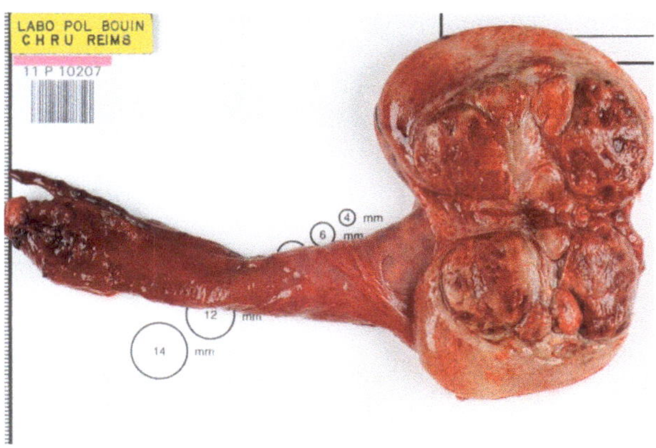

Fig. 18.1 Gross specimen of a radical orchiectomy showing a seminoma with areas of necrosis (Courtesy of A. Durlach, Pol Bouin Laboratory, University Hospital of Reims, France)

it has no ovarian homologue and is not associated with increase serum markers. It does not express PLAP, OCT3/4 (octamer-binding transcription factors), or i(12p), and it *is never found as part of mixed GCTs* [13]. It usually presents in older age groups with a peak incidence in the sixth decade (median age: 55 years). *It is considered a benign tumour as it virtually never metastasizes and is completely cured by orchiectomy* [13–15]. The cell size varies from that of a lymphocyte to that of a giant cell (100 μm). Following the discovery of polypoid populations of tumour cells in spermatocytic seminoma, it has been speculated that this tumour results from self-fertilization of germ cells [16]. This hypothesis may also explain why this pathological entity never occurs in the ovary. For all the above-mentioned reasons, *some authors have suggested not to consider spermatocytic seminoma as a variant of seminoma* [14]. Exceptional cases of a histological "transformation" of spermatocytic seminoma into testicular sarcoma have been reported with a high mortality rate within 2 years [17].

18.1.3 NSGCT

- *Embryonal carcinoma* (EC) occurs in a population estimated to be 10 years younger than that of the seminoma and comprises *2–3 % of GCT*. Its cells are undifferentiated with crowded pleomorphic nuclei and resemble primitive epithelial cells from early-stage embryos [13]. *EC is the second most aggressive GCT after choriocarcinoma and is associated with a high rate of metastasis, often with normal serum tumour markers* [2]. EC is the most undifferentiated cell type of NSGCT and has a *totipotent capacity,* i.e. is able to differentiate into other NSGCTs cell types. This differentiation capacity may be expressed in the primary tumour or in metastatic sites and would explain why a teratoma or other histological types may be identified in distant sites, while the primary type is an embryonal carcinoma. It was shown that 74 % of patients had nodal disease at presentation and half of these have also distant metastases [18].
- *Choriocarcinoma* (CC): Testicular CC is a rare and aggressive tumour with a very poor prognosis affecting mostly young subjects aged 25–30 years. Pure CC comprises only *0.3–0.5 % of GCT*. Mixed forms with a CC component are more frequent (8–16 % of GCT); however, a combination with spermatocytic seminoma or mature teratoma does not exist. The majority of patients at diagnosis have an advanced stage of the disease. CC may present with a disseminated form even if the primary lesion is small and *it spreads by hematogenous routes commonly to lungs, liver, gastrointestinal tract, adrenals and brain including the possibility of eye and skin metastases* [19, 20]. Histologically it contains *cytotrophoblasts and syncytiotrophoblasts*, the latter being responsible for the production of *βHCG* which is characteristically very elevated (>100,000 IU/L) in these tumours [21]. *Metastatic CCs are prone to bleed*, either spontaneously in a rapidly progressive advanced disease or immediately after initiation of chemotherapy. This bleeding can be catastrophic and fatal, particularly when it occurs in

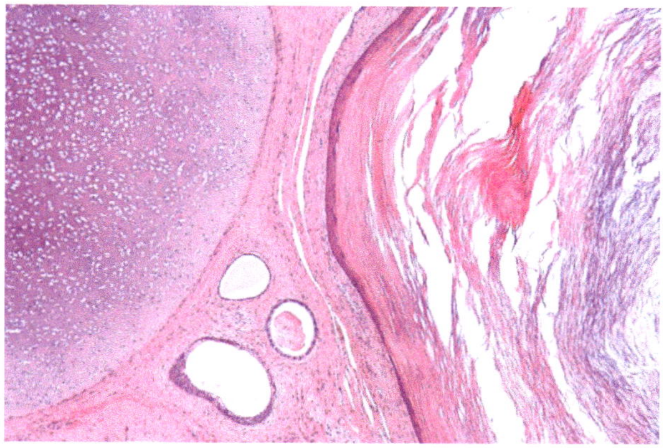

Fig. 18.2 Micrograph of a *teratoma* showing tissue from all three germ layers: *mesoderm* (immature cartilage – *left-upper corner of image*), *endoderm* (gastrointestinal glands – *centre-bottom of image*) and *ectoderm* (epidermis – *right of image*). H&E stain. CC BY-SA 3.0 (free of copy and share)

the lungs or brain [22]. Autopsy performed in patients who have died from this disease has revealed lung, liver and gastrointestinal metastases in 100, 86 and 71 % of cases respectively, while spleen, brain and adrenal metastases were encountered in 56 % [23].

- *Yolk sac tumour is also called endodermal sinus tumour and is the most common type of testicular GCT in the paediatric group below 15 years*. It is also commonly found as a component in the primary mediastinal mixed GCTs. *Schiller-Duval bodies*, embryonal bodies and hyaline globules may be seen in the yolk sac histology. *They almost always produce AFP (90 %) but not HCG*. 10–20 % are metastatic at presentation by lymphatic or hematogenous spread.
- *Teratoma*, from the Greek words teratos (monster) and oma (tumour), was coined by Rudolf Virchow in 1863 to this "strange" and "monstrous tumour" because of its gross appearance and its odd contents consisting of hair, bone, cartilage or teeth [24]. *Teratoma may be cystic or solid and contains all three germ cell layers in different stages of maturation*. These are endoderm (GI, respiratory), mesoderm (bone, muscle, cartilage) and ectoderm (squamous epithelium, neural tissue) (Fig. 18.2). Well-differentiated tumours are labelled *mature teratomas*, whereas the incompletely differentiated (i.e. similar to foetal or embryonal tissue) are called *immature teratomas*. Mature teratomas may include elements of mature bone, cartilage, tooth or hair. *They generally have normal tumour markers. Paediatric teratomas are benign and occur at a median age of 20 months.*

  In adults however, despite their benign histology, teratomas are frequently found at metastatic sites in patients with advanced NSGCT. As already stated above, non-teratomatous tumours (particularly EC) are thought to have the ability to mature into teratomas and the "teratomatous" metastases would most likely arise from these elements before their differentiation. In other words the absence of teratoma in the primary tumour does not preclude its presence in the retroperitoneum [25].

  Further clinical features contribute to the gravity of this tumour in the adult population which may have lethal consequences:

1. *Teratoma is resistant to chemotherapy and radiation. Therefore, any residual retroperitoneal mass after chemotherapy for NSGCT is highly suspicious of teratoma (40–50 %) and requires surgical resection.*
2. Teratomas may have *genetic abnormalities* in common with malignant GCT, including *aneuploidy, i(12p) and proliferative capacity* [26]. Their cystic forms may contain HCG and AFP, indicating their malignant potential [27, 28]. This genetic instability accounts for some important clinical implications: they may reach enormous sizes, compress or even invade surrounding structures and become inoperable, a phenomenon to which Logothetis has coined the term "*growing teratoma syndrome*" [29].
3. Rarely teratomas may transform into a somatic malignancy such as rhabdomyosarcoma, adenocarcinoma or primitive neuroectodermal tumour [30, 31]. These so-called teratomas with somatic-type malignancy or teratomas with malignant transformation *frequently have abnormalities of chromosome 12 or i(12p)*, indicating their origin from GCT [32]. *Malignant transformation is highly aggressive, resistant to conventional chemotherapy, and associated with a poor prognosis* [2].
4. Lastly unresected teratomas in the context of an advanced NSGCT have the potential to cause a late relapse [26].

- *Mixed GCTs* contain at least 2 of the above described histological types and make up 32–54 % of all GCTs. They are all clinically accompanied by an elevation of AFP and/or BHCG. The most common components are embryonal carcinoma (47 %), teratoma (47 %) and yolk sac tumour (41 %) (Fig. 18.3a, b). Choriocarcinoma component can also be seen. The seminomatous contents are found in a smaller proportion, but confer a better response to treatment with chemo or radiotherapy.
- *Primary carcinoid tumours of the testis* have also been described [33]. These are extremely rare tumours; they are not associated with ITGCN and may be pure or associated with cystic teratoma. In addition they affect patients of different ages from 12 to 65 years. They present with a testicular mass, but are sometimes incidentally discovered or may develop a carcinoid syndrome (diarrhoea, hot flush, palpitations). This form of the tumour typically has a benign course.

18.2 NGCTs Also Called Stromal Tumours

NGCTs include the sex cord/gonadal stromal tumours and the miscellaneous non-specific stromal tumours (see table). They account for 5–10 % of all testicular neoplasms.

- *Leydig and Sertoli cell tumours are the main histological types and the former is the most common NGCT.* Around 10 % of these tumours are malignant. *Leydig cell tumours secrete testosterone and oestrogen.* In addition to a testicular mass,

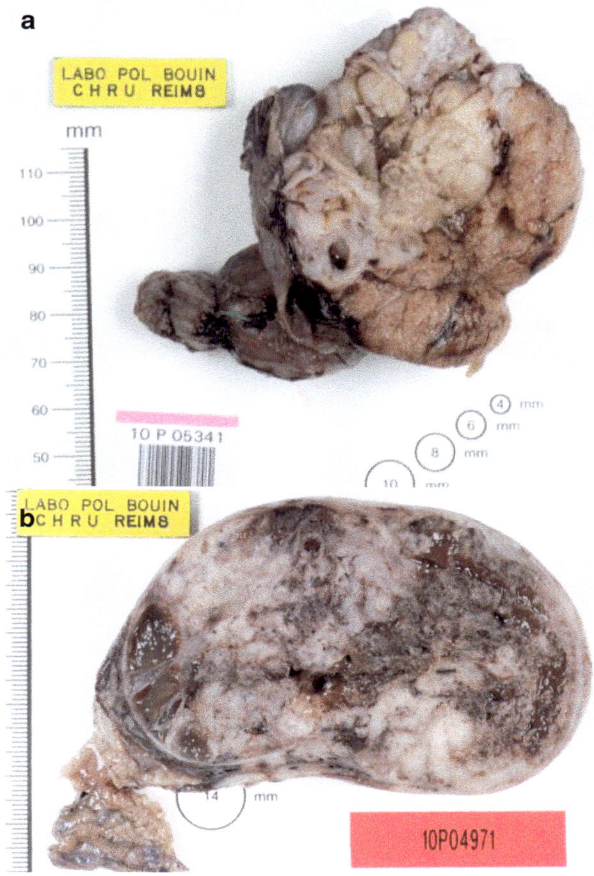

Fig. 18.3 (**a**, **b**) Mixed GCT: (**a**) A testicular teratocarcinoma : This tumour was made of 60 % of embryonal carcinoma and 40 % of mature cystic teratoma. (**b**) Mixed GCT made of 3 components: yolk sac tumour, seminoma and choriocarcinoma (Courtesy of A. Durlach, Pol Bouin Laboratory, University Hospital of Reims, France)

these tumours may present in childhood with *precocious puberty and virilization* and in adulthood with *gynaecomastia and impotence*. The primary treatment is orchiectomy. They are resistant to chemotherapy and radiation therapy; hence, metastatic LNs must be surgically removed.

- *Lymphoma of the testis can be primary or metastatic. It is the most common bilateral testicular neoplasm and its incidence peaks in the 5th decade.*
- *Granulosa cell tumours* are very rare benign tumours of gonads. They usually occur in the *neonatal period*. Orchiectomy is curative.
- *Gonadoblastoma* is a rare benign tumour that occurs *almost exclusively in patients with gonadal dysgenesis from intersex disorders* (*hermaphroditism*). Bilateral orchiectomy is advocated because two third of these tumours undergo transformation to malignant germ cell neoplasia.

Take-Home Message: Histological Classification

ITGCT (cis) is the common precursor for all GCTs except spermatocytic seminoma. The risk of transformation into invasive GCT is 50 % within 5 years and 70 % within 7 years.

GCTs comprise ±95 % of testicular cancers, are mostly unilateral and predominate on the right side in relation to cryptorchidism.

GCTs are classified as *seminoma* and *non-seminomatous germ cell tumours* (*NSGCT*), and the relative distribution of each is 55 and 45 %.

Seminomas include *classic seminoma* (95 %) and *spermatocytic seminoma* (5 %).

NSGCTs are teratoma, choriocarcinoma, embryonal carcinoma and *yolk sac tumour.*

Mixed GCTs contain at least 2 of the above described histological types (except spermatocytic seminoma) and make up 32–54 % of all GCTs

At presentation 75 % of classic seminoma are limited to the testes, 20 % have retroperitoneal extension and 5 % have supradiaphragmatic and/or visceral metastases.

Spermatocytic seminoma behaves differently from the classic one. *It is a rather benign tumour which virtually never metastasizes.*

Embryonal carcinomas have a *totipotent capacity* which allows them to transform into other GCTs types in primary or metastatic sites. They are *the second most aggressive GCT type after choriocarcinomas*, being associated with a *high rate of metastasis*

Choriocarcinoma (CC) is made of cytotrophoblasts and syncytiotrophoblasts which are responsible for the *high secretion of HCG*. It is *the most aggressive GCT* type with high propensity to metastasize through *hematogenous route. The metastases are very prone to bleed.*

Yolk sac tumour is the most common type of testicular GCTs in the paediatric group below 15 years. *It almost always produces AFP but not HCG.*

Teratomas are the second most common GCT after seminoma. They may be cystic or solid and *contain all three germ cell layers in different stages of maturation*. They are either *mature* (well-differentiated) or *immature* (incompletely differentiated). *Paediatric teratomas are benign* (*median age*: *20 months*) *and commonly pure*. Several features account for the gravity of teratomas in adults: frequent occurrence at metastatic sites in patients with advanced NSGCT, chemo- and radio-resistance, possible association with genetic abnormalities (aneuploidy, i(12p), and proliferative capacity) with subsequent capacity to induce the "*growing teratoma syndrome*", possible transformation into somatic malignancies and potential for late relapse.

NGCTs account for 5–10 % of all testicular tumours: Leydig (precocious puberty, gynaecomastia) and Sertoli cell tumours are the most frequent. Others are lymphomas in older men, granulosa cell tumours (benign), gonadoblastomas (benign).

References

1. La Vecchia C, Bosetti C, Lucchini F, et al. Cancer Mortality in Europe, 2000–2004, and an overview of trends since 1995. Ann Oncol. 2010;21(6):1323–60.
2. Stephenson AJ, Gilligan TD. Neoplasms of the testis. In: Wein AJ, Kavoussi LR, Novick AC, Partin AW, Peters CA, editors. Campbell-Walsh urology. Chapter 31, vol. 1. 10 ed. Philadelphia: Elsevier Saunders; 2012. p. 837–70.
3. McGlynn KA, Cook MB. Etiologic factors in testicular germ-cell tumours. Future Oncol. 2009;5(9):1389–402.

4. Powles TB, Bhardwa J, Shamash J, Mandalia S, Oliver T. The changing presentation of germ cell tumours of the testis between 1983 and 2002. BJU Int. 2005;95(9):1197–200.
5. Eble JN, Sauter G, Epstein JI, Sesterhenn IA. World Health Organization classification of tumours: pathology and genetics of tumours of the urinary system and male genital organs. Lyon: IARC; 2004. p. 218.
6. Dieckmann KP, Skakkebaek NE. Carcinoma in situ of the testis: review of biological and clinical features. Int J Cancer. 1999;83(6):815–22.
7. Berthelsen JG, Skakkebaek NE, von der Maase H, Sørensen BL, Mogensen P. Screening for carcinoma in situ of the contralateral testis in patients with germinal testicular cancer. Br Med J (Clin Res Ed). 1982;285(6356):1683–6.
8. Skakkebaek NE, Berthelsen JG, Müller J. Carcinoma-in-situ of the undescended testis. Urol Clin North Am. 1982;9(3):377–85.
9. Montironi R. Intratubular germ cell neoplasia of the testis: testicular intraepithelial neoplasia. Eur Urol. 2002;41(6):651–4.
10. Durand X, Rigaud J, Avancès C, et al. Les membres du CCAFU. CCAFU recommendations 2013: testicular germ cell cancer. Prog Urol. 2013;23(Supple 2):S145–60.
11. Motzer RJ, Bolger GB, Boston B, et al. Testicular cancer. Clinical practice guidelines in oncology. National Comprehensive Cancer Network. J Natl Compr Canc Netw. 2006;4(10):1038–58.
12. Ulbright TM. Testicular and paratesticular tumours. In: Mills SE, Greenson JK, Oberman HA, editors. Sternberg's diagnostic surgical pathology. 4th ed. Philadelphia: Lippincott Williams & Wilkins; 2004. p. 2168–90.
13. Ulbright TM. *Germ cell tumours* of the *gonads*: a selective review emphasizing problems in differential diagnosis, newly appreciated, and controversial issues. Mod Pathol. 2005;18 Suppl 2:S61–79.
14. Eble JN. Spermatocytic seminoma. Hum Pathol. 1994;25(10):1035–42.
15. Chung PW, Bayley AJ, Sweet J, Jewett MA, Tew-George B, Gospodarowicz MK, Warde PR. Spermatocytic seminoma: a review. Eur Urol. 2004;45(4):495–8.
16. Kraggerud SM, Berner A, Bryne M, et al. Spermatocytic seminoma as compared to classical seminoma: an immunohistochemical and DNA flow cytometric study. APMIS. 1999;107:297–302.
17. True LD, Otis CN, Delprado W, Scully RE, Rosai J. Spermatocytic seminoma of testis with sarcomatous transformation. A report of five cases. Am J Surg Pathol. 1988;12(2):75–82.
18. Vugrin D, Chen A, Feigl P, Laszlo J. Embryonal carcinoma of the testis. Cancer. 1988;61(11):2348–52.
19. Tinkle LL, Graham BS, Spillane TJ, Barr RJ. Testicular choriocarcinoma metastatic to the skin: an additional case and literature review. Cutis. 2001;67(2):117–20.
20. Osada K, Iijima H, Imasawa M, Takahashi H, Kobori Y, Nakagomi H, Takihana Y, Takeda M. Metastatic uveal tumour secondary to testicular choriocarcinoma. Jpn J Ophthalmol. 2004;48(1):85–7.
21. Cheville JC. Classification and pathology of testicular germ cell and sex cord-stromal tumours. Urol Clin North Am. 1999;26(3):595–609.
22. Motzer RJ, Bosl GJ. Hemorrhage: a complication of metastatic testicular choriocarcinoma. Urology. 1987;30(2):119–22.
23. Mostofi FK, Price EB. Tumours of the male genital system: atlas of tumour pathology. 2nd ed. Washington, DC: Armed Forces Institute of Pathology; 1973.
24. Virchow R. Die krankhaften Geschwulste. Dreissing Vorlesungen gehalten wahrend des Wintersemesters 1862–1867 an der Universitat zu Berlin, vol 1–3. Berlin: A. Hirschwald; 1863–1865.
25. Sheinfeld J, Motzer RJ, Rabbani F, McKiernan J, Bajorin D, Bosl GJ. Incidence and clinical outcome of patients with teratoma in the retroperitoneum following primary retroperitoneal lymph node dissection for clinical stages I and IIA nonseminomatous germ cell tumours. J Urol. 2003;170(4 Pt 1):1159–62.
26. Castedo SM, de Jong B, Oosterhuis JW, Idenburg VJ, Seruca R, Buist J, te Meerman GJ, Schraffordt Koops H, Sleijfer DT. Chromosomal changes in mature residual teratomas following polychemotherapy. Cancer Res. 1989;49(3):672–6.

27. Sella A, el Naggar A, Ro JY, Dexeus FH, Amato RJ, Lee JS, Finn L, Logothetis CJ. Evidence of malignant features in histologically mature teratoma. J Urol. 1991;146(4):1025–8.
28. Beck SD, Patel MI, Sheinfeld J. Tumour marker levels in post-chemotherapy cystic masses: clinical implications for patients with germ cell tumours. J Urol. 2004;171:168–71.
29. Logothetis CJ, Samuels ML, Trindade A, Johnson DE. The growing teratoma syndrome. Cancer. 1982;50(8):1629–35.
30. Comiter CV, Kibel AS, Richie JP, Nucci MR, Renshaw AA. Prognostic features of teratomas with malignant transformation: a clinicopathological study of 21 cases. J Urol. 1998;159(3): 859–63.
31. Little Jr JS, Foster RS, Ulbright TM, Donohue JP. Unusual neoplasms detected in testis cancer patients undergoing post-chemotherapy retroperitoneal lymphadenectomy. J Urol. 1994; 152(4):1144–9.
32. Motzer RJ, Amsterdam A, Prieto V, Sheinfeld J, Murty VV, Mazumdar M, Bosl GJ, Chaganti RS, Reuter VE. Teratoma with malignant transformation: diverse malignant histologies arising in men with germ cell tumours. J Urol. 1998;159(1):133–8.
33. Wang WP, Guo C, Berney DM, Ulbright TM, Hansel DE, Shen R, Ali T, Epstein JI. Primary carcinoid tumours of the testis: a clinicopathologic study of 29 cases. Am J Surg Pathol. 2010;34(4):519–24.

Chapter 19
Clinical Presentation of Testicular Tumours and Spreading Patterns

Qais Mohamed Al-Hooti and Said Abdallah Al-Mamari

The most common presentation of testicular cancers is a painless and firm testicular mass. However in 20–27 % of cases, the first symptom is *scrotal pain* [1] caused by the stretching of the tunica albuginea by intratumour infarction or haemorrhage from a rapidly growing vascular tumour. This presentation is more common with NSGCTs than with seminoma. Occasionally, trauma to the scrotum may incidentally bring into attention the presence of a testicular mass. In about 10 % of cases, *a testicular tumour can mimic epididymo-orchitis*, with consequent delay of the correct diagnosis.

Hydrocele is seen in a minority of cases and may obscure the presence of the mass.

Approximately 7 % of men with testicular cancer have *gynaecomastia* resulting from either elevated serum HCG levels, decreased androgen production or increased oestrogen [1]. *About 30 % of patients with Leydig and Sertoli cell tumours have gynaecomastia* [2]. *Subfertility* is found in a large proportion of men with GCT and occasionally can be the main complaint at presentation.

While only approximately 15 % of pure seminomas present with regional or distant metastasis, as much as 2/3 of NSGCTs are reported to be diagnosed in the advanced stages and 10–20 % present with symptoms consistent with metastatic disease [3]. Compression of the ureters, psoas muscle or nerve roots by bulky retroperitoneal metastases can cause flank and back pain which was reported to occur in about 11 % of cases [4]. Oedema of the lower extremity may also occur when there is compression of the inferior vena cava. Pulmonary and mediastinal metastasis may present by dyspnea, chest pain, cough or hemoptysis.

GCTs usually spread by the lymphatic route but can also metastasize haematogenously like choriocarcinomas and yolk sac tumours.

Q.M. Al-Hooti • S.A. Al-Mamari (✉)
Urology Department, The Royal Hospital, Muscat, Oman
e-mail: sabdal67@yahoo.com

S.A. Al-Mamari, S.S. Al-Busaidy (eds.), *Urological Cancer Management*,
DOI 10.1007/978-3-319-16301-7_19

With the exception of choriocarcinomas, the most common site for metastasis of testicular neoplasms is the retroperitoneal lymph nodes. Right and left testicular tumours spread mainly to the inter aortico-caval and para-aortic lymph nodes, respectively, at L2 vertebral level. Additionally a crossover spreading can occur mostly with right testicular tumours metastasizing to the left para-aortic lymph node group; however left-to-right crossover is also seen [5]. Sacrococcygeal, pelvic and even supraclavicular regions are other possible sites for lymphatic dissemination.

Tumour involving the epididymis or spermatic cord can spread to iliac lymph nodes. The necessity to perform a high ligation of the spermatic cord during radical orchidectomy in order to prevent this event has been reemphasized by a large population study [6]. This study which included 695 patients revealed that 2 % of them have inguinal nodal disease with approximately ¾ arising through spermatic cord metastases. It also showed that NSGCTs are more prone to develop inguinal LN than seminomas affecting 4 and 0.5 % of patients, respectively.

Inguinal lymph nodes can also be directly involved in case of previous inguinal or scrotal surgery including testicular biopsy and scrotal violation [7]. Inguinal LNs can also be invaded theoretically through retrograde lymph flow from retroperitoneal lymph nodes.

Distant non-nodal metastases commonly occur to the lungs, liver, brain and bone.

References

1. Durand X, Rigaud J, Avancès C, et al. Les membres du CCAFU. CCAFU recommendations 2013: testicular germ cell cancer. Prog Urol. 2013;23(Suppl 2):S145–60.
2. Conkey DS, Howard GC, Grigor KM, McLaren DB, Kerr GR. Testicular sex cord-stromal tumours: the Edinburgh experience 1988–2002, and a review of the literature. Clin Oncol (R Coll Radiol). 2005;17(5):322–7.
3. Stephenson AJ, Gilligan TD. Chapter 31. Neoplasms of the testis. In: Wein AJ, Kavoussi LR, Novick AC, Partin AW, Peters CA, editors. Campbell-Walsh urology, vol. 1. 10th ed. Philadelphia: Elsevier Saunders; 2012. p. 837–70.
4. Wanderås EH, Tretli S, Fosså SD. Trends in incidence of testicular cancer in Norway 1955–1992. Eur J Cancer. 1995;31A(12):2044–8.
5. Paño B, Sebastià C, Buñesch L, Mestres J, Salvador R, Macías NG, Nicolau C. Pathways of lymphatic spread in male urogenital pelvic malignancies. Radiographics. 2011;31(1):135–60.
6. Daugaard G, Karas V, Sommer P. Inguinal metastases from testicular cancer. BJU Int. 2006;97:724–6.
7. Wheeler Jr JS, Babayan RK, Hong WK, Krane RJ. Inguinal node metastases from testicular tumours in patients with prior orchiopexy. J Urol. 1983;129:1245–7.

Chapter 20
Diagnostic Approaches of Testicular Cancers

Qais Mohamed Al-Hooti and Said Abdallah Al-Mamari

20.1 Physical Examination

A firm testicular mass must be considered malignant until proven otherwise and should be further evaluated with relevant laboratory and radiological means. The differential diagnoses of a scrotal swelling include epididymoorchitis, hydrocoele, haematoma, torsion, spermatocele and paratesticular tumours. The delay in diagnosis can occur either because of the patient's negligence or due to the physician's mismanagement. It is therefore important that men are taught to perform *testicular self-examination* periodically in order to detect early changes, thereby reducing morbidity and mortality to the patients and costly management to the society [1].

Up to one-third of testicular tumours are initially misdiagnosed as epididymitis or hydrocoele and a mean delay of 3.9 months was found from the onset of symptoms to the time of the orchidectomy [2]. The delay in diagnosis was shown by some authors to negatively impact on the patient's survival [3]. Exploratory laparotomy performed for an unsuspected metastatic GCT was also pointed out as an important delaying and complicating factor in the management of GCT [4].

Nowadays, the clinical decision has greatly been improved by modern investigative tools and diagnostic delay has become rare.

Q.M. Al-Hooti • S.A. Al-Mamari (✉)
Urology Department, The Royal Hospital, Muscat, Oman
e-mail: sabdal67@yahoo.com

S.A. Al-Mamari, S.S. Al-Busaidy (eds.), *Urological Cancer Management*,
DOI 10.1007/978-3-319-16301-7_20

20.2 Laboratory Tests

20.2.1 Tumour Markers

Beta-human chorionic gonadotropin (βHCG) and alpha-fetoprotein (AFP) are extensively used for diagnosis, tagging, prognosis, surveillance and follow-up after chemotherapy or radiotherapy of germ cell tumours.

- HCG is a glycoprotein produced by syncytiotrophoblast and comprises 2 subunits: alpha and beta. The molecular weight of intact HCG, αHCG and βHCG are approximately 36.7, 14.5 and 22.2 kDa, respectively [5].

  Alpha subunit's structure is made of 92 amino acids and is common to all the gonadotropins (FSH, LH) and TSH. Beta subunit has 145 amino acids and is responsible of the specific biological activity of the molecule. Therefore the βHCG is the most commonly used subunit for normal or molar pregnancy diagnosis, as well as for choriocarcinoma in females and germ cell tumours of the testis. *It is normally undetectable in men. Its half-life in the serum is 1–2 days.*
- AFP is a 70 kDa glycoprotein encoded by the AFP gene which is located on the long or q arm of the chromosome 4 (4q11-22) along with the serum albumin-coding gene [6]. *AFP is the major plasma protein during fetal life* where it is produced by the yolk sac, the liver and the gastrointestinal tract. *With a concentration of 3 g/L, it is believed to be the fetal form of serum albumin.* Its plasma levels decrease rapidly after birth to reach normal adult levels usually by the age of 8–12 months. The normal adult values are generally undetectable by routine laboratory assays and are merely reported as being *less than 10 ng/ml (0.83 IU/ml)*. However, a very sensitive radioimmunoassay has allowed a more accurate determination of the normal adult AFP level of *3.04 ng/ml ± 1.9* and this has shown variations with sex (men > women) and age (older > younger) [7]. Any significant raise in adulthood (>10 ng/ml) indicates a need for further clinically oriented investigations to rule out GCT, liver diseases or gastrointestinal malignancies. *The AFP half-life in the serum is 5–7 days.*
- *Lactate dehydrogenase* (*LDH*) is another serum marker introduced in the clinical armamentarium. This is more of a *tissue destruction marker used to evaluate the whole bulk of the disease specifically in the metastatic stage*. Indeed, studies have revealed increased levels of serum LDH in about 80 % of advanced seminomas and 60 % of NSGCT [8]. LDH can also be raised in other pathological conditions: myocardial infarction, myopathies, haemolysis, megaloblastic anaemia, renal infarction. Normal value of plasmatic LDH is 190–390 IU/L.

  It is important to note that high marker levels are not necessary for the diagnosis of GCT and their presence largely depends on the histological type (Table 20.1). All choriocarcinomas and 10 % of pure seminomas secrete βHCG but they never produce AFP. On the other hand, yolk sac tumours secrete AFP but not βHCG while pure teratomas do not secrete either βHCG or AFP.

Table 20.1 Correlation between histology and tumours markers

Histological types	Markers	
	βHCG	AFP
Choriocarcinoma	+++100 %	No
Pure seminoma	+ 10 %	No
Yolk sac tumour	No	++
Embryonal carcinoma	No	++
Pure teratoma	No	No

Table 20.2 Prognostic groups based on serum tumor markers [13]

S (serum markers) staging	βHCG (mIU/ml)	AFP (ng/ml)	LDH (IU/L)
SX	Marker studies not available or not performed		
S0	Normal	Normal	Normal (190–390 IU/L)
S1	<5,000	<1,000	<1.5×*n* (*n*=upper limit of the normal range)
S2	5,000–50,000	1,000–10,000	1.5–10×*n*
S3	>50,000	>10,000	>10×*n*

Used with the permission of the American Joint Committee on Cancer (AJCC), Chicago, IL. The original source for this material is the AJCC Cancer Staging Manual, Seventh Edition (2010), published by Springer Science and Business Media LLC, www.springer.com

One must be cautious when interpreting these markers (AFP, βHCG and LDH) not only because of their lack of specificity, but also because of their limited sensitivity. A Spanish study has shown that *markers are only detected in approximately 64 % of men with testicular cancer, while they remain 'normal' in about 38 % of men with disease recurrence* [9].

- Other markers: Placental alkaline phosphatase (PLAP) has been known for over 30 years as a marker for seminoma [10]. However, the usefulness of serum PLAP assay has been questioned when used alone and this marker is not widely available [11]. Cytogenetic and molecular markers (immunohistochemistry of c-kit, OCT 3/4 and determination of gain of chromosome 12, high mobility group proteins HMGA1 and HMGA2, SOX17, CDK10) are presently only utilized in research studies in specialized centres [12].

Staging by the serum markers: *The use of staging by post-orchiectomy serum marker has been standardized and carries an important prognostic value* (Table 20.2) [13]. Following orchiectomy, the time interval repeating measurements depends on the marker's half-life. In practical terms a 6-week period is sufficient for both AFP and βHCG to normalize. A high value persisting beyond 6 weeks should raise suspicion of distant micro or macroscopic disease.

Possible causes of *false positive results* are marijuana abuse, hypoandrogenemia with consecutively raised LH and BHCG, liver diseases, gastric, pancreatic or lung carcinomas, ataxia-telangiectasia syndrome and familial AFP persistence [14]. Finally as for all statistical data, one should remember that the calculated normal values are based on a 95 % confidence interval, which means that up to 5 % of healthy men may be found to have a raised AFP.

For all these reasons, a moderately raised AFP >10 ug/L after surgery which *remains stable without chemo- or radiotherapy* may be compatible with clinical remission. Conversely normal levels do not mean tumour-free status [9].

20.2.2 Other Laboratory Investigations

Blood tests should also be done for haemoglobin and WBC when infection is suspected. The presence of a large retroperitoneal mass with associated symptoms of abdominal colicky pain should instigate investigations to assess the high possibility of obstructive uropathy, that is, the renal function tests. This is also important before and during chemotherapy in view of the nephrotoxic potential of the drugs used, especially cisplatin.

Liver function tests and bone profile may be deranged in case of liver or bony metastases, respectively. Moreover, as noted above, liver dysfunction may cause a high AFP and it may be difficult for the clinician to recognize this as a false positive result during the investigations or follow-up of GCTs.

Semen analysis and hormonal profile should also be performed before orchidectomy and the initiation of chemotherapy.

20.3 Radiological Procedures

20.3.1 Primary Disease

Imaging studies are used to confirm the presence of intratesticular mass, to exclude paratesticular tumours and to evaluate the contralateral testicle for any significant lesions. *Scrotal ultrasound is the radiological investigation of choice in assessing testicular pathologies.* It is fast, inexpensive and easily available in health services. In addition, it is accurate with about 100 % sensitivity [15, 16].

Scrotal ultrasound also allows surveillance of the contralateral testis where it may detect microlithiasis which is associated with an increased risk of subsequent testicular cancer in the follow-up [17]. Testicular microlithiasis is categorized as follows: grade 1: 5–10 microliths/image, grade 2: 10–20 microliths/image and grade 3: >20 microliths/image. Grade 3 is regarded by some expert panels as most prone to subsequent GCT development [18]; however, other authors have shown that this grading has no effect on the prevalence of associated testicular tumours [19]. MRI is an excellent tool for soft tissue masses. *It gives detailed information about the tumour and its extension. Compared to ultrasound, MRI is more specific but does not add much to clinical applications or decisions with regard to scrotal pathologies.*

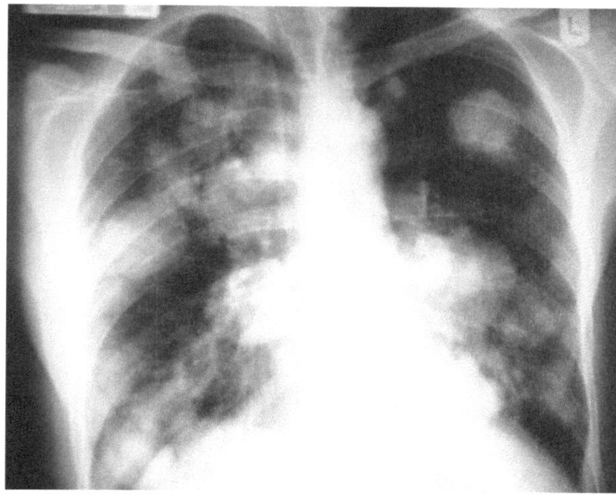

Fig. 20.1 Chest X-ray of the patient seen in Fig. 17.1 showing multiple roundish chest metastases ('canon balls') (Courtesy of Kurian George, Urology, Royal Hospital, Muscat, Oman)

20.3.2 Disease Extension Studies

If not contraindicated, chest, abdomen and pelvic CT scan with contrast is the standard imaging means for disease-extension evaluation. It is very useful in assessing the retroperitoneum and the mediastinum for staging of the testicular GCT. However, it harbours a false negative rate of 20–30 % in GCT. When using CT scan, the threshold of metastatic lymph node detection is 8 mm diameter [20, 21]. The efficacy of abdominal MRI is equal to CT scanning in detecting retroperitoneal metastases. However, being more expensive and less widely available, MRI is only used when CT scan is contraindicated. CT scan of the head is recommended when there is clinical suspicion of brain secondaries or in cases of choriocarcinoma due to its high possibility of haematogenous spread. A simple chest X-ray in the metastatic workup may be sufficient in some cases to detect chest secondary lesions (Fig. 20.1), but a CT scan must be performed to confirm any suspicious finding on X-ray or in cases of a bulky tumour. When CT scan has revealed retroperitoneal residual masses *after chemotherapy for seminoma*, further evaluation can be performed by a *FDG-PET scan* to assess hypermetabolic or necrotic lesions [22]. The presence of viable tissue among the residual tumours is an indication for retroperitoneal lymph nodes dissection (RPLND) (see pictures). It is important to note that *teratomas do not show hyperactivity in a FDG-PET scan; therefore, the presence of a viable carcinoma or mature teratoma cannot be differentiated from necrosis or fibrosis*. This fact was histologically confirmed by a prospective German trial which showed FDG-PET sensitivity and specificity of 70 % and 48 %, respectively, in detecting NSGCTs. FDG-PET was unable to provide clear additional clinical benefit compared to the standard diagnostic means with positive predictive values of 59, 55 and 61 % for FDG-PET, CT and serum markers, respectively [23].

Take-Home Message: Diagnostic Approaches of Testicular Cancers

Physical examination	*A firm testicular mass must be considered malignant until proven otherwise*. Up to one-third of testicular tumours are initially misdiagnosed as epididymitis or hydrocoele
Lymphatic spread pattern	With the exception of choriocarcinoma, *the most common site for metastasis of testicular neoplasms is the retroperitoneal lymph nodes*. Right and left testicular tumours spread mainly to the inter-aortico-caval and left para-aortic lymph nodes, respectively, at L2 vertebral level.
Laboratory examinations	AFP, βHCG and LDH are the most frequently used testicular tumour markers: AFP is positive in yolk sac tumours, embryonal carcinoma and mixed tumours βHCG is positive in 100 % of choriocarcinoma, 10 % of pure seminoma and in mixed tumours Pure teratomas and most pure seminomas do not express any tumour marker LDH is used to evaluate the whole bulk of the disease specifically in metastatic stage *These markers are used for diagnosis, follow-up and prognostic grouping after orchiectomy*. None of the markers is specific and caution should apply in their interpretation
Imaging investigations	*Scrotal ultrasound is the radiological investigation of choice in assessing testicular pathologies* *CT scan is the standard means for disease extension study*. MRI is indicated when CT scan is contraindicated and FDG-PET-scan can evaluate the activity of a CT-diagnosed mass, but it *is not sensitive for teratomas*

References

1. Aberger M, Wilson B, Holzbeierlein JM, Griebling TL, Nangia AK. Testicular self-examination and testicular cancer: a cost-utility analysis. doi:10.1002/cam4.318. © 2014 The Authors. Cancer Med. Published by John Wiley & Sons Ltd.
2. Chilvers CED, Saunders M, Bliss JM, Nicholls J, Horwich A. Influence of delay in diagnosis on prognosis in testicular teratoma. Br J Cancer. 1989;59:126–8.
3. Bosl GJ, Vogelzang NJ, Goldman A, Fraley EE, Lange PH, Levitt SH, Kennedy BJ. Impact of delay in diagnosis on clinical stage of testicular cancer. Lancet. 1981;2(8253):970–3.
4. Stephenson AJ, Russo P, Kaplinsky R, Sheinfeld J. Impact of unnecessary exploratory laparotomy on the treatment of patients with metastatic germ cell tumour. J Urol. 2004;171(4): 1474–7.
5. Gam LH, Latiff A. SDS-PAGE electrophoretic property of human chorionic gonadotropin (hCG) and its β-subunit. Int J Biol Sci. 2005;1(3):103–9.
6. Harper ME, Dugaiczyk A. Linkage of the evolutionarily-related serum albumin and alpha-fetoprotein genes within q11-22 of human chromosome 4. Am J Hum Genet. 1983;35(4): 565–72.
7. Ball D, Rose E, Alpert E. Alpha-fetoprotein levels in normal adults. Am J Med Sci. 1992;303(3):157–9.

8. Gori S, Porrozzi S, Roila F, Gatta G, De Giorgi U, Marangolo M. Germ cell tumours of the testis. Crit Rev Oncol Hematol. 2005;53:141–64.
9. Trigo JM, Tabernero JM, Paz-Ares L, García-Llano JL, Mora J, Lianes P, et al. Tumour markers at the time of recurrence in patients with germ cell tumours. Cancer. 2000;88:162–8.
10. Lange PH, Millan JL, Stigbrand T, Vessella RL, Ruoslahti E, Fishman WH. Placental alkaline phosphatase as a tumour marker for seminoma. Cancer Res. 1982;42(8):3244–7.
11. Nielsen OS, Munro AJ, Duncan W, Sturgeon J, Gospodarowicz MK, Jewett MA, Malkin A, Thomas GM. Is placental alkaline phosphatase (PLAP) a useful marker for seminoma? Eur J Cancer. 1990;26(10):1049–54.
12. Vilar E, Calvo E, Tabernero J. Molecular biology of testicular germ cell tumours. Clin Transl Oncol. 2006;8(12):846–50.
13. Testis. In: Edge SB, Byrd DR, Compton CC, Fritz AG., Greene FL, Trotti A, editors. AJCC cancer staging manual. 7th ed. New York: Springer; 2010. p. 472.
14. Schefer H, Mattman S, Joss RA. Hereditary persistence of alpha-fetoprotein. Case report and review and review of the literature. Ann Oncol. 1998;9:667–72.
15. Kim W, Rosen MA, Langer JE, et al. US-MR Imaging correlation in pathologic conditions of the scrotum. Radiographics. 2007;27(5):1239–53.
16. Lenz S. Cancer of the testicle diagnosed by ultrasound and the ultrasonic appearance of the contralateral testicle. Scand J Urol Nephrol Suppl. 1991;137:135–8.
17. Tan IB, Ang KK, Ching BC, Mohan C, Toh CK, Tan MH. Testicular microlithiasis predicts concurrent testicular germ cell tumours and intratubular germ cell neoplasia of unclassified type in adults: a meta-analysis and systematic review. Cancer. 2010;116(19):4520–32.
18. Durand X, Rigaud J, Avancès C, et al. Les membres du CCAFU. CCAFU recommendations 2013: testicular germ cell cancer. Prog Urol. 2013;23(Suppl 2):S145–60.
19. Sanli O, Kadioglu A, Atar M, Acar O, Nane I, Kadioglu A. Grading of classical testicular microlithiasis has no effect on the prevalence of associated testicular tumours. Urol Int. 2008;80(3):310–6.
20. Leibovitch L, Foster RS, Kopecky KK, Donohue JP. Improved accuracy of computerized tomography based clinical staging in low stage nonseminomatous germ cell cancer using size criteria of retroperitoneal lymph nodes. J Urol. 1995;154(5):1759–63.
21. Jing B, Wallace S, Zornoza J. Metastases to retroperitoneal and pelvic lymph nodes: computed tomography and lymphangiography. Radiol Clin North Am. 1982;20(3):511–30.
22. De Santis M, Becherer A, Bokemeyer C, et al. 2-18fluoro-deoxy-D-glucose positron emission tomography is a reliable predictor for viable tumour in postchemotherapy seminoma: an update of the prospective multicentric SEMPET trial. J Clin Oncol. 2004;22:1034–9.
23. Oechsle K, Hartmann M, Brenner W, et al. [^{18}F]Fluorodeoxyglucose positron emission tomography in nonseminomatous germ cell tumours after chemotherapy: the German Multicenter Positron Emission Tomography Study Group. J Clin Oncol. 2008;26(36):5930–5.

Chapter 21
Staging and Risk Categories

Qais Mohamed Al-Hooti and Said Abdallah Al-Mamari

21.1 Staging

Once the histology of the primary tumour has been defined after orchiectomy and the disease extension has been evaluated by imaging, the tumour can be given a TNM staging in accordance with the 2010 AJCC cancer staging (identical to the 2009 UICC classification) [1] (Table 21.1).

The stage grouping given on Table 21.2 incorporates the available post-orchiectomy tumor marker kinetics data.

Q.M. Al-Hooti • S.A. Al-Mamari (✉)
Urology Department, The Royal Hospital, Muscat, Oman
e-mail: sabdal67@yahoo.com

S.A. Al-Mamari, S.S. Al-Busaidy (eds.), *Urological Cancer Management*,
DOI 10.1007/978-3-319-16301-7_21

Table 21.1 The 2010 AJCC staging for testicular cancer [1]

Primary tumour (T). Except for pTis and pT4, the extent of primary tumour is usually classified after radical orchiectomy, and for this reason, a pathologic stage is assigned. Tx may be used for other categories in the absence of radical orchiectomy	
pTx	Primary tumour cannot be assessed
pT0	No evidence of primary tumour (e.g. histologic scar in the testis)
pTis	Intratubular germ cell neoplasia (testicular intraepithelial neoplasia or carcinoma in situ)
pT1	Tumour limited to the testis and epididymis *without vascular/lymphatic invasion*: tumour may invade into the tunica albuginea *but not the tunica vaginalis*
pT2	Tumour limited to testis and epididymis *with vascular/lymphatic invasion*, or tumour extending through the tunica albuginea with *involvement of the tunica vaginalis*
pT3	Tumour invades the *spermatic cord* with or without vascular/lymphatic invasion
pT4	Tumour invades *scrotum* with or without vascular/lymphatic invasion
Regional lymph nodes (N). The following nodes are considered regional: interaortocaval, para-aortic (periaortic), paracaval, preaortic, precaval, retroaortic, retrocaval. Nodes along the spermatic vein are also considered regional. The intrapelvic, external iliac and inguinal nodes are considered regional only after scrotal or inguinal surgery prior to the presentation of the testis tumour. All nodes outside the regional nodes are distant	
Clinical (after radiological imaging)	
Nx	Regional lymph nodes cannot be assessed
N0	No regional lymph node metastasis
N1	Metastasis with a *lymph node mass 2 cm or less* in greatest dimension; *or multiple lymph nodes, none more than 2 cm in greatest dimension*
N2	Metastasis with a *lymph node mass more than 2 cm but not more than 5 cm* in greatest dimension; or multiple lymph nodes, any one mass greater than 2 cm but not more than 5 cm in greatest dimension
N3	Metastasis with a *lymph node mass more than 5 cm* in greatest dimension
Pathologic (after lymph nodes dissection)	
pNX	Regional lymph nodes cannot be assessed
pN0	No regional lymph node metastasis
pN1	Metastasis with a *lymph node mass 2 cm or less* in greatest dimension and *less than or equal to 5 nodes positive, none more than 2 cm in greatest dimension*
pN2	Metastasis with a *lymph node mass more than 2 cm but not more than 5 cm* in greatest dimension; or *more than 5 nodes positive, none more than 5 cm*; or evidence or *extranodal extension of tumour*
pN3	Metastasis with a *lymph node mass more than 5 cm* in greatest dimension
Distant metastasis (M)	
M0	No distant metastasis
M1	Distant metastasis
M1a	Nonregional nodal or pulmonary metastasis
M1b	Distant metastasis other than to nonregional lymph nodes and lung

Used with the permission of the American Joint Committee on Cancer (AJCC), Chicago, Illinois. The original source for this material is the AJCC Cancer Staging Manual, Seventh Edition (2010), published by Springer Science and Business Media LLC, www.springer.com

Table 21.2 Anatomic stage/prognostic groups [1]

Group	T	N	M	S (Serum tumour markers)
Stage 0	pTIS	N0	M0	S0
Stage I	*pT1-T4*	*N0*	*M0*	*Sx*
Stage IA	pT1	N0	M0	S0
Stage IB	pT2-pT4	N0	M0	S0
Stage IS	Any pT	N0	M0	S1-3
Stage II	*Any pT*	*N1-N3*	*M0*	*Sx*
Stage IIA	Any pT	N1	M0	S0
	Any pT	N1	M0	S1
Stage IIB	Any pT	N2	M0	S0
	Any pT	N2	M0	S1
Stage IIC	Any pT	N3	M0	S0
	Any pT	N3	M0	S1
Stage III	*Any pT*	*Any N*	*M1*	*Sx*
Stage IIIA	Any pT	Any N	M1a	S0
	Any pT	Any N	M1a	S1
Stage IIIB	Any pT	N1-N3	M0	S2
	Any pT	Any N	M1a	S2
Stage IIIC	Any pT	N1-N3	M0	S3
	Any pT	Any N	M1a	S3
	Any pT	Any N	M1b	Any S

21.2 Risk Categories

(a) *Localized tumours*

- *Seminoma*: *Pure seminoma is never in the bad prognosis group whatever the disease stage at the time of diagnosis*, but there are few factors which can help in predicting the risk of distant recurrence after orchiectomy: *tumour size >4 cm and presence of rete testis invasion* [2, 3]. In stage I seminoma, the 4-year relapse-free survival rates are 94, 82 and 64 % for tumours <3, 3 to <6 and ≥6 cm, respectively [3]. Secondarily, other factors have been advocated including lymphatic or vascular invasion and younger age (≤33 years old) [4].
- *NSGCT*: The presence of *embryonal carcinoma* is consistently associated with a relapse risk [5–7]. *Lymphovascular invasion* has also been advocated as a predictor of recurrence [7, 8], while *yolk sac tumour* [9] and *mature teratoma* [10] were shown to be associated with a low rate of disease relapse. Other unfavourable prognostic factors are tumoural involvement of the spermatic cord and scrotal violation.

(b) *Metastatic disease*: The risk stratification is established according to the International Germ Cell Cancer Collaborative Group (IGCCCG) [11] (Table 21.3).

Take-Home Message: Staging and Risk Factors
Pure seminoma is never in the bad prognosis group whatever the disease stage at the time of diagnosis
Seminomatous tumour size >4 cm and presence of rete testis invasion are associated with high distant relapse rate when managed with surveillance alone and chemotherapy should be anticipated
For NSGCT, presence of embryonal carcinoma histology or lymphovascular invasion are unfavourable factors, while yolk sac tumour and pure teratoma histologies are good factors

Table 21.3 International Germ Cell Consensus Classification Group (IGCCCG) [11]: a prognostic factor-based staging system for metastatic germ cell cancers

Risk status	Seminoma	Nonseminoma
Good	*90 % of seminomas* *All of the following criteria*: Any primary site M0, M1a. No visceral metastasis except lung Normal AFP Any hCG Any LDH 5-year progression-free survival: 82 % 5-year overall survival: 86 %	*56 % of nonseminomas* *All of the following criteria*: Testis/retroperitoneal primary M0, M1a. No visceral metastasis except lung S0, S1 (AFP <1,000 ug/L, βHCG <5,000 IU/L and LDH <1.5 times the upper normal value) 5-year progression-free survival: 89 % 5-year overall survival: 92 %
Intermediate	*10 % of seminomas* *All of the following criteria*: Any primary site M1b. No extrapulmonary visceral metastasis Normal AFP Any hCG Any LDH 5-year progression-free survival: 67 % 5-year overall survival: 72 %	*28 % of nonseminomas* *All of the following criteria*: Testis/retroperitoneal primary M0, M1a. No extrapulmonary visceral metastasis S2. AFP ≥ 1,000 and ≤10,000 ug/L, βHCG ≥5,000 and ≤ 50,000IU/L and LDH ≥ 1.5 and ≤ 10 times the upper normal value 5-year progression-free survival: 75 % 5-year overall survival: 80 %
Poor	*There is no poor risk for seminoma*	*16 % of nonseminomas* *Any of the following criteria*: Mediastinal primary Non-pulmonary visceral metastasis (M1b) S3. AFP > 10,000 ug/L, βHCG >50,000IU/L (10,000 ng/mL) and LDH >10 times the upper normal value 5-year progression-free survival (PFS): 41 % 5-year overall survival: 48 %

References

1. Testis. In: Edge SB, Byrd DR, Compton CC, Fritz AG, Greene FL, Trotti A, editors. AJCC cancer staging manual. 7th ed. New York: Springer; 2010. p. 469–78.
2. Warde P, Specht L, Horwich A, Oliver T, Panzarella T, Gospodarowicz M, et al. Prognostic factors for relapse in stage I seminoma managed by surveillance: a pooled analysis. J Clin Oncol. 2002;20:4448–52.
3. von der Maase H, Specht L, Jacobsen GK, Jakobsen A, Madsen EL, Pedersen M, et al. Surveillance following orchidectomy for stage I seminoma of the testis. Eur J Cancer. 1993;29A:1931–4.
4. Parker C, Milosevic M, Panzarella T, Banerjee D, Jewett M, Catton C, et al. The prognostic significance of the tumour infiltrating lymphocyte count in stage I testicular seminoma managed by surveillance. Eur J Cancer. 2002;38:2014–9.
5. Atsu N, Eskicorapci S, Uner A, Ekici S, Güngen Y, Erkan I, et al. A novel surveillance protocol for stage I nonseminomatous germ cell testicular tumours. BJU Int. 2003;92:32–5.
6. Nicolai N, Pizzocaro G. A surveillance study of clinical stage I nonseminomatous germ cell tumours of the testis: 10-year follow-up. J Urol. 1995;154:1045–9.
7. Moul JW, McCarthy WF, Fernandez EB, Sesterhenn IA. Percentage of embryonal carcinoma and of vascular invasion predicts pathological stage in clinical stage I nonseminomatous testicular cancer. Cancer Res. 1994;54(2):362–4.
8. Dunphy CH, Ayala AG, Swanson DA, Ro JY, Logothetis C. Clinical stage I nonseminomatous and mixed germ cell tumours of the testis: a clinicopathologic study of 93 patients on a surveillance protocol after orchiectomy alone. Cancer. 1988;62:1202–6.
9. Read G, Stenning SP, Cullen MH, Parkinson MC, Horwich A, Kaye SB, et al. Medical Research Council prospective study of surveillance for stage I testicular teratoma: Medical Research Council Testicular Tumours Working Party. J Clin Oncol. 1992;10:1762–8.
10. Alexandre J, Fizazi K, Mahe C, Culine S, Droz JP, Théodore C, et al. Stage I non-seminomatous germ-cell tumours of the testis: identification of a subgroup of patients with a very low risk of relapse. Eur J Cancer. 2001;37:576–82.
11. International germ cell consensus classification: a prognostic factor-based staging system for metastatic germ cell cancers. J Clin Oncol. 1997;15:594–603 (no author listed).

Chapter 22
Treatment of Testicular Tumours

Qais Mohamed Al-Hooti and Said Abdallah Al-Mamari

Semen abnormalities are frequently found in patients with testicular tumours and are consistent with low volume or low sperm concentration and low motility [1, 2]. Endocrine abnormalities consistent with elevated serum HCG and estradiol, and relative decrease in FSH may also be encountered.

Chemotherapy and radiation therapy are factors which further impair the fertility. For all these reasons, patients in the reproductive age group should have a pre-treatment fertility profile assessment including semen analysis, blood testosterone, LH and FSH levels. *Sperm cryopreservation is mandatory and should be performed prior to chemotherapy treatment and optimally before orchiectomy*, since the semen concentration was found to deteriorate after the procedure [3, 4].

Retroperitoneal lymph nodes dissection (*RPLND*) also negatively impacts the fertility potency of the patient because of the anejaculation which is associated with sympathetic nerves and ganglia damage. This complication was almost constant until 1980s when Donohue proposed to replace the classical bilateral RPLND by a template unilateral procedure [5].

Finally, it is important to emphasize here that in addition to the negative effect on fertility, the *teratogenicity of chemotherapy* was shown in the offspring of treated rats in the laboratory [6, 7]. Although this fact was not confirmed in humans [8, 9], precaution is recommended and advice is given to the patient to use *effective contraceptive measures* from the initiation of chemotherapy up to 1 year following the end of the treatment [10].

Q.M. Al-Hooti • S.A. Al-Mamari (✉)
Urology Department, The Royal Hospital, Muscat, Oman
e-mail: sabdal67@yahoo.com

S.A. Al-Mamari, S.S. Al-Busaidy (eds.), *Urological Cancer Management*,
DOI 10.1007/978-3-319-16301-7_22

22.1 Primary Treatment: Radical Orchiectomy

Radical orchiectomy through inguinal approach and section of the spermatic cord at the internal inguinal ring is the initial treatment of a testicular tumour (Fig. 18.1). *Scrotal violation must be avoided to prevent the risk of local recurrence.*

Orchiectomy provides an accurate diagnosis and local staging upon which further management is decided. When a benign lesion is clinically suspected a frozen section biopsy can be performed after clamping the spermatic cord. *Cold ischaemia is not always necessary*, since the testicular parenchyma can sustain warm ischaemia without damage during the relatively short time needed until the biopsy report is available in the operating theater. This knowledge was gained from clinical experience of successful surgical procedures performed within 6 h of onset of a testicular torsion [11, 12]. Moreover, a very recent preclinical study did not demonstrate any benefit for cold ischaemia over warm ischaemia during a 30-min partial orchiectomy in the rat model [13].

Patients with unilateral or bilateral orchiectomy should be offered *size-matched testicular prostheses* to preserve the bodily image.

Chemotherapy may sometimes be indicated in life-threatening disseminated disease prior to orchiectomy [14–16].

Testis sparing surgery (*partial orchiectomy*) may be decided in selected cases: for instance, *a young patient with normal androgen function who wishes to preserve his fertility and has a small localized lump of less than 2 cm* (*or* <*30 % of the testis volume*), *with a solitary testis or with synchronous bilateral tumours*. Here also a frozen section biopsy is mandatory to ensure removal of the tumour with negative surgical margins. The patient should be informed about the high risk of developing malignancy in the remaining tissue due to the reported presence of ITGCN in 80–90 % of the cases. A frozen biopsy of the apparently healthy remaining testicular tissue is also advocated by expert panel [17] to confirm the presence of ITGCN which may justify adjuvant radiotherapy with the risk of further impairing the androgen production and causing infertility with long-term exposure [18].

> Close observation, local radiotherapy or orchiectomy are possible options in the management of ITGCN.

Controversy exists regarding whether it is necessary to treat ITGCT or not, since it is still not clear that active treatment improves survival compared to observation and treating only when a subsequent GCT develops. Moreover, this controversy is nourished by the morbidity accompanying ITGCT treatment and the fact that most of the associated metachronous tumours present at a low stage [19]. All these facts preclude recommending a systematic contralateral biopsy in all patients.

Life-long testosterone supplementation is necessary in patients undergoing bilateral orchidectomy or developing low testosterone levels after radiotherapy for ITGCT.

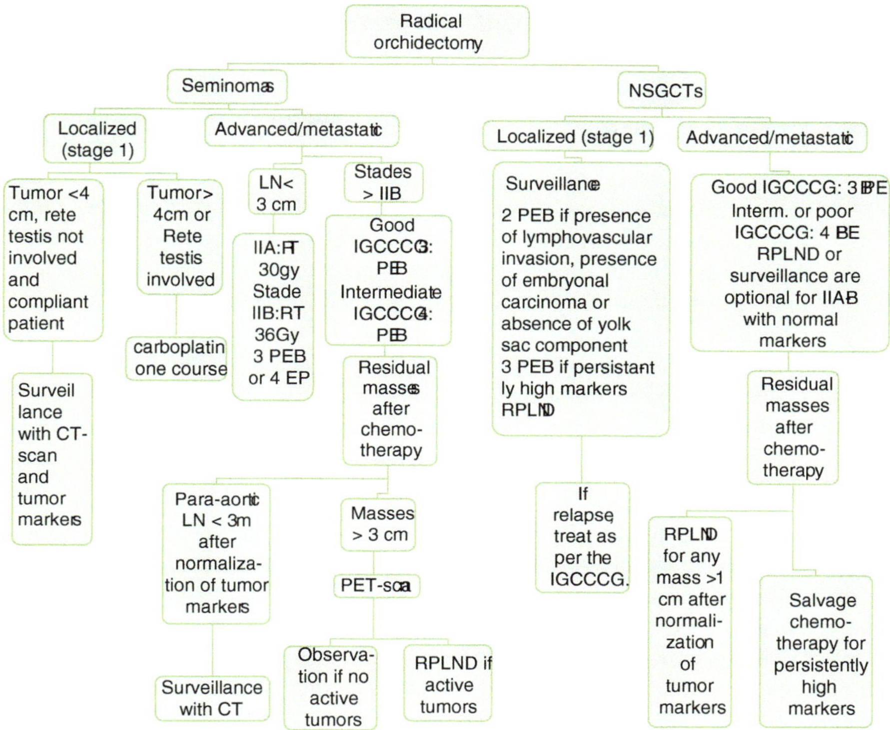

Fig. 22.1 Algorithm of the management of testicular tumor

22.2 Management After Orchiectomy (Fig. 22.1)

There is an excellent survival rate of GCTs owing to careful staging at diagnosis, efficacy of early adequate treatment based on chemotherapeutic combinations, with or without radiotherapy or surgery and the possibility of salvage therapies on subsequent follow-up. The 5-year overall survival of GCTs is estimated to be approximately 96–97 % in Germany and the United States, with spermatocytic seminoma having the best outcome (near 100 % 5-year survival rate) and choriocarcinoma portraying the worst relative survival rate (around 80 %) [20].

As already stated, *testicular histopathology, tumour markers and radiological imaging form an essential clinical tripod in establishing the risk categories and deciding further treatment.*

1. *For localized diseases*, the modality of treatment will depend on the prognostic risk factors for relapse.

   (a) *Seminoma*: Two options are possible for stage I seminoma and include surveillance and adjuvant chemotherapy with carboplatin [21]. Up to few years back adjuvant RT using 20 Gy was an option but is no more recommended due to the efficacy of carboplatin with less side effects as stated in a recent prospective randomized trial [22]. Active treatment with chemotherapy is considered in patients with *testicular tumours greater than 4-cm diameter or when the rete testis is involved*. Surveillance in this situation is associated with high relapse rate compared to active treatment. *Surveillance is recommended in compliant patients with tumours of less than 4-cm diameter* as they are associated with a low recurrence rate of 15–20 % which is manageable by an effective salvage therapy when it occurs. Therefore, unnecessary treatment is avoided in as much as 80 % of patients with low risk [23].

(b) *NSGCT: Three options are possible: Surveillance, chemotherapy with 2 cycles of PEB or RPLND* [21] *for patients with normalized serum markers*. Patients with persistently high markers should receive 3 cycles of PEB: combination of cis*p*latin, *e*toposide and *b*leomycin (see the following section).

A prospective study found a 73 % relapse-free rate during surveillance of teratoma after radical orchidectomy alone [24] and identified a high-risk group for disease relapse (lymphovascular invasion and/or presence of embryonal element and absence of a yolk sac component) for which chemotherapy is advocated. There is an interest in performing a diagnostic and eventually therapeutic primary RPLND in clinical stage I NSGCTs as the only reliable staging method. Around 28 % of patients clinically labelled stage I or N0 disease were found to have retroperitoneal LN metastases [25].

A strict follow-up after chemotherapy and/or RPLND is mandatory to decide for further treatment depending on tumour marker response and residual tumours.

2. *Metastatic disease* [17, 21]: In advanced disease, risk categories will determine the type and duration of chemotherapy, in addition to the prognosis and survival (Table 21.3).

   (a) Seminoma: For low volume disease (LN <3 cm): RT with 30 Gy for stage IIA and 36 Gy for IIB. Technically, the radiation should be unilateral and cover the hockey-stick field including the para-aortic area and the ipsilateral iliac region. Alternatively, chemotherapy (3 PEB or 4 EP) for stage IIB. Above stage IIB: chemotherapy with 3 cycles of PEB for the good prognostic group and 4 cycles for the intermediate risk group.
   (b) NSGCTs: Despite a study having shown that primary RPLND should better be restricted to clinical stages I and IIA patients with normal tumour markers after orchiectomy and stable retroperitoneal disease [26], the European expert panel extend that option to IIB disease patients with normal tumour markers and unwilling to undergo primary chemotherapy [21] which is mandatory for all higher stages. Practically, the following protocol is recommended: Good prognosis: 3 PEB cycles. Intermediate and bad prognosis: 4 PEB cycles. Surveillance is also an option for IIA-B patients.

Drugs Used in Chemotherapy for GCTs

Presently the most commonly used drugs are cisplatin, etoposide and bleomycin (PEB). Secondarily, ifosfamide (Holoxan) and carboplatin are also used whenever one of the BEP components is contraindicated. New proposed drugs are epirubicin, taxanes (paclitaxel), oxaliplatin, gemcitabine (Gemzar), etc.

- *Cisplatin* or cis-diamminedichloroplatinum(II) or CDDDP (Platinol®) is *nephrotoxic* (reversible dose-dependant tubular necrosis), *hematotoxic, ototoxic and neurotoxic*. It may also induce azoospermia and gastrointestinal upset. A randomized trial has shown that adjunction of the cytoprotective agent amifostine (Ethyol) alleviated the nephrotoxicity of a platinum-based chemotherapy [27]. The usual dose is 20 mg/m^2/day IV over 20–60 min for 5 days; repeated q21d for 3–4 cycles. The drug is contraindicated in documented hypersensitivity, pre-existing renal insufficiency (creatinine clearance <60 mL/min), myelosuppression or hearing impairment.
- *Etoposide* or VP-16 (Toposar®, VePesid®, Etopophos®) is *haematotoxic* (pancytopenia, possibility of late leukaemia). It also induces hypotension which may be severe, mucositis and gastrointestinal upset. More toxicity was found in patients with serum creatinine >130 umol/L, serum albumin <35 g/L, age >65 years and elevated liver enzymes. It appears to be caused by an increased concentration of free plasmatic etoposide found in these conditions [28]. The usual dose is 100 mg/m^2/day IV for 5 days; repeated q21d for 3–4 cycles and adjusted in hepatic or renal function impairment. Documented hypersensitivity to the drug is an absolute contraindication.
- *Bleomycin* (Blenoxane®) is a glycopeptide antibiotic produced by the bacterium Streptomyces verticillus. It has a high toxicity rate causing hyperthermia, *interstitial pneumonitis followed by lung fibrosis* and Raynaud's syndrome. The rate of pneumonitis varies with publications from 0 to 46 % of the patients depending on the definition criteria used [29]. Mortality rate also varies with publication and was shown to reach 14 % of the patients developing bleomycin pulmonary toxicity [30]. Pulmonary fibrosis characteristically appears after a cumulative dose >300,000 IU[1] (equivalent of 300 USP units[2] or 300 mg), mostly after radiation therapy. It affects mostly older patients (>40 years) as well as subjects with GFR <80 ml/min or stage IV disease at presentation. Patients respond poorly to steroids and are worse after oxygenation [30]. Lung toxicity occurs after a median time of 4.2 months from the start of bleomycin, but longer periods have been reported including an exceptional occurrence 10 years after cessation of the treatment [31]. Optionally a test dose can be given 1–2 mg IV/IM before starting the standard dose of 30 mg IV bolus every week on days 2, 9 and 16; repeated every 21 days (q21d) for 3–4 cycles. Documented hypersensitivity, significant renal function impairment and pre-existing compromised pulmonary function are absolute contraindications for this drug.

[1] IU: International Units

[2] USP units: United States Pharmacopeia Units

Due to the high toxicity of these drugs, supportive care is necessary with erythropoietin, G-CSF (Neupogen, Eprex.), anti-emetic and anti-allergic drugs, steroids, neuroleptic (chlorpromazine), etc. However, beware of a reported synergistic effect between bleomycin and G-CSF in promoting pulmonary toxicity [32]. Nowadays, *the protocol PEB has become the international standard therapy* since 1987 when Williams et al. demonstrated that it is less toxic and provides a better survival rate than the former PVB combination (cisplatin, vinblastine, bleomycin) [33]. This combination is credited with a higher than 85 % overall cure rate and the treatment duration has now been reduced to 3–4 months. It was shown that *a 3-day cycle and a total of 3 PEB cycles* carried less toxicity while maintaining same efficacy as a 5-day cycle and a total of 4 cycles for GCTs with a good prognosis [34].

Other protocols are EP (without bleomycine) and VIP: Etoposide, ifosfamide (Ifex), cisplatine.

Salvage protocols: VIP, VeIP (vinblastine, ifosfamide, and cisplatin), CARBOPEC (carboplatin, etoposide, cyclophosphamide).

Note: A transient elevation of βHCG and AFP can occur after the initiation of chemotherapy. AFP surge, as opposed to βHCG elevation, appears to be an adverse prognostic factor [35, 36].

22.3 Management of Residual Metastatic Masses After Chemotherapy (Fig. 22.1)

- Seminomas: If para-aortic lymphadenopathy <3 cm is present after normalization of tumour markers, the patient can be put under careful surveillance and followed-up with repeat CT scan and/or PET scan [17, 21]. The rationale is the known slow regression of this tumour which may take months or even years to be completed [37]. However, if the masses are >3 cm, a PET scan is indicated to detect active tissue which is an indication for a RPLND.
- NSGCTs: RPLND applies to any supracentimetric residual mass after normalization of serum markers [17, 21]. In case of persistently high serum markers after chemotherapy, a salvage second chemotherapy can be given. If the latter fails, a 'desperation surgery' can be attempted aiming at removing all resectable tumours [21]. When >10 % viable tumour is seen in the resected LN, this may be an indication for a postsurgical repeat chemotherapy with the same regimen used in the induction, that is, PEB protocol, but beware of the cumulative bleomycin dose. This so-called 'consolidation chemotherapy' is performed with 2 PEB cycles and is mostly justified when there is an incomplete resection of NSGCTs other than teratoma [21]. However, it was shown that the benefit of this post-surgical redo-chemotherapy is found only in patients with IGCCC intermediate prognostic group [38]. The completeness of the resection which is better performed by experienced surgeons is of paramount importance as it has been shown to be the strongest predictor of both progression-free survival and overall-survival [39]. Other predictors are <10 % viable malignant cells and favourable IGCCC group.

Take-Home Message: Treatment of Testicular Cancer

Close observation, local radiotherapy or orchiectomy is a possible option in the management of ITGCN

Sperm cryopreservation is mandatory and should be performed prior to chemotherapy treatment and optimally even before orchiectomy

Radical orchiectomy through inguinal approach and section of the spermatic cord at the internal inguinal ring is the initial treatment of a testicular tumour

Chemotherapy may sometimes be indicated in life-threatening disseminated disease prior to orchiectomy

After orchiectomy, testicular histopathology, tumour markers and imaging form an essential clinical tripod in establishing the risk categories and deciding further treatment:

- In localized disease (stage I):
  - *Seminomatous tumours greater than 4-cm diameter or when the rete testis is involved should not be managed with surveillance alone* and patients should be offered chemotherapy with carboplatin. Due to the efficacy of carboplatin, RT is not recommended anymore in localized seminoma
  - Around 30 % of NSGCTs will relapse on surveillance alone and *chemotherapy with 2 cycles of PEB should be anticipated when lymphovascular invasion and/or embryonal elements are present and when a yolk sac component is absent*. A primary RPLND is an interesting option for clinical stage I with normalized serum markers after orchidectomy for accurately staging the disease. Patients with persistently high serum markers should be treated with 3 cycles of PEB
- Advanced diseases (stages II-III):
  - *Seminoma*: *If LN <3 cm: RT with 30 (stage IIA) and 36 Gy (stage IIB). The radiation must be unilateral and cover the para-aortic and the ipsilateral iliac areas in a hockey stick fashion. Stage IIB patients can also be given 3 PEB or 4 EP cycles. Above stage IIB, all patients must receive 3 PEB cycles for good prognostic group or 4 cycles for intermediate risk group*
  - *NSGCTs*: RPLND and surveillance are options for Stage IIA-B patients with normal tumour markers after orchiectomy and stable retroperitoneal disease. However, the standard treatment for all NSGCT patients with advanced disease is *3 PEB cycles for good prognostic group and 4 PEB cycles for intermediate and bad prognostic groups*

At present PEB is the most commonly used combination with a standard protocol of 5-day cycle and a total of 3–4 cycles according to the risk group. Secondarily, ifosfamide and carboplatin can be used whenever one of the PEB components is contraindicated. *The most striking side effect of bleomycin is lung toxicity (interstitial pneumonitis followed by lung fibrosis)*, while haematologic side effects and nephrotoxicity should be closely monitored for etoposide and cisplatin, respectively

Diagnostic and eventually therapeutic primary RPLND is advocated for clinical stage I NSGCTs as the only reliable staging method. This disease is not well assessed by a PET scan

When serum markers have been normalized following chemotherapy, RPLND is indicated in residual seminomatous LN >3 cm after confirmation with PET-CT scan and in all supracentimetric NSGCT residual masses

References

1. Carroll PR, Whitmore Jr WR, Herr HW, et al. Endocrine and exocrine profiles of men with testicular tumours before orchiectomy. J Urol. 1987;137(3):420–3.
2. Williams DH, Karpman E, Sander JC, Spiess PE, Pisters LL, Lipshultz LI. Pretreatment semen parameters in men with cancer. J Urol. 2009;181:736–40.
3. Petersen PM, Skakkebaek NE, Rørth M, Giwercman A. Semen quality and reproductive hormones before and after orchiectomy in men with testicular cancer. A J Urol. 1999;161(3): 822–6.
4. Liguori G, Trombetta C, Bucci S, Benvenuto S, Amodeo A, Ocello G, Belgrano E. Semen quality before and after orchiectomy in men with testicular cancer. Arch Ital Urol Androl. 2008;80(3):99–102.
5. Donohue JP, Foster RS, Rowland RG, Bihrle R, Jones R, Geier G. Nerve sparing retroperitoneal lymphadenectomy with preservation of ejaculation. J Urol. 1990;144:287–92.
6. Auroux M, Dulioust EJ, Nawar NN, Yacoub SG, Mayaux MJ, Schwartz D, David G. Antimitotic drugs in the male rat. Behavioral abnormalities in the second generation. J Androl. 1988;9:153–9.
7. Auroux M, Dulioust E, Selva J, Rince P. Cyclophosphamide in the F0 male rat: physical and behavioral changes in three successive adult generations. Mutat Res. 1990;229:189–200.
8. Senturia YD, Peckham CS. Children fathered by men treated with chemotherapy for testicular cancer. Eur J Cancer. 1990;26(4):429–32.
9. Dodds L, Marrett LD, Tomkins DJ, Green B, Sherman G. Case-control study of congenital anomalies in children of cancer patients. BMJ. 1993;307(6897):164–8.
10. Schmoll HJ, Souchon R, Krege S, et al.; European Germ Cell Cancer Consensus Group. European consensus on diagnosis and treatment of germ cell cancer: a report of the European Germ Cell Cancer Consensus Group (EGCCCG). Ann Oncol. 2004;15(9):1377–99.
11. Rampaul MS, Hosking SW. Testicular torsion: most delay occurs outside hospital. Ann R Coll Surg Engl. 1998;80(3):169–72.
12. Cattolica EV, Karol JB, Rankin KN, Klein RS. High testicular salvage rate in torsion of the spermatic cord. J Urol. 1982;128(1):66–8.
13. McNamara ER, Madden-Fuentes RJ, Routh JC, Rouse D, Madden JF, Wiener JS, Rushton Jr HG, Ross SS. Evaluation of cold ischemia for preservation of testicular function during partial orchiectomy in the rat model. J Pediatr Urol. 2014;10(4):593–7.
14. Reddy BV, Sivakanth A, Naveen Babu G, Swamyvelu K, Basavana Goud YG, Madhusudhana BA, Challa VR. Role of chemotherapy prior to orchiectomy in metastatic testicular cancer—is testis really a sanctuary site? Ecancermedicalscience. 2014;8:407.
15. Geldart TR, Simmonds PD, Mead GM. Orchidectomy after chemotherapy for patients with metastatic testicular germ cell cancer. BJU Int. 2002;90(4):451–5.
16. Ondrus D, Horňák M, Breza J, Mat'oska J, Schnorrer M, Belan V, Kausitz J. Delayed orchiectomy after chemotherapy in patients with advanced testicular cancer. Int Urol Nephrol. 2001;32(4):665–7.
17. Durand X, Rigaud J, Avancès C, Les membres du CCAFU, et al. CCAFU recommendations 2013: testicular germ cell cancer. Prog Urol. 2013;23 Suppl 2:S145–60.
18. Heidenreich A, Weissbach L, Höltl W, Albers P, Kliesch S, Köhrmann KU, DIeckmann KP, German Testicular Cancer Study Group. Organ sparing surgery for malignant germ cell tumour of the testis. J Urol. 2001;166(6):2161–5.
19. Albers P, Göll A, Bierhoff E, et al. Clinical course and histopathologic risk factor assessment in patients with bilateral testicular germ cell tumours. Urology. 1999;54(4):714–8.
20. Stang A, Jansen L, Trabert B, Rusner C, Eberle A, Katalinic A, Emrich K, Holleczek B, Brenner H, GEKID Cancer Survival Working Group. Survival after a diagnosis of testicular germ cell cancers in Germany and the United States, 2002-2006: a high resolution study by histology and age. Cancer Epidemiol. 2013;37(4):492–7.
21. Albers P, Albrecht W, Algaba F, Bokemeyer C, Cohn-Cedermark G, Fizazi K, Horwich A, Laguna MP, European Association of Urology. EAU guidelines on testicular cancer:

2011 update. Eur Urol. 2011;60(2):304–19. doi:10.1016/j.eururo.2011.05.038. Epub 2011 May 25.
22. Oliver RT, Mead GM, Rustin GJ, Joffe JK, Aass N, Coleman R, Gabe R, Pollock P, Stenning SP. Randomized trial of carboplatin versus radiotherapy for stage I seminoma: mature results on relapse and contralateral testis cancer rates in MRC TE19/EORTC 30982 study (ISRCTN27163214). J Clin Oncol. 2011;29(8):957–62.
23. Porcaro AB, Antoniolli SZ, Schiavone D, Maffei N, Bassetto MA, Curti P. Management of clinical stage I testicular pure seminoma. Report on 42 patients and review of the literature. Arch Ital Urol Androl. 2002;74(2):77–80.
24. Read G, Stenning SP, Cullen MH, Parkinson MC, Horwich A, Kaye SB, Cook PA, Medical Research Council Testicular Tumours Working Party. Medical Research Council prospective study of surveillance for stage I testicular teratoma. J Clin Oncol. 1992;10(11):1762–8.
25. Heidenreich A, Albers P, Hartmann M, et al. Complications of primary nerve sparing retroperitoneal lymph node dissection for clinical stage I nonseminomatous germ cell tumours of the testis: experience of the German Testicular Cancer Study Group. J Urol. 2003;169:1710.
26. Stephenson AJ, Bosl GJ, Motzer RJ, Kattan MW, Stasi J, Bajorin DF, Sheinfeld J. Retroperitoneal lymph node dissection for nonseminomatous germ cell testicular cancer: impact of patient selection factors on outcome. J Clin Oncol. 2005;23(12):2781–8.
27. Hartmann JT, Fels LM, Knop S, Stolt H, Kanz L, Bokemeyer C. A randomized trial comparing the nephrotoxicity of cisplatin/ifosfamide-based combination chemotherapy with or without amifostine in patients with solid tumours. Invest New Drugs. 2000;18(3):281–9.
28. Joel SP, Shah R, Clark PI, Slevin ML. Predicting etoposide toxicity: relationship to organ function and protein binding. J Clin Oncol. 1996;14(1):257–67.
29. Sleijfer S. Bleomycin-induced pneumonitis. Chest. 2001;120(2):617–24.
30. O'Sullivan JM, Huddart RA, Norman AR, Nicholls J, Dearnaley DP, Horwich A. Predicting the risk of bleomycin lung toxicity in patients with germ-cell tumours. Ann Oncol. 2003;14(1):91–6.
31. Tashiro M, Izumikawa K, Yoshioka D, et al. Lung fibrosis 10 years after cessation of bleomycin therapy. Tohoku J Exp Med. 2008;216(1):77–80.
32. Matthews JH. Pulmonary toxicity of ABVD chemotherapy and G-CSF in Hodgkin's disease: possible synergy. Lancet. 1993;342:988.
33. Williams S, Birch R, Einhorn LH, et al. Treatment of dissiminated germ cell tumours with cisplatin, bleomycin and either vinblastin or etoposide. N Engl J Med. 1987;316(23): 1435–40.
34. de Wit R, Roberts JT, Wilkinson PM, de Mulder PH, Mead GM, Fosså SD, Cook P, de Prijck L, Stenning S, Collette L. Equivalence of three or four cycles of bleomycin, etoposide, and cisplatin chemotherapy and of a 3- or 5-day schedule in good-prognosis germ cell cancer: a randomized study of the European Organization for Research and Treatment of Cancer. Genitourinary Tract Cancer Cooperative Group and the Medical Research Council. J Clin Oncol. 2001;19(6):1629–40.
35. Horwich A, Peckham MJ. Transient tumour marker elevation following chemotherapy for germ cell tumours of the testis. Cancer Treat Rep. 1986;70(11):1329–31.
36. de Wit R, Collette L, Sylvester R, de Mulder PH, Sleijfer DT, ten Bokkel Huinink WW, Kaye SB, van Oosterom AT, Boven E, Stoter G. Serum alpha-fetoprotein surge after the initiation of chemotherapy for non-seminomatous testicular cancer has an adverse prognostic significance. Br J Cancer. 1998;78(10):1350–5.
37. Peckham MJ, Horwich A, Hendry WF. Advanced seminoma: treatment with cis-platinum-basedcombination chemotherapy or carboplatin (JM8). Br J Cancer. 1985;52:7–13.
38. Fizazi K, Tjulandin S, Salvioni R, et al. Viable malignant cells after primary chemotherapy for disseminated nonseminomatous germ cell tumours: prognostic factors and role of postsurgery chemotherapy–results from an international study group. J Clin Oncol. 2001;19(10): 2647–57.
39. Fizazi K, Oldenburg J, Dunant A. Assessing prognosis and optimizing treatment in patients with postchemotherapy viable nonseminomatous germ-cell tumours (NSGCT): results of the sCR2 international study. Ann Oncol. 2008;19(2):259–64.

Chapter 23
Extragonadal Germ Cell Tumours (EGGCTs)

Said Abdallah Al-Mamari and Qais Mohamed Al-Hooti

One question should always be borne in mind while dealing with an EGGCT: *Is it truly a primary extragonadal or a secondary of an occult testicular tumour?* Hence, every effort must be made to confirm a possible testicular primary since this differentiation has direct clinical, therapeutic and prognostic consequences. Therefore, the testes are carefully examined by palpation, high-definition ultrasound and even random biopsy. It is generally accepted now that "primary" *retroperitoneal EGGCTs* arise from occult or burnt-out testicular GCTs because they behave clinically in a manner very similar to that of the primary testicular cancers [1]. However, this is not true for mediastinal, pineal or sacrococcygeal EGGCTs which show major differences in clinical behaviour compared to testicular tumours. Hypothetically ruling out a testicular primary with absolute certainty can only be achieved by performing bilateral orchidectomy and a careful histopathological examination of the testes. Clearly, this extreme approach is neither ethical nor clinically acceptable. However, it does illustrate the point that when a clinician is talking about a primary testicular tumour, he should only state "not confirmed" rather than "ruled out".

Primary extragonadal tumours are very rare with less than 1,000 published cases. Klinefelter syndrome is a risk factor associated with these tumours [2]. They are characterized by their *midline localization from the pineal gland to the coccyx* and generally have a *bad prognosis which is associated with* their site, size and propensity to metastasize. The presence of liver metastases and two or more metastatic sites negatively influences the survival [3]. A multicentric study involving 635 cases has found NSGCTs and seminomas in 524 (*83 %*) and 104 (*16 %*) patients, respectively, the remaining 7 cases (1 %) being unidentified [4].

S.A. Al-Mamari (✉) • Q.M. Al-Hooti
Urology Department, The Royal Hospital, Muscat, Oman
e-mail: sabdal67@yahoo.com

S.A. Al-Mamari, S.S. Al-Busaidy (eds.), *Urological Cancer Management*,
DOI 10.1007/978-3-319-16301-7_23

The same study also found mediastinal and retroperitoneal localizations in 54 and 45 %, respectively. Other localizations were the sacrococcygeal region, the pineal gland (epiphysis), the thyroid, the nasal sinuses, the rectum, the prostate, the orbits, the liver and the gastrointestinal tract [1, 4]. Adverse prognostic factors included nonseminomatous histology, the presence of non-pulmonary visceral metastases, primary mediastinal location and elevated βHCG.

Several theories have attempted to explain the pathogenesis of these tumours:

- *Embryologic theories*: persistence of pluripotent cells in extragonadal areas and abnormal migration of germ cells from the endodermic sinus between the 4th and 6th week. Nonetheless, histological studies from murine and human embryos did not find abnormally located primitive germ cells [5, 6].
- *Cytogenetic theories*: the pathogenesis is explained by the finding of identical genetic abnormalities such as the isochromosome of the short arm of chromosome 12 – i(12p) in both the mediastinal primary tumours and testicular GCTs [7]. The hypothesis of reverse migration of testicular occult carcinoma in situ was also advocated, suggesting that extragonadal tumours could be of gonadal origin [8].
- *Clinical data*: patients with EGGCT are at an increased risk to develop a metachronous testicular GCT especially for NSGCT and retroperitoneal localization despite a platinum-based chemotherapy [4].

EGGCTs insidiously develop until they reach a high volume and produce local and regional symptoms.

- The presenting symptoms depend on the localization.
  - For mediastinal localization, the patient may present with rapidly progressive chest pain, dyspnoea, cough, fever, weight loss and superior vena cava compression syndrome.
  - For retroperitoneal site, the presenting complains may be non-specific: fever, weight loss and abdominal and back pain [4].

Progressive symptoms prompt investigations such as chest-abdomen-pelvis CT scan or MRI which reveal unexpected *space-occupying mediastinal or retroperitoneal lesions* (Fig. 23.1). Tumour markers should be routinely performed (βHCG, AFP, LDH) as well as a percutaneous CT-guided biopsy to get a histological diagnosis.

- The metastatic pattern of EGCCT also depends on the site and the histological type [4]:
  - Mediastinum: Seminomas to cervical LN and nonseminoma to lungs (27 %).
  - Retroperitoneum: Seminomas to retroperitoneal LN (26 %) and then to mediastinal and cervical LN. Nonseminomas to the lungs (49 %), abdominal LN (34 %) and liver (25 %). Metastases to the brain and bone have also been reported.

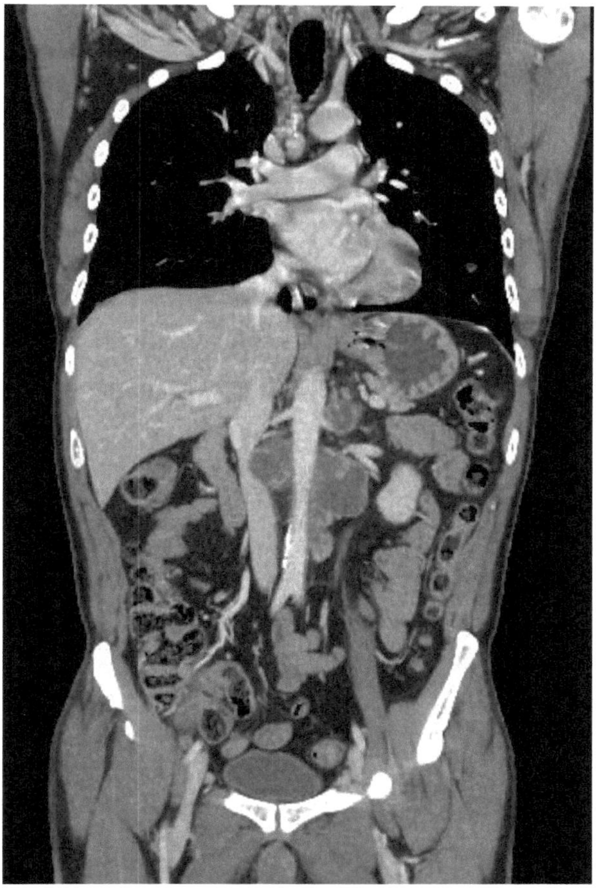

Fig. 23.1 CT scan showing multiple left paraaortic and interaortico-caval LNs consistent with EGGCT. Teratoma was seen in most of them (Courtesy of Dr J-L Hoepffner, Onco-Urologist, Saint-Augustin Clinic and Bergonié Oncological Institute, Bordeaux, France)

23.1 Treatment of EGGCT

- Retroperitoneal GCTs should be treated in a similar fashion as testicular tumours.
  - Seminomatous EGGCT: Cisplatin-based chemotherapy is the standard treatment and is credited for >90 % 5-year survival rate. Radiotherapy harbours a high rate of disease relapse; it carries a 5-year progression-free survival rate of 33 % compared with 87 % for chemotherapy [3]. Surgery is indicated if active residual masses are diagnosed, applying similar criteria as in testicular GCTs.
  - Nonseminomatous EGGCT: PEB chemotherapy has a median survival rate of 34 months. Surgery is indicated for residual masses or persistently high tumour markers (Fig. 23.2a, b).

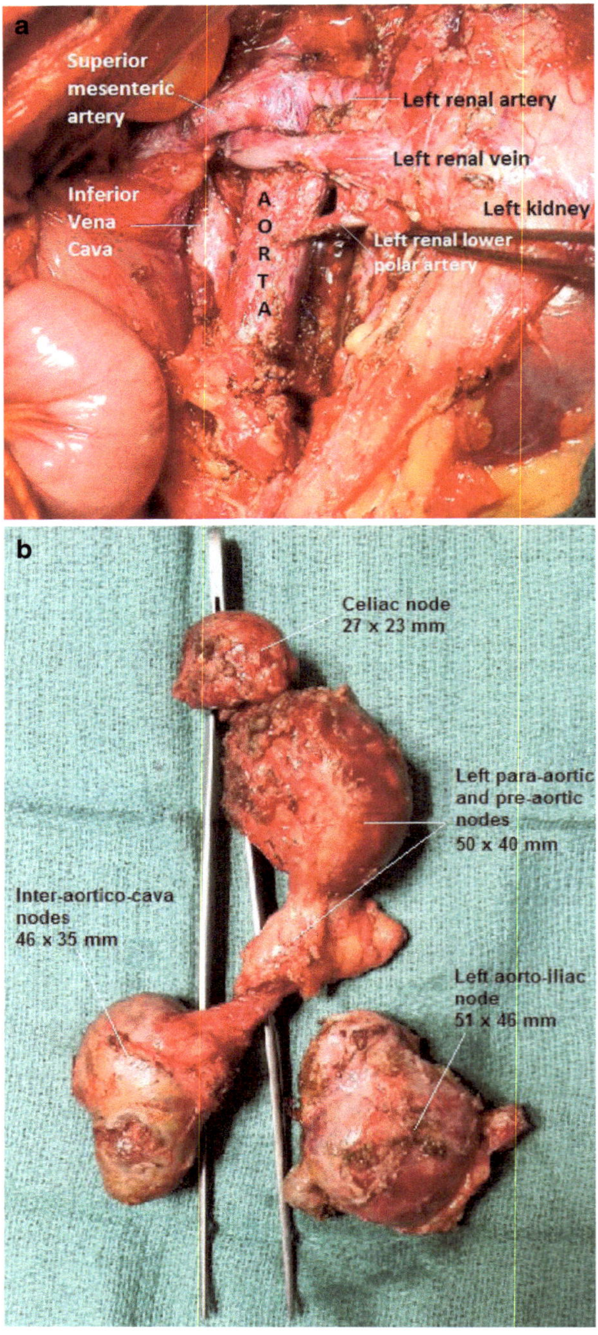

Fig. 23.2 (**a**, **b**) View of the retroperitoneum after an RPLND (same patient on Fig. 23.1) and the removed LNs (the forceps in Figure b reproduces the relative position of the aorta) (Courtesy of Dr J-L Hoepffner, Onco-Urologist, Saint-Augustin Clinic and Bergonié Oncological Institute, Bordeaux, France)

- Mediastinal nonseminomatous EGGCTs have an overall 5-year survival rate of 45 and 17 % for intermediate- and poor-risk groups, respectively, defined as per the same IGCCCG criteria seen on Table 21.3 [4]. A study recently performed at Indiana University suggests replacing bleomycin by ifosfamide for patients with mediastinal nonseminomatous EGGCTs to prevent pulmonary complications, as these patients generally require extensive thoracic surgical resection [9].

Take-Home Message: EGGCTs

In the presence of apparently primary EGGCTs, every *effort must be done to rule out an occult primary testicular tumour*
EGGCTs are characterized by their *midline localization from the pineal gland to the coccyx, but mediastinal and retroperitoneal localizations predominate*
Nonseminomatous EGGCTs are more frequently encountered than seminomatous EGGCTs. The majority of seminomatous EGGCTs are found in the retroperitoneal location
The pattern of EGGCT presentation and metastases depends on their sites and histological types
Generally, EGGCTs have a worse prognosis compared to equivalent stage of GCTs with documented testicular primaries. Retroperitoneal EGGCTs should be treated in similar fashion as testicular tumours. *Mediastinal nonseminomatous EGGCTs have the worst prognosis* and should be treated more aggressively

References

1. Schmoll H-J. Extragonadal germ cell tumours. Ann Oncol. 2002;13 Suppl 4:265–72.
2. Hasle H, Jacobsen BB, Asschenfeldt P, et al. Mediastinal germ cell tumour associated with Klinefelter syndrome. A report of case and review of the literature. Eur J Pediatr. 1992;151(10):735–9.
3. Bokemeyer C, Droz JP, Horwich A, Gerl A, Fossa SD, Beyer J, Pont J, Schmoll HJ, Kanz L, Einhorn L, Nichols CR, Hartmann JT. Extragonadal seminoma: an international multicenter analysis of prognostic factors and long term treatment outcome. Cancer. 2001;91(7): 1394–401.
4. Bokemeyer C, Nichols CR, Droz JP, Schmoll HJ, Horwich A, Gerl A, Fossa SD, Beyer J, Pont J, Kanz L, Einhorn L, Hartmann JT. Extragonadal germ cell tumours of the mediastinum and retroperitoneum: results from an international analysis. J Clin Oncol. 2002;20(7):1864–73.
5. Chiquoine AD. The identification, origin, and migration of the primordial germ cells in the mouse embryo. Anat Rec. 1954;118:135–46.
6. Witschi E. Migration of the germ cells of human embryos from the yolk sac to the primitive gonadal folds. Contr Embryol Carnegie Inst. 1948;32:67–80.
7. Chaganti RSK, Houldsworth J. Genetics and biology of adult human male germ cell tumours. Cancer Res. 2000;60(6):1475–82.
8. Chaganti RS, Rodriguez E, Mathew S. Origin of adult male mediastinal germ-cell tumours. Lancet. 1994;343(8906):1130–2.
9. Albany C, Einhorn LH. Extragonadal germ cell tumours: clinical presentation and management. Curr Opin Oncol. 2013;25(3):261–5.

Chapter 24
Penile Cancer

Said Abdallah Al-Mamari and Qais Mohamed Al-Hooti

24.1 Epidemiology

Penile tumour is very rare in the western community where its incidence is less than 1 new case/100,000 population per year, accounting only for 0.5 % of male malignancies [1]. However, it is more frequent in Latin America (Paraguay) and in Africa (Uganda) where incidences of more than 4 new cases/100,000 year have been recorded [2–4]. It affects mostly old men.

24.2 Aetiology

Reported aetiological factors associated with penile cancer are *poor genital hygiene*, *human papillomavirus (HPV) types 16 and 18*, condyloma acumunata, balanitis xerotica obliterans (BXO) (penile equivalent of lichen sclerosus et atrophicus), smoking and treatment with psoralen and ultraviolet A photochemotherapy (PUVA). Precancerous lesions are *erythroplasia of Queyrat* which refers to a CIS involving the glans penis, prepuce or shaft and *Bowen's disease* which is a CIS involving the remainder of the genitalia or perineal region. *The hygienic factor is corroborated by the fact that neonatal circumcision is highly protective against this cancer* [5, 6] *and by the strong association of phimosis with this tumour* [7]. This raises suspicion about the long-term effect of the smegma as a carcinogenic agent, but valid supportive evidence is lacking. The role of human papillomavirus (HPV) types 16 and 18 is potentiated by sexual contact at an early age and increased number of sexual intercourse and partners. This viral infection has been consistently advocated since

S.A. Al-Mamari (✉) • Q.M. Al-Hooti
Urology Department, The Royal Hospital, Muscat, Oman
e-mail: sabdal67@yahoo.com

S.A. Al-Mamari, S.S. Al-Busaidy (eds.), *Urological Cancer Management*,
DOI 10.1007/978-3-319-16301-7_24

it is present in about 42 % of cases of penile carcinoma, 90 % of cases of dysplasia and 100 % of cases of condyloma [4]. Cost-effectiveness of the HPV vaccine tried for cervix cancer is also being evaluated for penile cancer [8].

24.3 Histopathology

Penile cancers are squamous cell carcinomas in 95 % of cases. The tumour is categorized as per the modified Broders grading system [9]:

- Grade I: Well-differentiated cells, prominent keratin pearls
- Grade II to III: Nuclear atypia and increased mitotic activity, decreased keratin pearls
- Grade IV: deeply invasive, marked nuclear pleomorphism, nuclear mitosis, necrosis, lymphatic and perineural invasion, no keratin pearls

24.4 TNM Classification 2010

See AJCC cancer staging Table 24.1 [10].

24.5 Diagnosis of the Primary Lesion

The patient presents generally after several weeks or months due to negligence or denial. Sometimes the lesion remains unnoticed being hidden by the prepuce in 25–75 % cases. *Overall 30 % of penile cancer are diagnosed at advanced stage* [11]. The presenting complaints are consistent with a painless non-healing ulcer. This can be associated with itching, burning sensation and oozing. Sometimes there is intermittent bleeding (either spontaneously or after a scratch), foul-smelling discharge and even dysuria in advanced cases. *The diagnostic approach is initiated by a physical examination to assess the primary tumour and evaluate inguinal metastatic lymph nodes when present. A penile lesion that does not resolve after 2–3 weeks of careful observation and skin care requires biopsy*. Preferably excision biopsies should include enough tissue to determine the depth of invasion for accurate staging and subsequent planning of treatment. An incisional biopsy is recommended for large lesions [12].

At presentation, squamous cell carcinoma is found in the glans in 48 % of cases, in the prepuce in 21 %, in both glans and prepuce in 9 %, on the coronal sulcus in 6 % and in the shaft in <2 % [13].

Table 24.1 2010 AJCC staging for penile cancer [10]

Primary tumour (T)	
TX	Primary tumour cannot be assessed
T0	No evidence of primary tumour
Tis	Carcinoma in situ
Ta	Non-invasive verrucous carcinoma
T1	*Tumour invades subepithelial connective tissue*
T1a	Tumour invades subepithelial connective tissue without lymph vascular invasion and is not poorly differentiated
T1b	Tumour invades subepithelial connective tissue with lymph vascular invasion and is poorly differentiated
T2	*Tumour invades corpus spongiosum or cavernosum*
T3	*Tumour invades urethra*
T4	*Tumour invades other adjacent structures*
Regional lymph nodes (N)	
Clinical stage (palpation + imaging)	
cNX	Regional lymph nodes cannot be assessed
cN0	No palpable or visibly enlarged inguinal LN
cN1	Palpable mobile unilateral inguinal LN
cN2	Palpable mobile multiple or bilateral inguinal LN
cN3	Palpable fixed inguinal LN mass or pelvic lymphadenopathy unilateral or bilateral
Pathologic stage (biopsy or surgical excision)	
pTNX	Regional lymph nodes cannot be assessed
pTN0	No regional lymph node metastasis
pTN1	Metastasis in a single inguinal lymph node
pTN2	Metastasis in a multiple or bilateral inguinal lymph nodes
pTN3	Extranodal extension of lymph node metastasis or pelvic lymph node(s) unilateral or bilateral
Distant metastasis	
M0	No distant metastasis
M1	Distant metastasis (LN metastasis outside of the true pelvis in addition to visceral or bone sites)
Anatomic stage/prognostic groups	
Stage 0	TisN0M0 or TaN0M0
Stage I	T1aN0M0
Stage II	T1bN0M0 or T2N0M0 or T3N0M0
Stage IIIa	T1–3N1M0
Stage IIIb	T1–3N2M0
Stage IV	T4, any N, M0 or any T, N3, any M or any T, any N, M1

Used with the permission of the American Joint Committee on Cancer (AJCC), Chicago, Illinois. The original source for this material is the *AJCC Cancer Staging Manual*, Seventh Edition (2010), published by Springer Science and Business Media LLC. www.springer.com

In the past about 50 % of palpable inguinal LN (cN1–cN2) at presentation were considered to be inflammatory [13], *and it was common practice to first treat the patient with fluoroquinolones for 4–6 weeks. Only after that period were persistent LNs considered as metastatic and managed accordingly. Nowadays expert panels consider this old dogma no longer valid because metastatic disease is highly likely to be present in these patients. It is now recommended to proceed to fine needle aspiration cytology (FNAC) in all patients without delay, even in those with non-palpable LN where US guidance should be used* [14, 15]. *Furthermore, ILND should be considered for all diseases higher than pT1G2 even in N0 patients* [14]. Histopathology of the primary lesion is of paramount importance in *predicting the risk of locoregional extension*: this is increased by the presence of *vascular, neural or lymphatic invasion*, a *deep or high-grade tumour* or a *sarcomatoid variant* which has a 90 % risk of nodal extension. A study has shown that almost all patients with tumour depth of invasion *greater than 6 μm* and all patients with vascular invasion developed cancer progression after a mean follow-up of 28 months [16]. Conversely *Tis, pTa and verrucous carcinomas are never associated with nodal disease* [17]. Buschke-Löwenstein lesion or giant condyloma acumunata is a variant of verrucous carcinoma, a well-differentiated form of SCC representing about 5 % of penile SCC. It does not metastasize, but it is clinically important due to its ability to spread by local extension and eventually to destroy part or all the penile tissues if left untreated [18].

MRI imaging after intracavernosal contrast has shown great potential in local staging, accurately predicting corpora cavernosa invasion compared to histopathology, and was proven to be a reliable tool in selecting patients for partial penectomy [19].

Tomoscintigraphy, a combination of CT scan with scintigraphy after technetium 99, also called SPECT (single-photon emission computed tomography) is being evaluated for early sentinel lymph node detection [20].

Note: A difficult differential diagnosis may exist with an extramammary Paget's disease of the penis. This lesion presents as a penoscrotal erythematous lesion progressing for several months and resistant to antifungal drugs. It is in fact an intraepithelial adenocarcinoma often associated with a regional malignancy (prostate, bladder, colon, rectum) and readily diagnosed by biopsy. Isolated Paget's disease of the penis is extremely rare [21].

24.6 Disease Extension Imaging

Despite having low sensitivity for detecting pelvic or para-aortic LN metastases of a penile cancer, *CT scan remains the standard investigation because MRI does not perform any better* [22]. *Nonetheless CT is only indicated if inguinal LNs are positive, because there is no pelvic or aortic LNs invasion without initial involvement of the inguinal LNs* [23, 24].

PET-TDM using ^{18}F-FDG has been shown to have good sensitivity in N1 disease or higher and excellent specificity with an overall diagnostic accuracy of 89 % in detecting nodal and distant metastases of a penile cancer. It is recommended as a second imaging modality if inguinal LNs are clinically palpable when a suspicion of pelvic or distant disease persists after an inconclusive or negative CT scan [25, 26].

24.7 Treatment

24.7.1 Tis and Ta

If isolated small preputial lesion, a *circumcision* can be sufficient. *Systematic circumcision is recommended even in balanic localization.* An associated *partial glansectomy* remains a possibility for relatively large lesion provided there is a *1–2 mm healthy margin. Mohs technique* (serial progressive excision + histopathology) is preferable in such cases in order to ensure negative margins with minimal excision [27]. CO2 and Nd-Yag (neodymium-doped yttrium aluminium garnet) lasers are also suggested as organ-sparing tools [28]. Other conservative measures are cytotoxic cream (5-fluorouracil, imiquimod 5 %) and dynamic phototherapy. Surveillance is essential after these conservative procedures with reassessment every 3 months for 2 years. Complete removal of a non-invasive verrucous carcinoma can be achieved by thorough "shaving" of the lesion with optimal organ preservation (Fig. 24.1a–c).

24.7.2 T1

Same, but with a *3 mm margin*. CO2 and Nd-Yag laser can be applied. Beware of the 32 % recurrence rate following organ preservation procedures [29].

24.7.3 T2

- Involving solely the glans: partial glansectomy if the lesion occupies less than 50 % of the glans, otherwise total glansectomy.
- Extending proximal to the glans: partial penectomy is advocated provided a *2-cm negative margin* can be obtained and *a minimum 3 cm penile length* can be preserved to allow the patient to urinate without permanently soaking his scrotum. Otherwise, it is advised to proceed to a *total penectomy and perineal urostomy*. A total amputation can also be performed if the patient is not compliant with regular follow-up.

High-dose-rate ^{192}Iridium brachytherapy (*>60 Gy*) can also be given as conservative management in T1–T2 disease, but it harbours a high risk of urethral stenosis (20–40 %), necrosis and painful ulcerations (26 %) [30, 31].

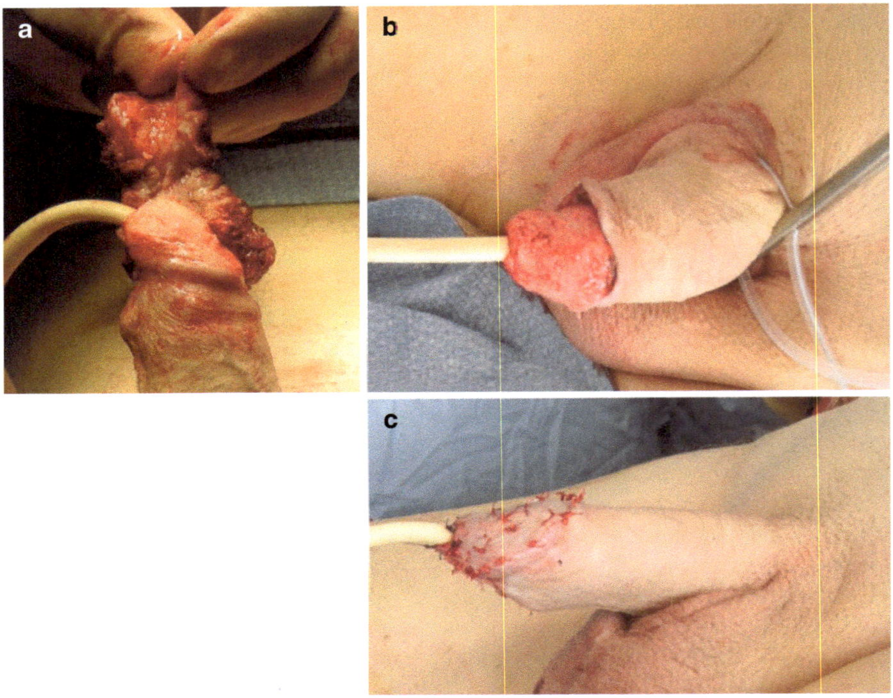

Fig. 24.1 (**a–c**) Shaving of a non-invasive verrucous carcinoma developed onto the glans. The growth was removed with a complete organ preservation. Figure (**c**) shows a split-thickness skin graft harvested from the thigh using a 0.5 mm dermatome (Courtesy N. Morel-Journel, Urology, CHU Lyon, France)

24.7.4 Management of Lymph Nodes

Ultrasonography and CT scan may be useful in the presence of an obese patient with LNs that are not palpable but in whom there is a strong clinical and pathological suspicion of nodal extension. If enlarged nodes are found by US, they should be needle-biopsied. *If biopsy is positive, LN dissection is indicated. If biopsy is negative, tomoscintigraphy should be performed to exclude a sentinel node*. If this is found, it should be removed along with the palpable LNs.

Accurate LN assessment is essential for prognosis and treatment [12].

- N0 : 100 % 5-year overall survival rate
- N1 : 92 % 5-year overall survival rate
- N2 : 68 % 5-year overall survival rate
- N3 : 31 % 5-year overall survival rate (Fig. 24.2a, b)

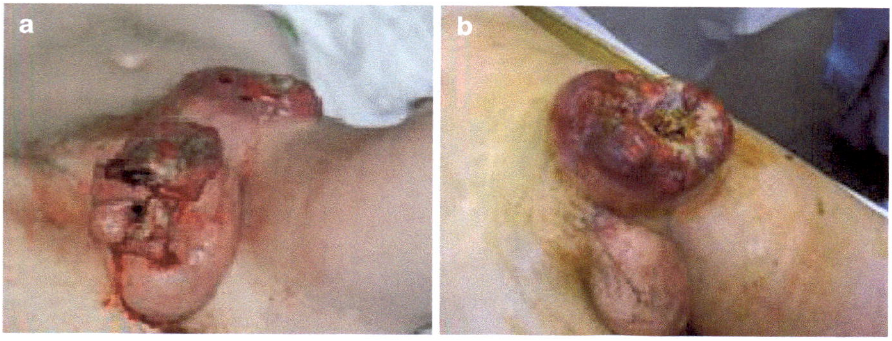

Fig. 24.2 (**a**, **b**) Extreme case of a penile SCC with fixed necrotic and ulcerated inguinal LN (Courtesy N. Morel-Journel, Urology, CHU Lyon, France)

Surveillance after primary tumour surgery is recommended only in patients with pTis, pTa and T1G1N0 disease and requires to have a well-informed, compliant patient [14].

A study has shown that 62 % of patients with N0 disease have inguinal nodal relapse with ¾ of the recurrence manifesting within 3 years after treatment of the primary lesion [23]. The only predicting factor for nodal relapse was shown to be the primary tumour grade at initial treatment. *In the long term, half of the patients with grade I disease and 100 % of all higher grades relapse* [23]. Consequently *while grade I patients may be offered surveillance or inguinal lymph nodes dissection (ILND), all higher grades patients must be treated with bilateral ILND.*

Hence, the importance of bilateral ILND despite the associated morbidity: Deep venous thrombosis, pulmonary embolism, wound infection, lymphocele, lymphoedema, bleeding and skin necrosis [32]. To reduce this morbidity, Catalona has suggested a controversial template for bilateral ILND where the sartorius muscles are not transpositioned, the saphenous veins are preserved and only deep LNs medial to them are dissected [33]. However, this was proven to bear a large number of false-negative results [34].

Therefore, the classic ILND remains the recommended approach [15]: The skin is incised parallel to and 2 cm above the inguinal ligament. The superficial LNs (8–25 in number, found between superficial fascia and fascia lata) and deep LNs (3–5 in number, deep to fascia lata around the fossa ovalis) are removed. *The saphenous veins are sacrificed, and the sartorius muscles are transpositioned to cover the femoral vessels* (Fig 24.3a, b). *Lymphostasis is meticulously performed with suture materials, and cautery is avoided.* The skin should be preserved as much as possible. When large skin and subcutaneous tissues have been removed, the wound can be covered using scrotal skin. In extreme cases, it may be necessary to mobilize a transverse or a vertical rectus abdominis muscle (TRAM or VRAM) myocutaneous

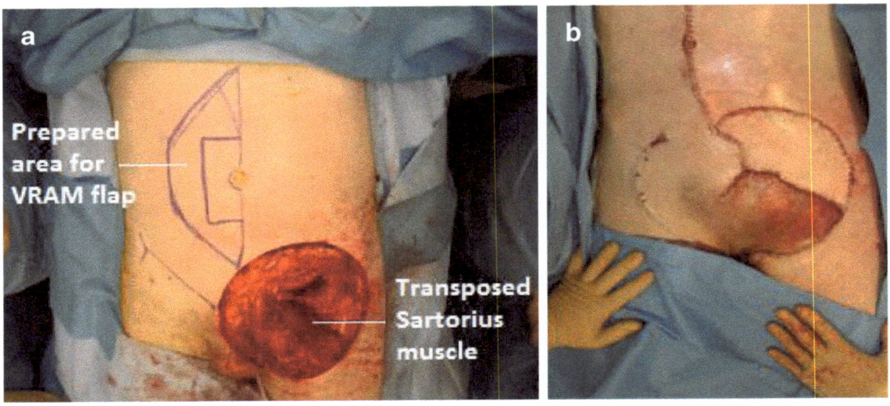

Fig. 24.3 (**a**, **b**) Use of a scrotal and a vertical rectus abdominis muscle (VRAM) flaps to cover a large wound left after ILND (Same patient in Fig. 24.2). Sartorius muscle was transpositioned to cover the iliac vessels (Courtesy N. Morel-Journel, Urology, CHU Lyon, France)

flaps to cover the wound (Fig. 24.3a, b). The patient is given *anticoagulant therapy* + anti-embolism compression stockings commonly referred to as thromboembolism-deterrent (*TED*) stockings + *prophylactic antibiotics*.

Standard or robotic-assisted laparoscopic approaches are emerging techniques successfully performed by some pioneers as an effective and less mutilating method to perform the ILND [35–37].

Surgery alone involving removal of the primary lesion with ILND may be considered curative in pN1 patients. For N2–3 disease, a multimodal approach combining surgery and chemotherapy or radiotherapy must be undertaken after multidisciplinary discussions [24].

Take-Home Message: Penile Cancer

Epidemiology	Penile cancers are very rare with higher incidence recorded in Latin America and Africa than in western countries. It generally affects old men.
Risk factors	*Poor genital hygiene* and *human papillomavirus (HPV) types 16 and 18 with condyloma acumunata are the most commonly reported aetiological factors*. Others are balanitis xerotica obliterans (BXO) (penile equivalent of lichen sclerosis et atrophicus), smoking, phimosis and treatment with psoralen and ultraviolet A photochemotherapy.
Prevention	*Hygiene, neonatal circumcision* and *HPV vaccine (on trial).*
Histopathology	Erythroplasia of Queyrat and Bowen's disease are CIS and differ only by their anatomical locations. *Squamous cell carcinoma (SCC) is encountered in 95 % of cases of invasive penile cancer.*

Presentation	*A painless non-healing ulcer is the commonest complaint.*
	Overall 30 % of penile cancer are diagnosed at advanced stage.
Diagnosis of the primary lesion	*Excision biopsy must be performed for any suspicious penile cancer.*
	MRI with intracavernosal contrast can reliably define intracavernosal invasion and helps in selecting patients for partial penectomy.
	Once the positive diagnosis of the primary lesion has been reached, it is recommended to proceed to FNAC of the inguinal LNs, even for patients with non-palpable LNs. In the latter group, US guidance should be used.
Nodal disease risk factors	*Unfavourable factors: presence of vascular, neural or lymphatic invasion, deep (>6 μm) or high-grade tumour or a sarcomatoid variant.*
	Favourable factors: Tis, pTa and verrucous carcinomas which are never associated with nodal disease.
Disease extension investigations	*CT scan is the standard method to evaluate pelvic, abdominal and chest disease extension.* However, its sensitivity is low for LN metastasis. It should not be requested when inguinal LNs are negative.
	PET-TDM using ^{18}F-FDG has a better specificity and sensitivity and is recommended as a second-line imaging method in highly suspicious patients with initially negative CT.
Treatment of the primary lesion	Conservative management is possible with T1 and selected T2 cases but requires close follow-up.
	MOHS technique is the best technique for all organ-sparing surgeries to ensure negative margin with the least amount of tissue as possible sacrificed.
	High-dose-rate ^{192}iridium brachytherapy (>60 Gy) can also be offered to T1–T2 patients for organ-sparing purpose but is associated with many local complications (urethral stenosis, necrosis and painful ulcerations)
Management of inguinal LN	After a negative biopsy in highly suspicious cases, a tomoscintigraphy is indicated to locate an eventual sentinel node which should be removed along with the associated LN group.
	Surveillance after primary tumour surgery is recommended only in patients with pTis, pTa and T1G1N0 disease, but a well-informed, compliant patient is essential. For all other stages, the control of nodal disease is paramount in the management of penile cancer.
	ILND should be considered for all patients higher than pT1G2 even in N0 patients.
	Classic bilateral ILND is the standard despite the associated morbidity.

References

1. Chaux A, Netto GJ, Rodríguez IM, et al. Epidemiologic profile, sexual history, pathologic features, and human papillomavirus status of 103 patients with penile carcinoma. World J Urol. 2013;31(4):861–7.
2. Parkin DM, Whelan SL, Ferlay J, et al. Cancer incidence in five continents, vol. VIII. IARC Scientific Publications No. 155. Lyon: IARC; 2002.
3. Wabinga H, Parkin D, Wabwire-Mangen F, Nambooze S. Trends in cancer incidence in Kyadondo County, Uganda 1960–1997. Br J Cancer. 2000;82:1585–92.
4. Rubin M, Kleter B, Zhou M, Ayala G, Cubilla A, Quint W, et al. Detection and typing of human papillomavirus DNA in penile carcinoma: evidence for multiple independent pathways of penile carcinogenesis. Am J Pathol. 2001;159:1211–8.
5. Licklider S. Jewish penile carcinoma. J Urol. 1961;86:98.
6. Schoen EJ, Oehrli M, Colby C, et al. The highly protective effect of newborn circumcision against invasive penile cancer. Pediatrics. 2000;105:E36.
7. Tsen HF, Morgenstern H, Mack T, et al. Risk factors for penile cancer: results of a population-based case-control study in Los Angeles County (United States). Cancer Causes Control. 2001;12:267–77.
8. Shabbir M, Barod R, Hegarty PK, Minhas S. Primary prevention and vaccination for penile cancer. Ther Adv Urol. 2013;5(3):161–9.
9. Broders AC. Squamous-cell epithelioma of the skin: a study of 256 cases. Ann Surg. 1921;73(2):141–60.
10. Penis. In: Edge SB, Byrd DR, Compton CC, editors. AJCC Cancer Staging Manual. 7th ed. New York: Springer, 2010. p. 447–55.
11. Culkin DJ, Beer TM. Advanced penile carcinoma. J Urol. 2003;170(2 Pt 1):359–65.
12. Pow-Sang MR, Benavente V, Pow-Sang JE, et al. Cancer of the penis. Cancer Control. 2002;9(4):305–14.
13. Sufrin G, Huber R. Benign and malignant lesions of the penis. In: Gillenwater JY, Howards SS, Duckett JW, editors. Adult and pediatric urology. 2nd ed. St Louis: Mosby-Year Book; 1991; 1943.
14. Hakenberg OW, Comperat E, Minhas S, Necchi A, Protzel C, Watkin N. Guinelines on Penile Cancer. Eur Urol. 2015;67(1):142–50.
15. Heyns CF, Fleshner N, Sangar V, Schlenker B, Yuvaraja TB, van Poppel H. Management of the lymph nodes in penile cancer. Urology. 2010;76(2 Suppl 1):S43–57.
16. Emerson RE, Ulbright TM, Eble JN, Geary WA, Eckert GJ, Cheng L. Predicting cancer progression in patients with penile squamous cell carcinoma: the importance of depth of invasion and vascular invasion. Mod Pathol. 2001;14(10):963–8.
17. Guimarães GC, Lopes A, Campos RS, Zequi Sde C, Leal ML, Carvalho AL, da Cunha IW, Soares FA. Front pattern of invasion in squamous cell carcinoma of the penis: new prognostic factor for predicting risk of lymph node metastases. Urology. 2006;68(1):148–53.
18. Lynch Jr DF. Cancer of the penis. In: Kufe DW, Pollock RE, Weichselbaum RR, Bast RC, Gansler TS, Holland JF, Frei E, editors. Holland-Frei cancer medicine. 6th ed. Hamilton: BC Decker; 2003.
19. Kayes O, Minhas S, Allen C, Hare C, Freeman A, Ralph D. The role of magnetic resonance imaging in the local staging of penile cancer. Eur Urol. 2007;51(5):1313–8; discussion 1318–9.
20. Brouwer OR, van den Berg NS, Mathéron HM, Wendler T, van der Poel HG, Horenblas S, Valdés Olmos RA, van Leeuwen FW. Feasibility of intraoperative navigation to the sentinel node in the groin using preoperatively acquired single photon emission computerized tomography data: transferring functional imaging to the operating room. J Urol. 2014;192:1810–6. pii: S0022-5347(14)04046-4.
21. Ekwueme KC, Zakhour HD, Parr NJ. Extramammary Paget's disease of the penis: a case report and review of the literature. J Med Case Reports. 2009;3:4.

22. Vapnek JM, Hricak H, Carroll PR. Recent advances in imaging studies for staging of penile and urethral carcinoma. Urol Clin North Am. 1992;19(2):257–66.
23. Cabanas RM. An approach for the treatment of penile carcinoma. Cancer. 1977;39(2): 456–66.
24. Theodorescu D, Russo P, Zhang ZF, Morash C, Fair WR. Outcomes of initial surveillance of invasive squamous cell carcinoma of the penis and negative nodes. J Urol. 1996;155(5): 1626–31.
25. Rigaud J, C. Avancès C, Camparo P et al. CCAFU members. Recommandations en onco-urologie 2013 du CCAFU: tumeurs malignes du pénis. Prog Urol. 2013;23 Suppl 2:S135–4.
26. Souillac I, Rigaud J, Ansquer C, Marconnet L, Bouchot O. Prospective evaluation of (18) F-fluorodeoxyglucose positron emission tomography-computerized tomography to assess inguinal lymph node status in invasive squamous cell carcinoma of the penis. J Urol. 2012;187(2):493–7.
27. Mohs FE, Snow SN, Larson PO, et al. Mohs micrographic surgery for penile tumours. Urol Clin North Am. 1992;19:291–304.
28. Horenblas S, van Tinteren H, Delemarre JF, et al. Squamous cell carcinoma of the penis. II. Treatment of the primary tumour. J Urol. 1992;147:1533–8.
29. Gerber GS. Carcinoma in situ of the penis. J Urol. 1994;151:829–33.
30. Rozan R, Albuisson E, Giraud B, et al. Interstitial brachytherapy for penile carcinoma: a multicentric survey (259 patients). Radiother Oncol. 1995;36(2):83–93.
31. De Crevoisier R, Slimane K, Sanfilippo N, Bossi A, Albano M, Dumas I, et al. Long-term results of brachytherapy for carcinoma of the penis confined to the glans (N-or NX). Int J Radiat Oncol Biol Phys. 2009;74:1150–6.
32. Horenblas S, van Tinteren H. Squamous cell carcinoma of the penis. IV. Prognostic factors of survival: analysis of tumour, nodes and metastasis classification system. J Urol. 1994;151:1239–43.
33. Catalona WJ. Modified inguinal lymphadenectomy for carcinoma of the penis with preservation of saphenous veins: technique and preliminary results. J Urol. 1988;140:306–10.
34. Marconnet L, Rigaud J, Bouchot O. Long-term follow-up of penile carcinoma with high risk for lymph node invasion treated with inguinal lymphadenectomy. J Urol. 2010;183(6): 2227–32.
35. Sotelo R, Sánchez-Salas R, Carmona O, Garcia A, Mariano M, Neiva G, et al. Endoscopic lymphadenectomy for penile carcinoma. J Endourol. 2007;21:364–7.
36. Josephson DY, Jacobsohn KM, Link BA, Wilson TG. Robotic-assisted endoscopic inguinal lymphadenectomy. Urology. 2009;73:167–71.
37. Dogra PN, Saini AK, Singh P. Robotic-assisted inguinal lymph node dissection: a preliminary report. Indian J Urol. 2011;27(3):424–7.

Part VI
Adrenal Gland Cancer

Said Abdallah Al-Mamari and Salim Said Al-Busaidy

Introduction

Primary malignant adrenal tumours usually occur in the cortex and are referred to as *adrenocortical carcinomas (ACC), which comprise of 90 % of all adrenal cancers* [1]. Other cancers encountered in the adrenal glands include malignant phaeochromocytomas (MPC) which occur in the medullar part of the gland, and secondary tumours from other organs. In this part, we will mainly consider the primary adrenocortical carcinoma, giving only a brief account of the MPC.

Reference

1. Correa P, Chen VW. Endocrine gland cancer. Cancer (Phila). 1995;75:338–52.

Chapter 25
Epidemiology, Aetiological Factors, Symptoms and Signs of ACC

Said Abdallah Al-Mamari and Salim Said Al-Busaidy

25.1 Epidemiology and Aetiological Factors

The annual incidence of ACC is *1–2 in a 1,000,000 population* [1] with a *bimodal age incidence* peaking in the first and fifth decades of life [2]. In fact the disease mostly occurs in children below 5 years of age and in adults aged between 40 and 50 years. There is a slight female predominance with a F/M ratio of 3/2, and it has been observed that more women develop functioning ACCs in contrast to men who develop more nonfunctioning ACC [3].

The vast majority of cases are sporadic, but there are some genetically linked syndromes which predispose to adrenal tumours especially in the paediatric age group: Beckwith-Wiedemann syndrome, Li-Fraumeni syndrome, familial adenomatous polyposis (FAP), multiple endocrine neoplasia (MEN1) and hereditary non-polyposis colorectal cancer (Lynch syndrome). Smoking and use of oral contraceptives have also been incriminated [4] but there are few randomized studies to support these associations.

At presentation only 30 % of ACC are confined to the gland. Fortunately, this is a very rare tumour, accounting for *only 3 % of all endocrine cancers* [5]. However, adrenal tumours are among the most frequent tumours discovered incidentally at autopsy, being present in at least 3 % of individuals over the age of 50. Nonetheless most adrenal masses have no clinical consequences, and *approximately 1 out of every 4,000 adrenal tumours is malignant* [6]. ACCs have a *poor prognosis* with reported overall 5-year survival rates varying from 10.3 % in older series [7] to 37 % in newer studies [8]. Cortisol-secreting tumours in particular have the worse prognosis.

S.A. Al-Mamari (✉)
Urology Department, The Royal Hospital, Muscat, Oman
e-mail: sabdal67@yahoo.com

S.S. Al-Busaidy
Senior Consultant and HOD, Urology Department, The Royal Hospital, Muscat, Oman
e-mail: salimalbusaidy@hotmail.com

S.A. Al-Mamari, S.S. Al-Busaidy (eds.), *Urological Cancer Management*,
DOI 10.1007/978-3-319-16301-7_25

25.2 Symptoms and Signs

Malignant features of adrenal tumours are consistent with the presence of:

- *Virilizing symptoms in women* (mostly associated with Cushing's syndrome) or, more rarely, *feminization in men*. 62 % of adrenocortical carcinoma are functional (i.e. have hormonal activity), while 38 % are non-functional [9].
- *Ipsilateral loin or abdominal pain, fever, anorexia, weight loss.*
- *Palpable mass* on physical examination, which is consistent with a large tumour burden.

The different syndromes caused by an excess of adrenocortical hormone secretion are Cushing's syndrome or hypercortisolism, adrenogenital syndrome with virilization (excess testosterone production in females) or feminization (excess oestrogen production in males), precocious puberty and Conn's syndrome (hyperaldosteronism).

Exceptionally the tumour may present as an acute abdomen due to a rupture with extensive retroperitoneal haemorrhage [10, 11] or renal vein thrombosis and varicocele [12].

Unlike the paediatric population, ACCs in adults present more commonly as *a mixed clinical picture with features of both Cushing and virilizing syndromes* due to the overproduction of corticoids and androgens. The tumour runs a far *more aggressive course* leading to a rapid death within months or a few years [2].

A number of patients are discovered to have unsuspected adrenal tumours during investigations for unrelated medical conditions. *These tumours are called "incidentalomas" because they are discovered incidentally and without any clinical presentation related to them. They are reported to occur in about 5 % of abdominal CT scans* [13]. Once discovered, these tumours have to be evaluated to determine whether they are hormonally active or nonfunctioning and whether they are malignant or benign. Secretion of sexual hormones (mainly androgens) by an adrenal incidentaloma is in favour of a malignancy; however, the majority of them are benign adenomas and *less than 5 % will be proven to be malignant.*

Take-Home Message. ACC: Epidemiology, Symptoms, Signs

Epidemiology	ACC = 90 % of all adrenal cancers
	The annual incidence is *1–2 in a 1,000,000 population*
	Bimodal age incidence: below 5 years in children and between age 40 and 50 years
	Vast majority are sporadic. Some genetically linked associations
	At presentation, only 30 % of ACC are confined to the adrenal gland
	Only about 1 ACC out of every 4,000 adrenal tumours
	Poor prognosis
Symptoms and signs	In functioning tumours (62 % of cases): Virilization in females and feminization of males
	Ipsilateral loin or abdominal pain, fever, anorexia, weight loss
	Palpable mass on physical examination, which means a large tumour burden
	Rarely varicocoele, acute abdominal signs
	Incidental findings (incidentaloma)

References

1. Lombardi G, Rossi R. Adrenocortical carcinoma: 12 years prospective experience. World J Surg. 2004;28:896–903.
2. Wajchenberg BL, Albergaria Pereira MA, Medonca BB, et al. Adrenocortical carcinoma: clinical and laboratory observations. Cancer. 2000;88(4):711–36.
3. Crucitti F, Bellantone R, Ferrante A, Boscherini M, Crucitti P. The Italian Registry for Adrenal Cortical Carcinoma: analysis of a multiinstitutional series of 129 patients. The ACC Italian Registry Study Group. Surgery. 1996;119(2):161–70.
4. Hsing AW, Nam J-M, Co Chien HT, McLaughlin JK, Fraumeni Jr JF. Risk factors for adrenal cancer: an exploratory study. Int J Cancer. 1996;65(4):432–6.
5. Correa P, Chen VW. Endocrine gland cancer. Cancer. 1995;75:338–52.
6. Grumbach MM, Biller BMK, Braunstein GD, et al. NIH state-of-the-science statement on management of the clinically inapparent adrenal mass ("incidentaloma"). NIH Consens State Sci Statements. 2002;19(2):1–25.
7. Favia G, Lumachi F, D'Amico DF. Adrenocortical carcinoma: is prognosis different in nonfunctioning tumours? results of surgical treatment in 31 patients. World J Surg. 2001;25:735–8.
8. Abiven G, Coste J, Groussin L, et al. Clinical and biological features in the prognosis of adrenocortical cancer: poor outcome of cortisol-secreting tumours in a series of 202 consecutive patients. J Clin Endocrinol Metab. 2006;91(7):2650–5.
9. Ng L, Libertino J. Adrenocortical carcinoma: diagnosis, evaluation and treatment. J Urol. 2003;169:5–11.
10. Jagtap SV, Desai S, Halder S, Jagtap SS, Badwe AS. Adrenocortical carcinoma presenting as a rupture and extensive retroperitoneal haemorrhage. J Clin Diagn Res. 2014;8(3):117–8.
11. Symeonidis D, Chatzinikolaou I, Koukoulis G, Mamaloudis I, Tepetes K. Adrenocortical carcinoma presenting with signs of acute abdomen. Case Rep Surg. 2013;2013:132726.
12. Cheungpasitporn W, Horne JM, Howarth CB. Adrenocortical carcinoma presenting as varicocele and renal vein thrombosis: a case report. J Med Case Rep. 2011;5:337.
13. Blake MA, Cronin CG, Boland GW. Adrenal imaging. AJR Am J Roentgenol. 2010;194(6):1450–60.

Chapter 26
Investigations

Said Abdallah Al-Mamari and Salim Said Al-Busaidy

26.1 Primary Diagnosis Means

CT scan is the standard imaging modality for diagnosing an adrenocortical carcinoma [1].

In most cases, it allows differentiation of benign tumours such as adenoma and myelolipoma (Fig. 26.1) from malignant growths.

Before IV contrast injection, a density ≤10 Hounsfield Units (HU), a homogenous appearance, and neat contours are features of a benign tumour, while malignant cortical adrenal tumours generally have a consistent *density value ≥18 HU*. Another characteristic feature seen in primary ACC, pheochromocytomas and metastatic tumours is the relatively *slow contrast wash out* [2]. *A decrease of more than 40 % of the maximal enhancement 10 min after the injection has been reported to be pathognomonic of an adenoma* [3].

The tumour size is another important feature to differentiate between a benign mass and an ACC. According to statistical data collected from a large series, the likelihood of malignancy doubles (to 10 %) at a threshold of ≥*4 cm* and rises to more than ninefold (47 %) for tumours ≥*8 cm* [4, 5] (Fig. 26.2a, b).

Gadolinium-enhanced MRI may be an alternative in patients allergic to iodinated contrast.

Once suspicion of an ACC is raised by other investigations, *18F-FDG PET appears to be the standard imaging means to "ascertain" the diagnosis* because of its reported 100 % sensitivity and negative predictive value (Fig. 26.3a–d) [6]. A threshold ratio of 1.8 between the maximum standardized uptake values (SUVmax)

S.A. Al-Mamari (✉)
Urology Department, The Royal Hospital, Muscat, Oman
e-mail: sabdal67@yahoo.com

S.S. Al-Busaidy
Senior Consultant and HOD, Urology Department, The Royal Hospital, Muscat, Oman
e-mail: salimalbusaidy@hotmail.com

S.A. Al-Mamari, S.S. Al-Busaidy (eds.), *Urological Cancer Management*,
DOI 10.1007/978-3-319-16301-7_26

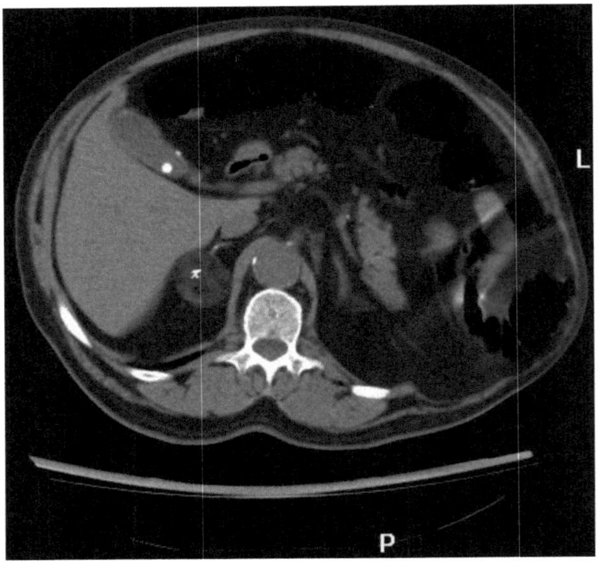

Fig. 26.1 CT scan showing a very rare case of adrenal myelolipoma on the right side. This is a low-density benign tumour consistent with fat content (Courtesy of S. Novellas, Radiology, Arnault-Tzanck Institute, Saint-Laurent- du- Var and CHU Nice, Nice, France)

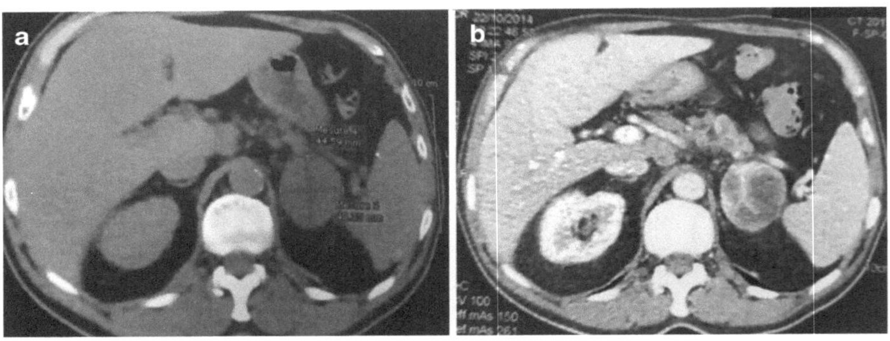

Fig. 26.2 (**a**, **b**) CT scan showing a 45 × 40 mm enhancing mass above the left kidney consistent with a left adrenal ACC in a 70-year-old man

of the tumour and that of the liver demonstrated 100 % sensitivity and specificity after correlation with the final histological diagnosis [6]. *A cutoff SUV of 3.1 was also proposed as a reliable demarcation point between malignant lesions and adrenal adenomas* with sensitivity, specificity, positive predictive value and negative predictive value of 98.5 %, 92 %, 89.3 %, 98.9 %, respectively [7].

Nine histological criteria of Weiss were used to predict tumour malignancy and prognosis: Fuhrman nuclear grade III or IV (see Chap. 13, Table 13.2), >5 mitosis/50 HPF, atypical mitosis, cytoplasm characteristics (less than 25 % of clear vacuolated cells being an unfavourable factor), diffuse architecture, tumour necrosis, venous invasion, sinusoid invasion and capsular invasion [8]. Each criterion is scored 1 when present. A total score >3 is predictive of malignancy. In view of the possible subjectivity inherent to the interpretation of some criteria of Weiss, a

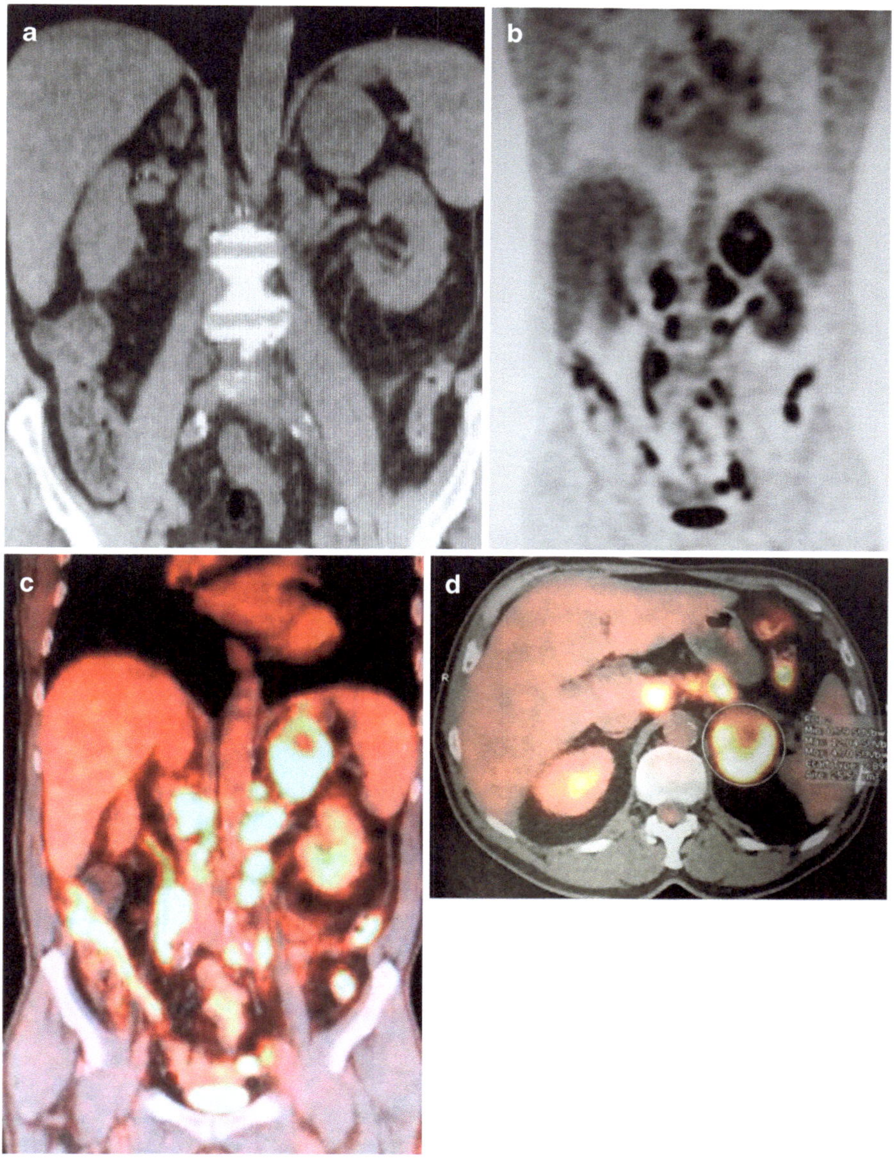

Fig. 26.3 (**a–d**) Same patient of Fig. 26.2. (**a**) Plain CT scan. (**b**) FDG-^{18}F-PET. (**c**) Fusion PET-TDM showing a 45 × 48 mm hypermetabolic left adrenal tumour with SUV max 12, consistent with a ACC. There is a necrotic centre. There are also multiple hyperactive associated LNs SUV max from 9.1 to 13.1. (**d**) PET-TDM in horizontal section

retrospective study proposed to double the weight of the 2 most reliable ones, i.e. the mitotic rate and the cytoplasm characteristics. In this *modified Weiss criteria*, presence of atypical mitosis, tumour necrosis and capsular invasion are still considered with a score 1 while the remaining has been abandoned [9].

However, *histopathological diagnosis of ACC remains challenging as the distinction from a benign adenoma is generally difficult.* A French study has identified *3 molecular predictors* using tumour RNA micro-arrays as novel tools for the detection of malignancy and for predicting survival [10]: the combination of DLG7 and PINK1 for malignancy signature and the combined expression of BUB1B and PINK1 as predictors of survival.

More recently a novel steroid metabolomics[1] approach was proposed to help in the differential diagnosis between an ACC and an adrenal adenoma [11]. This is a simplified diagnostic tool based on the identification of only 9 adrenal steroids from a 24-h urinary collection with properties that are most helpful in differentiating the malignant from the benign variety. This investigation is virtually equal in sensitivity and specificity to the currently used fastidious 32 steroid-based study.

Transcutaneous biopsy of the ACC is currently not recommended for the diagnosis of a primary ACC because of poor diagnostic value and possible complications (bleeding, tumour cell spillage), although a recent retrospective study has shown that it does not affect the recurrence-free or overall survival [12].

The use of a fine-needle biopsy should be restricted to [13]:

- A suspected secondary tumour in patients with a history of other cancers (particularly lung, breast, kidney), with no signs of other metastases
- A heterogeneous mass with high unenhanced attenuation value (>20 HU) after exclusion of pheochromocytoma

26.2 Disease Extension Investigations and Staging

These consist of the use of gadolinium-enhanced MRI and/or 18F-FDG PET scans.

Adrenal tumours metastasize most frequently to *the lungs (72 %) and liver (55 %).* Other sites include the peritoneum (33 %), bones (24 %), the contralateral adrenal gland (15 %) and brain (10 %) [14].

The first staging classification of ACC was proposed by MacFarlane over half century ago [15], which included four criteria: tumour size, lymph nodes, local invasion and metastases. This was later modified by Sullivan [16], and the first TNM classification was introduced in 2003 by the Union Internationale Contre le Cancer (UICC). More recently the European Network for the Study of Adrenal Tumours (ENSAT) developed a revised staging system [17] (Table 26.1). Its superiority in predicting cancer-specific mortality was corroborated by subsequent studies [18, 19].

---

[1] Bennett Daviss defines the term "Metabolomics" as "the systematic study of the unique chemical fingerprints that specific cellular processes leave behind". http://www.the-scientist.com/?articles.view/articleNo/16400/title/Growing-Pains-for-Metabolomics/

Table 26.1 New Staging System for adrenocortical carcinoma (European Network for the Study of Adrenal tumour Classification 2008). ENSAT 2008

Primary tumour (T)	T1, tumour ≤5 cm; T2, tumour >5 cm; T3, any size, tumour infiltration into surrounding tissue; T4, tumour invasion into adjacent organs or venous tumour thrombus in vena cava or renal vein
Lymph nodes (N)	N0, no positive lymph node; N1, positive lymph node(s)
Distant metastasis (M)	M0, no distant metastases; M1, presence of distant metastasis
Anatomic stages (prognostic groups)	
I	T1, N0, M0
II	T2, N0, M0
III	T1-T2, N1, M0 or T3-T4, N0-N1, M0
IV	T1-T4, N0-N1, M1
In summary:	
Stage I – tumour less than 5 cm; in adrenal gland	
Stage II – tumour greater than 5 cm; in adrenal gland	
Stage III – tumour of any size; has spread to lymph nodes near adrenal glands	
Stage IV – tumour of any size; has spread to lungs, bones, liver and/or abdominal wall	

Reproduced from Fassnacht et al. [17], with permission from John Wiley and Sons

Take-Home Message. ACC: Investigations

Primary diagnosis	*TDM is the standard means with two characteristic features:*
	Density ≥18 HU before contrast and slow wash out *Larger tumour size increases the likelihood of malignancy: 10 % if ≥4 cm, 47 % if ≥8 cm*
	Gadolinium-enhanced MRI is an alternative in patients allergic to iodinated contrast
	When suspicion is raised by TDM or MRI, *18F-FDG PET appears to be the standard imaging means to "ascertain" the diagnosis* (100 % sensitivity and negative predictive value). *A cutoff SUV of 3.1 can be used to differentiate ACC from adrenal adenomas*
	The histopathological distinction between ACC and adenoma remains challenging and the definitive diagnosis generally relies on the presence of distant metastasis and/or local invasion
	Transcutaneous biopsy of the ACC is currently not recommended
Disease extension investigations	*Based on gadolinium-enhanced MRI and/or 18F-FDG PET*
	Metastatic sites are *lungs (72 %), liver (55 %),* peritoneum (33 %), bones (24 %), contralateral adrenal gland (15 %) and the brain (10 %)
	The revised ENSAT classification appears to be the best today in predicting cancer-specific mortality

References

1. Sèbe P, Rigaud J, Avancès C et al. Les membres de l'AFCE; Les membres du CCAFU. CCAFU's contribution to the French National Cancer Institute's reference frame: adrenal malignant tumours. Prog Urol. 2013;23(Suppl 2):S167–74.
2. Szolar DH, Korobkin M, Reittner P, et al. Adrenocortical carcinomas and adrenal pheochromocytomas: mass and enhancement loss evaluation at delayed contrast-enhanced CT. Radiology. 2005;234:479–85.
3. Slattery JM, Blake MA, Kalra MK, Misdraji J, Sweeney AT, Copeland PM, Mueller PR, Boland GW. Adrenocortical carcinoma: contrast washout characteristics on CT. AJR Am J Roentgenol. 2006;187(1):W21–4.
4. Sturgeon C, Shen WT, Clark OH, Duh QY, Kebebew E. Risk assessment in 457 adrenal cortical carcinomas : how much does tumour size predict the likelihood of malignancy ? J Am Coll Surg. 2006;202:423–30.
5. Mege D, Taieb D, Lowery A, Loundou A, DE Micco C, Castinetti F, Morange I, Henry JF, Sebag F. Contemporary review of large adrenal tumours in a tertiary referral center. Anticancer Res. 2014;34(5):2581–8.
6. Tessonnier L, Sebag F, Palazzo FF, Colavolpe C, De Micco C, Mancini J, Conte-Devolx B, Henry JF, Mundler O, Taïeb D. Does 18 F-FDG PET/CT add diagnostic accuracy in incidentally identified non-secreting adrenal tumours? Eur J Nucl Med Mol Imaging. 2008; 35(11):2018–25.
7. Metser U, Miller E, Lerman H, Lievshitz G, Avital S, Even-Sapir E. 18 F-FDG PET/CT in the evaluation of adrenal masses. J Nucl Med. 2006;47(1):32–7.
8. Weiss LM. Comparative histologic study of 43 metastasizing and nonmetastasizing adrenocortical tumours. Am J Surg Pathol. 1984;8(3):163–9.
9. Aubert S, Wacrenier A, Leroy X, Devos P, Carnaille B, Proye C, Wemeau JL, Lecomte-Houcke M, Leteurtre E. Weiss system revisited: a clinicopathologic and immunohistochemical study of 49 adrenocortical tumours. Am J Surg Pathol. 2002;26(12):1612–9.
10. de Reyniès A, Assié G, Rickman DS, et al. Gene expression profiling reveals a New classification of adrenocortical tumours and identifies molecular predictors of malignancy and survival. J Clin Oncol. 2009;27:7.
11. Arlt W, Biehl M, Taylor AE, et al. Urine steroid metabolomics as a biomarker tool for detecting malignancy in adrenal tumours. J Clin Endocrinol Metab. 2011;96(12):3775–84.
12. Williams AR, Hammer GD, Else T. Transcutaneous biopsy of adrenocortical carcinoma is rarely helpful in diagnosis, potentially harmful, but does not affect patient outcome. Eur J Endocrinol. 2014;170(6):829–35.
13. Schteingart DE, Doherty GM, Gauger PG, et al. Management of patients with adrenal cancer: recommendations of an international consensus conference. Endocr Relat Cancer. 2005; 12:667–80.
14. Proye CAG, Pattou FN, Armstrong J. Primary adrenocortical carcinoma. In: Linos DA, van Heerden JA, editors. Adrenal glands: diagnostic aspects and surgical therapy. Berlin/ Heidelberg: Springer; 2005. p. 136.
15. MacFarlane DA. Cancer of the adrenal cortex; the natural history, prognosis and treatment in a study of fifty-five cases. Ann R Coll Surg Engl. 1958;23(3):155–86.
16. Sullivan M, Boileau M, Hodges CV. Adrenal cortical carcinoma. J Urol. 1978;120(6):660–5.
17. Fassnacht M, Johanssen S, Quinkler M, et al. Limited prognostic value of the 2004 International Union Against Cancer staging classification for adrenocortical carcinoma: proposal for a Revised TNM Classification. Cancer. 2009;115(2):243–50.
18. Lughezzani G, Sun M, Perrotte P, Jeldres C, Alasker A, Isbarn H, Budäus L, Shariat SF, Guazzoni G, Montorsi F, Karakiewicz PI. The European Network for the Study of Adrenal Tumours staging system is prognostically superior to the international union against cancer-staging system: a North American validation. Eur J Cancer. 2010;46(4):713–9.
19. Fassnacht M, Wittekind C, Allolio B. Current TNM classification systems for adrenocortical carcinoma. Pathologe. 2010;31(5):374–8.

Chapter 27
Treatment

Said Abdallah Al-Mamari and Salim Said Al-Busaidy

A multidisciplinary approach is required in the management of these adrenocortical cancers which should include opinions from the endocrinologist, medical oncologist, radiologist, nuclear oncologist (radiotherapist), pathologist and either the endocrine surgeon or urologist. In the paediatric age group, opinion of the geneticist is also necessary. Nonfunctioning cortical adenomas <4–5 cm in size do not require any treatment, but should be followed up clinically and radiographically [1]. *Tumours greater than 5 cm should be regarded as potentially malignant and be treated accordingly.*

27.1 Surgery

All solid incidentalomas greater than 5 cm on CT or MRI should be removed surgically [2]. Many centres are now routinely performing total adrenalectomy through a laparoscopic approach, although open surgery remains a common practice.

27.2 Medical Treatment

Reserved for inoperable tumours or for secreting tumours requiring hormonal control before surgery. Two categories of drugs are used:

S.A. Al-Mamari (✉) • S.S. Al-Busaidy
Urology Department, The Royal Hospital, Muscat, Oman
e-mail: sabdal67@yahoo.com; salimalbusaidy@hotmail.com

S.A. Al-Mamari, S.S. Al-Busaidy (eds.), *Urological Cancer Management*,
DOI 10.1007/978-3-319-16301-7_27

27.2.1 Mitotane (Lysodren®)

This drug is also known as o,p'-DDD. It is an isomer of the DDD (dichlorodiphenyldichloroethane) which is derived from the well-known insecticide DDT (dichlorodiphenyltrichloroethane). The biochemical mechanism of action of this drug is not yet fully understood, but several studies have shown that it suppresses gene transcription of different enzymatic steps of the steroidogenetic pathway, and induces the cytochrome P450 3A4 (CYP3A4) expression, thus accelerating the metabolic clearance of a variety of drugs including steroids.

Mitotane is the standard treatment and indicated in the following situations where it has been reported to be beneficial in the overall and recurrence-free survival rates [3]:

- Unresectable or metastatic adrenocortical tumours
- Incompletely resected tumours as an adjuvant therapy
- Secreting tumours before surgery

Furthermore, a large multicentre Italian and German study has also suggested that the use of mitotane *as adjuvant treatment even when ACC is radically resected* will significantly improve the recurrence-free survival [4].

Mitotane has to be taken under specialized supervision following established protocols as seen in the following section:

2–3 Gr/day orally (Two 500 mg tablets twice or thrice per day) → Increase the dose progressively, every 2 weeks, to reach a target plasmatic concentration of 14 -20 mg/L

The target plasma concentration is generally attainable with a dose of 4–6 g day.

Note: When the control of an associated Cushing syndrome is urgently required, it may be necessary to initiate the treatment at higher doses (4–6 g per day) which may be increased more rapidly (weekly).

There is a wide range of side effects related to this drug [5, 6]:

- Gastrointestinal upsets (38–54 % of patients): anorexia, nausea, vomiting, diarrhoea
- Hepatic signs (25–47 %): increased transaminases and gamma-glutamyl transferase
- Neurologic signs (27–39 %): dysarthria, ataxia, confusion, dizziness, paresthesia
- Gynecomastia (18 %) and impotence

- Skin manifestations (10 %)
- Others: lipid profile disorders, mild neutropenia (between 1,000 and 1,500/mm^3), acute depression, ocular (diplopia, blurred vision), genitourinary (haematuria, hemorrhagic cystitis, albuminuria), cardiovascular signs (hypertension, orthostatic hypotension), generalized pain, hyperthermia

It is important to remember that a substantial percentage of patients taking mitotane will develop the adrenal insufficiency syndrome. Therefore, patients should be closely monitored to prevent or detect this event, and early substitution with corticosteroids should be initiated whenever indicated. Monitoring includes measuring the serum adrenocorticotropic hormone (ACTH), thyroid hormones, testosterone, electrolytes and lipids levels. Urinary free cortisol is also estimated and abnormalities corrected.

27.2.2 Chemotherapy

A randomized study comparing the combination of mitotane with EDP (etoposide, doxorubicin and cisplatin) and the combination of mitotane with streptozocin (streptozotocin) has shown that the former carries better rates of response and progression-free survival as a first-line therapy, but they have similar rates of toxic events and no significant difference in the overall survival [7].

27.3 EBRT

The efficacy of *adjuvant radiotherapy* in reducing the high rate of local recurrence in ACC has been shown by a large population-based German study [8]. Recently, the effectiveness of radiation therapy has been reported in the management of metastatic ACC for both palliation and preventing complications of large metastases [9]. However, EBRT did not improve the disease-free and overall survival, and *reoperation remains the most effective therapeutic option for recurrent adrenocortical carcinoma* [10].

27.4 Others

Radiofrequency ablation may be used in patients with a low tumour volume (<5 cm) who are also poor candidates for surgery. It may also be useful in some patients with metastatic ACC.

Follow-up After Surgery

As mentioned above, ACC is a very aggressive tumour with a high propensity to recur after surgical resection. Therefore, close follow-up is necessary since *a recurrence diagnosed at an early stage will generally be amenable to further surgical treatment*. The follow-up includes clinical assessment and the use of imaging such as abdominal and chest CT-scans *every 3 months for the first 2 years after surgery, then every 6–12 months for at least 5 years*. PET scans can be used as an alternative to CT scanning.

In symptomatic patients, isotope bone scans are indicated to rule out bony metastases. Moreover 3-monthly measurements of the hormone levels are necessary for patients with functional tumours to detect early tumour recurrence [11].

Management of Recurrent ACC

Certain criteria are proposed to clinically determine the aggressiveness of an ACC recurrence and to further adjust the treatment [12, 13]:

- The speed of symptoms exacerbation
- The time elapsed from surgical resection
- The lactate dehydrogenase (LDH) level at onset of the recurrence

Rapidly aggravating symptoms, or a short interval of recurrence of less than 6 months, or LDH levels of more than 1,000 units/L must be regarded as poor prognostic factors.

In keeping with the principles of other surgical malignancies, the management depends on the type of recurrence, that is, whether local or systemic (distant).

a. Repeat Surgery

Repeat surgery is the cornerstone for an isolated local recurrence and will consist of a second 'complete' resection. In this setting open surgery is recommended as opposed to the laparoscopic approach. If the tumour is unresectable, neoadjuvant combined chemotherapy should be initiated with the aim of rendering the tumour amenable to surgery for a second time [11].

b. EBRT

The use of radiotherapy for recurrent ACC is controversial and different studies have reported conflicting results.

c. Radiofrequency Ablation Therapy

This U/S-guided percutaneous therapy has been shown by several studies to be a valuable tool in selected patients with recurrent ACC, either alone, or in combination with surgery [12].

d. Mitotane

Mitotane is the cornerstone for managing systemic recurrences (metastases) of ACC. Its specific indications are as follows:

- A low tumour volume and slow progressive disease, or patient's unfitness for chemotherapy when mitotane may be given alone.
- A high tumour volume, or rapidly progressive disease: Mitotane should be combined with chemotherapy, either with EDP (etoposide-doxorubicin-cisplatin), or with streptozocine [14, 15].

To date no effective salvage therapy has evolved for advanced cases after failure of the above-mentioned therapies. Studies have shown no objective response with combinations of bevacizumab with capecitabine [16], paclitaxel with sorafenib [17] or docetaxel with cisplatin [18] and more supportive data are awaited for the role of gemcitabine combined with metronomic[1] fluoropyrimidines such as 5-fluorouracil or capecitabine [19].

[1] The expression 'Metronomic chemotherapy' was used for the first time by Douglas Hanahan et al. in 2000. It refers to the use of lower doses than the traditionally used 'maximum tolerated doses', but with shorter periods of rest aiming at increasing the anti-angiogenic potential of the chemotherapeutic drugs ('Less is more, regularly') [20].

Take-Home Message: Treatment of ACC

Surgery	*All solid incidentalomas greater than 5 cm on CT or MRI should be removed surgically*
Medical treatment	For inoperable tumours or for a secreting tumour requiring hormonal control before surgery
	1. *Mitotane. Standard treatment for:* *Unresectable or metastatic adrenocortical tumours* *Incompletely resected tumours as an adjuvant therapy* *Secreting tumours before surgery* Also suggested as *adjuvant treatment even for radically resected ACC*
	2. *Chemotherapy:* mitotane + EDP (etoposide, doxorubicin and cisplatin) or mitotane + streptozocin (streptozotocin)
EBRT	As adjuvant therapy after surgery
	Recently suggested for management of metastatic ACC, in palliating local symptoms and in preventing complications of large metastases
Others	Radiofrequency ablation may be used in patients with low tumour volumes (<5 cm) who are poor candidate for surgery
Follow-up after surgery	*Abdominal and chest TDM* every 3 months for the first 2 years after surgery and then every 6–12 months for at least 5 years
	3-monthly hormone level measurements for patients with functional tumours
Management of recurrent ACC	*Repeat surgery is the cornerstone of isolated local recurrence. It consists of a second "complete" resection*
	Mitotane is the cornerstone for systemic recurrences (metastases) of ACC.

References

1. Brunt LM, Moley JF. Adrenal incidentaloma. World J Surg. 2001;25:905–13.
2. Ng L, Libertino J. Adrenocortical carcinoma: diagnosis, evaluation and treatment. J Urol. 2003;169:5–11.
3. Jean-Dominique DOUBLET et les Membres du sous comité Rein. Tumeurs malignes de la surrénale de l'adulte. Recommandation. Progrès en Urologie. 2007;17:1147–50.
4. Terzolo M, Angeli A, Fassnacht M, et al. Adjuvant mitotane treatment for adrenocortical carcinoma. N Engl J Med. 2007;356:2372–80.
5. Terzolo M, Baudin AE, Ardito A, et al. Mitotane levels predict the outcome of patients with adrenocortical carcinoma treated adjuvantly following radical resection. Eur J Endocrinol. 2013;169(3):263–70.
6. Baudry C, Coste J, Bou Khalil R, et al. Efficiency and tolerance of mitotane in Cushing's disease in 76 patients from a single center. Eur J Endocrinol. 2012;167(4):473–81.
7. Fassnacht M, Terzolo M, Allolio B, et al. Combination chemotherapy in advanced adrenocortical carcinoma. N Engl J Med. 2012;366:2189–97.

8. Fassnacht M, Hahner S, Polat B, Koschker AC, Kenn W, Flentje M, Allolio B. Efficacy of adjuvant radiotherapy of the tumour bed on local recurrence of adrenocortical carcinoma. J Clin Endocrinol Metab. 2006;91(11):4501–4.
9. Ho J, Turkbey B, Edgerly M, Alimchandani M, Quezado M, Camphausen K, Fojo T, Kaushal A. Role of radiotherapy in adrenocortical carcinoma. Cancer J. 2013;19(4):288–94.
10. Miccoli P, Iacconi P. Recurrent adrenocortical carcinoma. In: Linos DA, van Heerden JA, editors. Adrenal glands: diagnostic aspects and surgical therapy. Berlin/Heidelberg: Springer; 2005. p. 145.
11. Glover AR, Ip JCY, Zhao JT, Soon PSH, Robinson BG, Sidhu SB. Current management options for recurrent adrenocortical carcinoma. Onco Targets Ther. 2013;6:635–43.
12. Datrice NM, Langan RC, Ripley RT, et al. Operative management for recurrent and metastatic adrenocortical carcinoma. J Surg Oncol. 2011;105(7):709–13.
13. Fassnacht M, Libé R, Kroiss M, Allolio B. Adrenocortical carcinoma: a clinician's update. Nat Rev Endocrinol. 2011;7(6):323–35.
14. Berruti A, Baudin E, Gelderblom H, et al. Adrenal cancer: ESMO clinical practice guidelines for diagnosis, treatment and follow-up. Ann Oncol. 2012;23 Suppl 7:vii131–8.
15. Sèbe P, Rigaud J, Avancès C, et al. Les membres de l'AFCE; Les membres du CCAFU. CCAFU's contribution to the French National Cancer Institute's reference frame: adrenal malignant tumours. Prog Urol. 2013;23(Suppl 2):S167–74.
16. Wortmann S, Quinkler M, Ritter C, Kroiss M, Johanssen S, Hahner S, Allolio B, Fassnacht M. Bevacizumab plus capecitabine as a salvage therapy in advanced adrenocortical carcinoma. Eur J Endocrinol. 2010;162(2):349–56.
17. Berruti A, Sperone P, Ferrero A, et al. Phase II study of weekly paclitaxel and sorafenib as second/third-line therapy in patients with adrenocortical carcinoma. Eur J Endocrinol. 2012;166(3):451–8.
18. Urup T, Pawlak WZ, Petersen PM, Pappot H, Rørth M, Daugaard G. Treatment with docetaxel and cisplatin in advanced adrenocortical carcinoma, a phase II study. Br J Cancer. 2013;108(10):1994–7.
19. Sperone P, Ferrero A, Daffara F, et al. Gemcitabine plus metronomic 5-fluorouracil or capecitabine as a second-/third-line chemotherapy in advancedadrenocortical carcinoma: a multicenter phase II study. Endocr Relat Cancer. 2010;17(2):445–53.
20. Hanahan D, Bergers G, Bergsland E. Less is more, regularly: metronomic dosing of cytotoxic drugs can target tumour angiogenesis in mice. J Clin Invest. 2000;105:1045–7.

Chapter 28
Malignant Phaeochromocytoma (MPC)

Said Abdallah Al-Mamari and Salim Said Al-Busaidy

The overall annual incidence of phaeochromocytoma is 6 per one million population [1]. MPCs account for only 10 % of all phaeochromocytomas and mostly occur in the 30–40-year age group. Clinically, MPCs like their benign counterparts present with paroxysmal hypertension, headaches, palpitations, etc. *The suspicion of malignancy will be raised by the persistence of the signs and symptoms, as well as the elevated values of plasma and urinary methoxyamines after surgical excision of the tumour. The histopathological features of malignancy are controversial and not specific.*

18 F-Dopa is used to diagnose the MPCs and to locate metastases. *Methoxytyramine* was recently introduced as a new biomarker and should be added to the current armamentarium in the investigation of metastatic MPC [2].

The treatment is adrenalectomy, associated with excision of metastases whenever possible. Radiofrequency ablation, cryotherapy and selective chemo-embolization have been proposed as the treatment of multiple secondaries especially in the liver [1].

For an inoperable tumour, chemotherapy can be initiated, combining cyclophosphamide, vincristine and dacarbazine.

Alternatively, metabolic scintigraphy using ^{131}I-meta-iodobenzylguanidine (MIBG) has been tried as adjuvant treatment after surgical resection, but the clinical response in seen in only one third of the patients.

S.A. Al-Mamari (✉) • S.S. Al-Busaidy
Urology Department, The Royal Hospital, Muscat, Oman
e-mail: sabdal67@yahoo.com; salimalbusaidy@hotmail.com

S.A. Al-Mamari, S.S. Al-Busaidy (eds.), *Urological Cancer Management*,
DOI 10.1007/978-3-319-16301-7_28

Take-Home Message: Management of Malignant Phaeochromocytoma	
Management of MPC	Clinically suspected when signs-symptoms-elevated values of plasma and urinary methoxyamines persist after surgical excision of a tumour believed to be a benign phaeochromocytoma
	18F-Dopa and methoxytyramine are valuable biomarkers used to diagnose MPCs and to detect metastases
	Treatment: adrenalectomy and excision of metastases

References

1. Scholz T, Eisenhofer G, Pacak K, Dralle H, Lehnert H. Clinical review: current treatment of malignant pheochromocytoma. J Clin Endocrinol Metab. 2007;92(4):1217–25.
2. Eisenhofer G, Lenders JW, Siegert G, Bornstein SR, Friberg P, Milosevic D, Mannelli M, Linehan WM, Adams K, Timmers HJ, Pacak K. Plasma methoxytyramine: a novel biomarker of metastatic pheochromocytoma and paraganglioma in relation to established risk factors of tumour size, location and SDHB mutation status. Eur J Cancer. 2012;48(11):1739–49.

Part VII Clinical Scenarios

Qais Mohamed Al-Hooti, Said Abdallah Al-Mamari, and Salim Said Al-Busaidy

The following scenarios are based on *true clinical cases* discussed in multidisciplinary tumour board meetings and the management proposed below is based on individual cases. *The answers provided are merely intended to initiate a discussion and are not rigid solutions to complex clinical scenarios which can often be arguably approached in different ways.* The learning process is continuous and lifelong, with that thought our readers are encouraged to digest the facts in this book and embellish their knowledge from the medical literature when dealing with similar live scenarios.

Like all professional healthcare providers, *Urologists should always take into account the individual circumstances of each patient and adapt their management decisions to the reality of the local environment and institutions.*

Chapter 29
Scenarios and Questions

Qais Mohamed Al-Hooti, Said Abdallah Al-Mamari, and Salim Said Al-Busaidy

29.1 Prostate Cancer

1. An 88-year-old man develops castration-resistant prostate cancer (CRPC) after bilateral orchidectomy and flutamide (Casodex®). Androgen withdrawal was attempted with no symptomatic or biochemical improvement. Magnetic resonance imaging (MRI) was performed for persistent back pain which revealed collapsed T8 and T9 vertebrae without neurological compression or evidence of bony or other metastases.
   - What will be your oncological management?
   - Does the skeletal status influence your management?
2. A 56-year-old man with a PSA of 1.22 ng/ml has a routine digital rectal examination (DRE) revealing a nodule in the apex of the left prostatic lobe. What is your management?
3. A 73-year-old man with a clinical prostate cancer T1b has a progressive rise of the PSA reaching 9 ng/ml. A robotic-assisted laparoscopic prostatectomy was performed and the histopathology was reported: pT3b (involving the right seminal vesicle). Surgical margins were negative (R0). The patient was warned about the risk of disease recurrence and advised immediate adjuvant radiotherapy but refuses. PSA 6 months post-operative was undetectable. What is your management?

Q.M. Al-Hooti • S.A. Al-Mamari (✉)
Urology Department, The Royal Hospital, Muscat, Oman
e-mail: sabdal67@yahoo.com

S.S. Al-Busaidy
Senior Consultant and HOD, Urology Department, The Royal Hospital, Muscat, Oman

S.A. Al-Mamari, S.S. Al-Busaidy (eds.), *Urological Cancer Management*,
DOI 10.1007/978-3-319-16301-7_29

4. A 68-year-old patient has a rapid increase of the PSA, rising to 8.7 ng/ml. He has no LUTS. The prostatic biopsy shows a core positive at the apex on the left lobe, GS: 6 (3+3).

   He is known to have a severe cardiomyopathy with echocardiography showing 20 % left ventricular ejection fraction. What is your management?
5. A 74-year-old man was treated with EBRT for PC confined to the prostate as defined by pelvic MRI (initial PSA 25 ng/ml). On follow-up his PSADT was 5 months and a salvage cryotherapy was performed after negative bone scan and F-choline-PET scans suggesting confined disease. What is your management?
6. A 67-year-old man had radical prostatectomy performed and this histopathological report (HPR): prostate adenocarcinoma pT3bN0, Gleason 3+4. His chest, abdomen and pelvis MRI was normal. Bone scan is also normal. What is your further management?
7. A 68-year-old patient is on active surveillance with a cT2a PC, Gleason 6 (3+3), and PSA 6. The PSA rises to 15 on follow-up. MRI: One LN metastasis. What is your management?
8. A 56-year-old man had RP with PLND. HPR: pT3bN0, negative surgical margins. His PSA was undetectable in the follow-up, but rose to 0.13 ng/ml 3 years post-surgery.

   What is your plan?
9. A 48-year-old man has PSA 10 ng/ml, GS 9 (4+5) and a cT3N1. MRI shows involvement of the right seminal vesicle (VS) and a pelvic CT-scan reveals enlargement of a pelvic LN. Isotope bone scan is normal. What is your management?
10. A 66-year-old man with PC GS 7 (3+4), PSA 15. MRI: T3b left seminal vesicle. Biopsy: All 12 biopsies are positive. What is your management?
11. A 60-year-old man with family history of PC comes for a screening which reveals a PSA of 4.5 ng/ml with F/T ratio of 25 %. He has a normal MRI. Does he require a prostatic biopsy?
12. A 65-year-old man has a PC with GS 7 (3+4), 2+/12 (2 biopsies positive out of 12), both at the right base, PSA 6.66 ng/ml. MRI: T3b (both VS are involved). Your management?
13. A 56-year-old man with a PSA of 1.22 ng/ml and a nodule felt in the apex on the left side has a TRUS-guided prostatic biopsy revealing a 6-mm tumour, Gleason's score 6 (3+3), 1+/12.

    The MRI shows a peripheral lesion on the left lobe. No regional extension.

    What are the possible treatment options?
14. A 70-year-old sexually active man has a PSA of 3. DRE: suspected nodule on the right lobe. Biopsy: 3+/12 right apex and left mid-pole, GS 7 (3+4). MRI: Lesion limited to the apex, no capsular infiltration.

    - What is the clinical stage of this tumour and the d'Amico risk group?
    - What is your management?
    - Does the patient need a PLND?

15. An 81-year-old man had radical prostatectomy in 2003 and the HPR was: pT2b, GS 6 (3+3), R0. Then he had biochemical and local failure in 2006 for which

an RT was done. Again he developed a local failure and biochemical recurrence in 2009. He was started on HT with Casodex®. Again Casodex® was given in 2013 because of elevated PSA. Despite Casodex® the PSA continued to rise again to 2.4 ng/ml. The testosterone level was 15 ng/dL. The patient had no pain. CT-scan: Iliac LN enlargement was seen. Bone scan: There is one lesion at the left sacro-iliac joint. What is your subsequent management?

16. A 65-year-old man is known to have a PC since 2007: 2 mm tumour of GS 5 (3+2). He was kept under AS since then and his PSA started to rise progressively from 3.96 → 12 → 18 → 19. He had a repeat biopsy in 2013 which showed no tumour! He has voiding difficulty due to a prostatic adenoma. A comparison of an MRI performed in 2007 and repeated in 2014 showed a similar sized (5 mm) tumour at the left base.
    - What is your conclusion?
    - What is your further management?
17. A 58-year-old man has a PSA 9 and prostatomegaly of 120 cc. Biopsy shows 2 microfoci of less than 2 mm each in the mid prostate and the apex and GS 6 (3+3). MRI shows a lesion in the left posterior aspect of the prostate. What is your management?
18. A 70-year-old man has a clinical T3b PC with PSA 16 and GS 9 (4+5). He has radio-hormonotherapy. A follow-up choline-PET showed a local recurrence 6 months later for which he had a salvage prostatectomy+PLND. The HPR is pT3b Nx, GS 9 (but now 5+4). The PSA 3 months after surgery was 3 (same level as pre-operatively).
    - Why does the report state Nx despite performing PLND?
    - What is the further management?
19. A 66-year-old patient is known with prostatic enlargement and a PSA of 3 which has risen to 6.89 on follow-up. The prostate volume is 60 ml. DRE is normal. He has a TRUS-guided biopsy of the prostate with the HPR: Gleason 6 (3+3) in 2 cores: 6 mm at the apex and 2 mm at the base. What is your management?
20. 73-year-old man with a rising PSA from 3 to 8.63 ng/ml over a 3-year period. No urinary symptoms. Past history: L3-L4 surgery for disc prolapse. Biopsy: GS 8 (4+4) with 9 mm total tumour length in all biopsies, perineural infiltration by the tumour, prostatic capsule involved. MRI: cT3a. Bone scan: L3 isotope hyperfixation. What is your management?
21. A 66-year-old man is a known case of PC: T3b, GS 7 (3+4), PSA 10; had combined RT+HT in 2005. The PSA fell. Then in 2007: the patient had urinary infection and the PSA rose to 8. The patient was treated with antibiotics and again the PSA fell to 4. He had TURP performed in 2007 for prostatomegaly and voiding difficulty. Now again PSA has reached 8. The patient develops recurrent retention of urine. What is your management?
22. A 73-year-old man is known to have a prostate cancer. GS 7 and PSA 11. Biopsy: 7+/12. He had RP done in 2005. On follow-up he had a rising PSA and a CT-scan showed a single costal metastasis as well as a 33-mm supra-pubic pre-vesical soft tissue mass at the midline, infiltrating the recti abdominis muscles (Fig. 29.1). Both lesions and the PSA progress on follow-up despite Casodex®+Decapeptyl. The patient is asymptomatic. What is your management?

Fig. 29.1

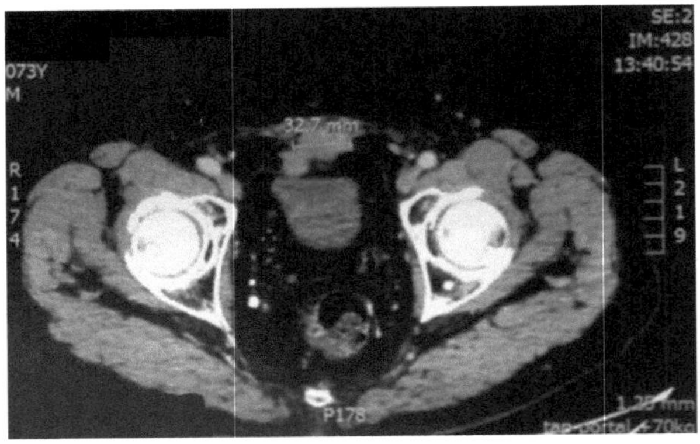

23. A 63-year-old man has a PC with PSA 9, GS 6 (3+3) and T2b right side. The capsule is invaded but no tumour beyond. What is the d'Amico risk group and what is your management?
24. A 68-year-old man had RP done in 2011. HPR: GS 7, pT3aR1NX (positive margin at the apex right side). No PLND done. Undetectable PSA following surgery. Then rose to 0.21 in August 2014 (confirmed on repeat test). A bone scan is negative. MRI is also negative. The patient is asymptomatic. What is your impression and management?
25. A 59-year-old man had RP with GS 7. He had a local failure after 1 year for which a salvage RT was performed. He is now developing bony and nodal metastases but he is still in good general condition. DRE was negative. He has already received five lines therapy: Abiraterone (Zytiga)® → docetaxel → estradiol (Estrana)® → estramustine (Estracyst)® → enzalutamide (Xtandi)®.

    The PSA is rising despite Xtandi and the patient remains asymptomatic. Now PSA is 355.

    Your management?
26. A 59-year-old man with PSA 6.7 has two biopsies +/12 in the apex on the right side with GS 6. IRM: 2 mm long tumour. What are the possible managements here?
27. A 75-year-old patient had RP 12 years ago. On follow-up he developed a biochemical failure after RP. MRI shows an isolated single 8-mm lesion in the prostatic bed near the urethral sphincter with no other metastases. What is your management?
28. A 64-year-old man is a regular long distance bicycle rider. He is found to have a PSA 7. He is asymptomatic. DRE: 50 g prostate, no nodule felt. He had a repeat PSA: 1.87. A third PSA was performed due to increased anxiety and was again high 6.5. He had an MRI which showed a 4-mm lesion in the left lobe. On biopsy there is a HGPIN in 2/12 at the base and apex. What is your management?

Fig. 29.2

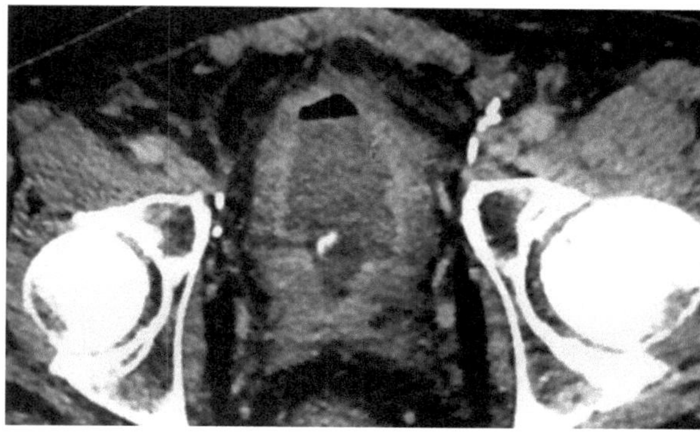

29. A 65-year-old man is a k/c/o PC with RT performed 1 year ago. Now complaining of dysuria for several months and found to have recurrent UTIs. Had pelvic CT shown in Fig. 29.2. What is your differential diagnosis? Discuss the further management.
30. A 52-year-old African gentleman with primary infertility for 15 years. His PSA was 4.12 ng/ml in 2011, then 6.15 in 2013. He had MRI showing prostatomegaly 90 g with a large median lobe with no suspicious lesion. No history of LUTS. PSA rose to 6.58 in 2014. He had a prostate biopsy showing: 2+/12, 1–3 mm right base and left mid-gland, GS 6 (3+3). A bone scan was negative. The patient is very anxious about his disease.
    Do you have any criticism about the management so far? Discuss further possible treatment options.

29.2 Bladder Cancer

1. A 72-year-old man has a known T2N1 BC for which he had chemoradiation therapy. On follow-up a CT-scan shows new liver lesions. What is your further management?
2. A 70-year-old female had radical cystectomy + adjuvant chemotherapy for a pT2b N2 tumour. On follow-up she complained of diplopia. She had an MRI of the head which revealed a solitary brain metastasis and a suspicious image of the glottis. An ENT opinion stated that there was no glottic lesion. What is your management?
3. An 80-year-old man had radical cystectomy with HPR: pT3aN0. He is found to have a loco-regional recurrence on a follow-up CT-scan 14 months later. The patient has multiple comorbidities. Chemotherapy was started with gemcitabine (Gemsar)®. However, the patient complained increasingly of bladder irritation syndrome, tenesmus and anal pain. He had an MRI shown in Fig. 29.3. Discuss the management of this patient.

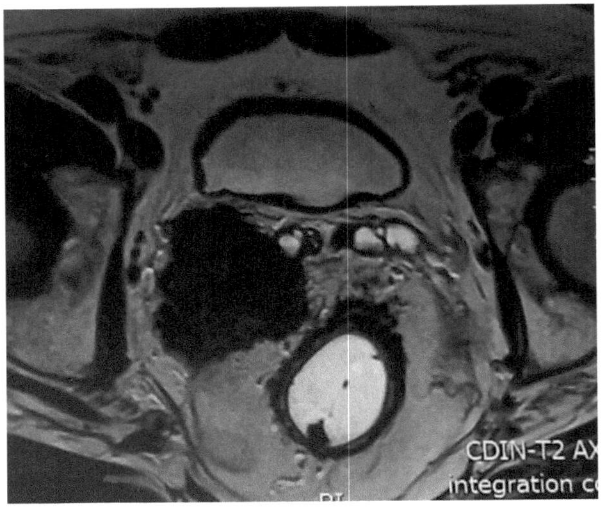

Fig. 29.3

4. A 79-year-old woman has recurrent UTI and haematuria. She has no comorbidities. A CT-scan showed a 5×4×7 cm thickened and calcified bladder wall at the dome, no LN enlargement. HPR of the TURBT specimen showed a high-grade MIBT. She had a partial cystectomy performed and the HPR revealed CIS lesions in addition to the high-grade MIBT, the surgical margins were negative. What is your plan?
5. A 45-year-old patient has a urachal tumour invading the vesical dome and lung metastases.
   - What is the most probable histopathology of this tumour?
   - What is your management?
6. A 65-year-old man has a TURBT for multifocal BC (4 foci). HPR: High-grade pT1.
   - What is the risk stratification of this disease?
   - If you choose to treat this patient with bladder instillations which agent should be used?
   - Follow-up cystoscopies performed after instillation show multifocal recurrence. A second TURBT was undertaken which again showed HPR: pT1a (superficial invasion of the lamina propria) but no CIS. What is your further management?
7. A 65-year old woman has an MIBT with a suspected nodal lesion in the pelvis. She receives neoadjuvant chemotherapy followed by radical cystectomy with ePLND and orthotopic replacement. HPR: pT3N+. There was one positive LN

out of 20 contained in the specimen. A PET shows no new lesion. The patient has not yet regained her continence. What is your future plan?

8. A 54-year-old female has TURBT performed for a 2.5–3 cm tumour located in the left lateral wall. HPR: High grade pT2. CT-scan is negative for disease extension and she has good renal function. What is your management?
9. An 85-year-old healthy man presents with haematuria. Cystoscopy revealed a bladder tumour which was resected. Histopathology was reported as high-grade MIBT. CT: No extra-vesical extension seen, normal upper tract, no LN enlargement, no distant metastases. Neoadjuvant chemotherapy was given and a radical cystoprostatectomy + PLND + Bricker diversion was performed. Incidentally a pT2c prostate cancer was found with 2LN+/15 with R0, but no tumour was found in the bladder. What is your management?
10. A 61-year-old man had a high-grade T1 low-grade NMIBT since 2011. He received MMC, then BCG because the tumours progressed to high-grade. Repeat cystoscopies showed multiple tumours which were resected and reported as high-grade disseminated Ta. Your management?
11. A 51-year-old man had a laparoscopic cystoprostatectomy + PLND with orthotopic bladder reconstruction. Histopathology: pT3N1. A follow-up PET-TDM scan performed few months after is shown in Fig. 29.4. What is your diagnosis and management?
12. A 44-year-old man from overseas presented with haematuria and was found to have a large bladder tumour. TURBT was performed and the tumour reported as high-grade pT2b, but no vascular embolus was seen. His renal function was normal. He had a CT-scan chest-abdomen-pelvis which showed prostate infiltration and two enlarged pelvic LN. There is a suspicious nodule seen in the right lung measuring 1 cm in diameter. No other lesions are seen.
    What is the stage of the disease?
    What is your management?

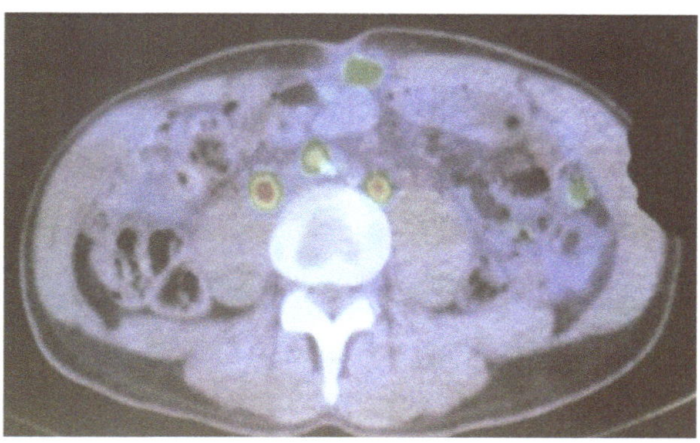

Fig. 29.4

29.3 Upper Tract TCC

1. A 76-year-old man had a nephroureterectomy for an extensive TCC of the lower ureter. HPR: High-grade diffuse TCC, pT3 NX, MX. He had adjuvant chemotherapy. A CT-scan showed a borderline positive right iliac node.
   - What is your best investigation to ascertain the positivity of that LN?
   - If positive, what would be your further management?
2. A 70-year-old man had total nephroureterectomy with HPR: Caliceal TCC high-grade, pT3, N0, with vascular emboli. The bladder surgical margin was healthy. Post-surgical chest-abdomen-pelvic CT at 3 months: no evidence of local or distant recurrence. The patient is seen in OPD and is about to be discharged by a young resident with an appointment after 1 year. What is your suggestion for the present and future plans?
3. A 72-year-old patient with h/o a right mid-ureteric 2-cm TCC for which he had a right ureteric segmentectomy performed followed by mitomycin C instillation. On follow-up he had recurrences in the bladder and the right renal pelvis. Then a right nephroureterectomy was performed. Then again he had a bladder recurrence for which he had TURBT for two tumours, one of them being at the left ureteric orifice. Then BCG instillations were given but failed. A recent CT-scan performed demonstrated dilated left pelvi-caliceal system and the whole length of the ureter. There is also a small left para-aortic LN.
   - What may be the possible causes for the left hydroureteronephrosis and impaired renal function?
   - What it your further management?

29.4 Renal Tumours

1. A 64-year-old lady has a U/S performed for a vague abdominal discomfort. This reveals a 4-cm calcified cystic lesion in the upper pole of the left kidney. Contrast-CT confirms a 39-mm lesion with an enhancing contour. There are internal non-enhancing septae. No renal vein thrombus, no extension to the perinephric fat or to the adrenals. No LN enlargement. The right kidney is normal.
   - What is the Bosniak classification of this lesion?
   - What is your management?
2. The precedent patient had a laparoscopic partial nephrectomy performed. The HPR is papillary oncocytoma. What is the next step in your management?
3. A 57-year-old man has a 7-cm tumour in the upper pole of the left kidney. Otherwise no perinephric fat infiltration, no LN and normal left adrenal gland and renal vein. He has a normal right kidney.

- What is the TNM classification of this tumour?
- What is your management?

4. An 80-year-old man had radical right nephrectomy. HPR: Clear cell carcinoma, Fuhrman grade 4, T3aN1. Follow-up CT-scan: Enlargement of retroperitoneal LN with appearance of a suspicious pulmonary mass.
   How would you manage him?
5. A 56-year-old man has a past history of laparotomy in 2010 for intestinal obstruction due to adhesions. Several months later he had a right partial nephrectomy for a 3-cm upper pole tumour: RCC, grade 3 Fuhrman. On follow-up, a CT-scan performed in 2012 showed multiple supra and infra-diaphragmatic LNs, all <1 cm. What is your management?
6. An 80-year-old man had bilateral radical nephrectomy for RCC. He is now on regular HD through a right arm perm-cath. He complains of right arm pain which is first believed to be due to the perm-cath. Two weeks later he gets a pathological fracture of the right humerus and a CT-scan revealed a metastatic deposit. What is your management?
7. A 61-year-old man is treated for a mandibular lymphoma. On follow-up abdomen CT, he is incidentally found to have an endophytic 3×2.5 cm tumour in the mid-pole of the right kidney near the hilum. No evidence of local or distant extension of this tumour. The left kidney is normal. A CT-guided biopsy confirmed an RCC. He had a right total nephrectomy performed which showed an RCC Fuhrman grade 3, RO. What is your management?
8. A 67-year-old woman is found to have a 3-cm Bosniak 2 left renal cyst in the upper pole in 2012. On a follow-up CT-scan, the cyst was upgraded to Bosniak 4 because of intra-lesion contrast enhancement of 20 HU and thick calcifications. The right kidney is normal.
   What is your management?
9. A 46-year-diabetic female receives chemotherapy for an oesophageal carcinoma with mediastinal metastases. She is fed through a gastrostomy tube. Subsequently, she developed pulmonary embolism and her general status deteriorated further. A routine CT-scan performed showed that the oesophageal tumour was unchanged but incidentally revealed a left renal 30×36 mm upper polar tumour. She had a repeat CT-scan 6 months later showing both lesions remained unchanged. The patient's GC continued to be poor and second-line chemotherapy was initially planned. What is your management with regard to the renal tumour?
10. A 37-year-old woman developed respiratory inflammatory syndrome 2 months earlier: dyspnoea, fever, generalized body ache, fatigue. Bacteremia was noted on blood cultures and a chest and abdomen CT performed incidentally revealed a 3-cm left mid-renal endophytic lesion. After 3 weeks of antibiotic treatment, the inflammatory episode settled and a percutaneous biopsy of the left renal lesion showed parenchymal inflammatory features. Discuss your management.

11. An 86-year-old gentleman with cardiomyopathy had right radical nephrectomy performed 3 years ago for a 6-cm tumour. A 3-cm pulmonary nodule was noted in the follow-up and was treated with RFA. A recent CT-scan revealed a 5-mm recurrent lesion in the right kidney bed. His cardiac failure has gradually worsened and he has developed pleural effusion and deranged renal function. What is your management?
12. A 55-year-old woman has an incidentally discovered right renal 3.4 cm tumour as shown on the Fig. 29.5a, b. What is your treatment plan?
13. A 47-year-old fit female has a CT performed which is shown in Fig. 29.6a–c. Describe the findings and discuss the treatment.
14. A 71-year-old woman presented with severe back pain. CT-scan showed an infiltrating mass at L4 vertebra and class IV left renal cystic tumour (See Figs. 16.8 and 16.9). Spinal fixation was performed as an emergency and a biopsy of spinal tumour during the surgery showed a poorly differentiated adenocarcinoma. Later on she underwent a left radical nephrectomy

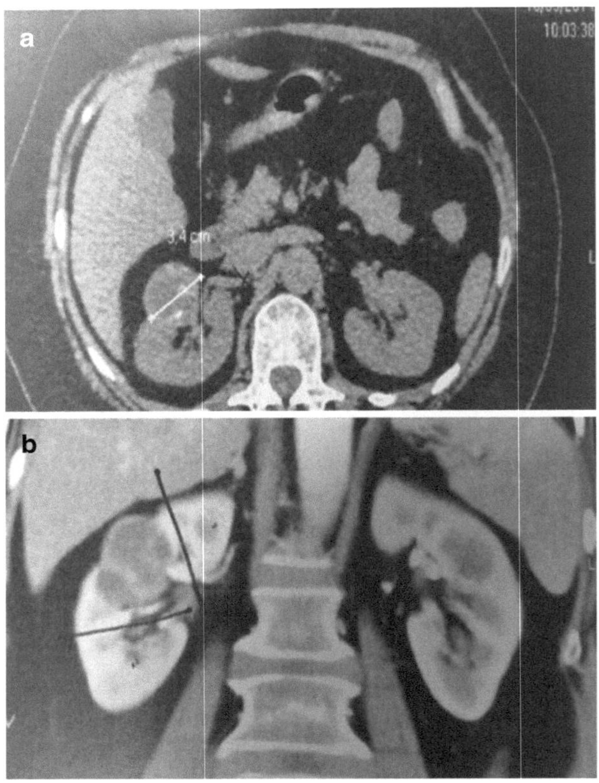

Fig. 29.5

revealing a clear cell RCC Fuhrman's grade 3. What is your further management?

15. A 62-year-old man was incidentally found to have a left renal mass shown in Fig. 29.7a–c. Describe the lesion and suggest possible diagnoses and the treatment of choice.

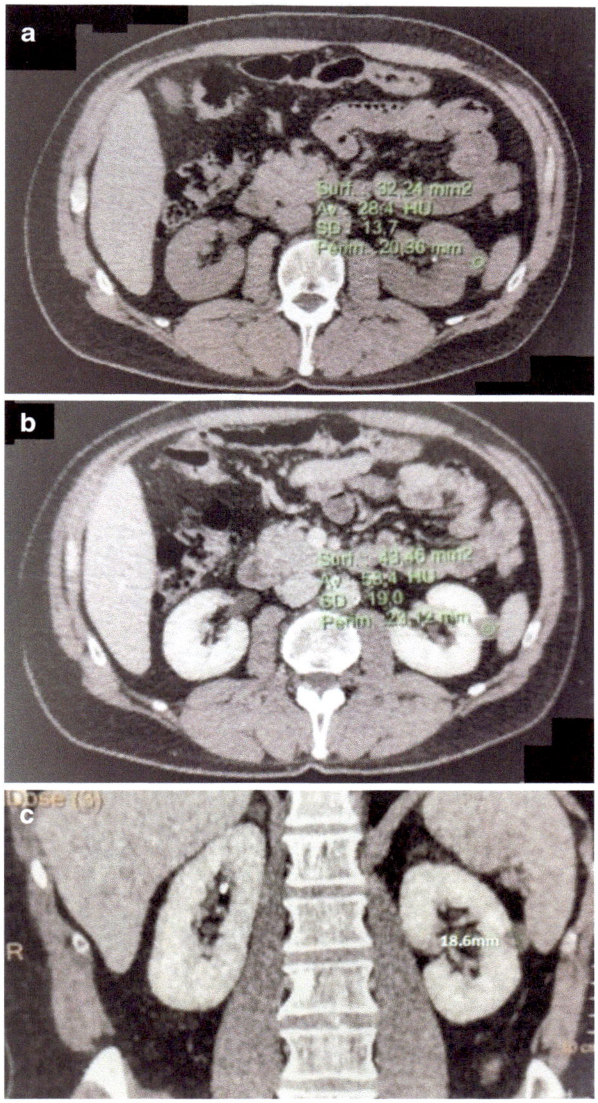

Fig. 29.6

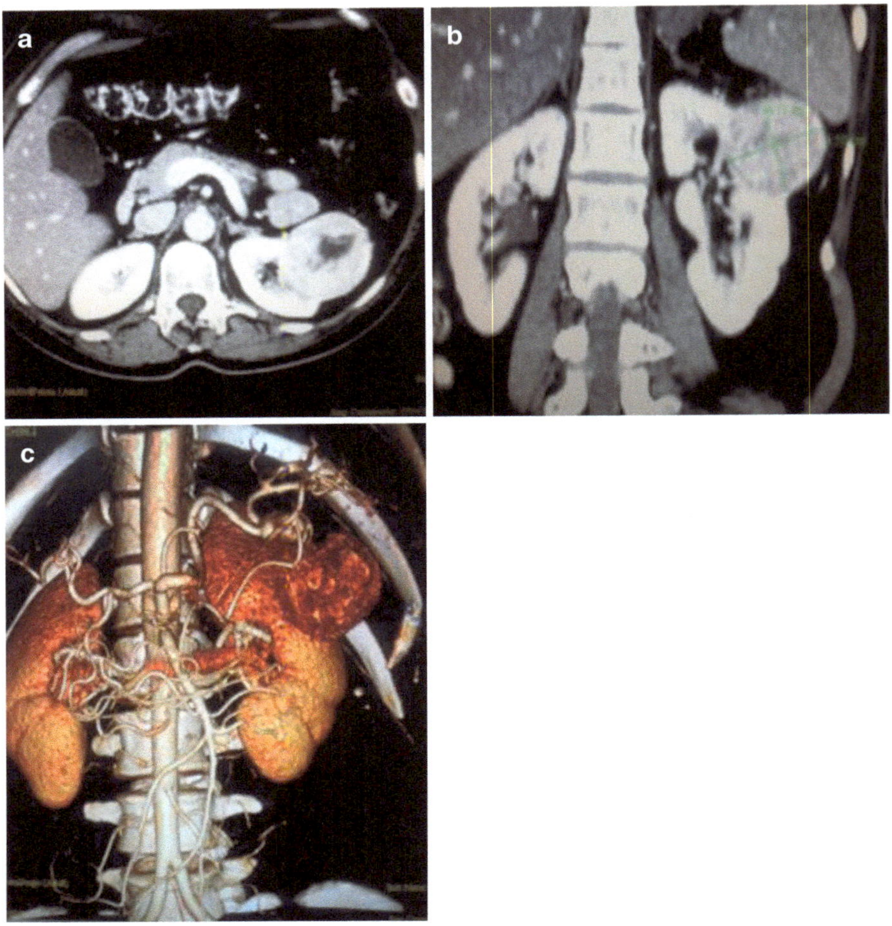

Fig. 29.7 (**a–c**) Contrast CT (horizontal, sagittal and 3D-reconstructed) showing a left renal mass

29.5 Male Genital Cancers

1. A 30-year-old man had a right orchidectomy for a testicular tumour. HPR: Seminoma. AFP was elevated 3 months after surgery, but β-HCG was normal. PET-scan was also normal.
   What is your management?
2. A 46-year-old man had a left testicular tumour. Radical orchidectomy revealed a testicular seminoma. On follow-up the TDM showed 1-cm left para-aortic LN.
   What is your management?

3. A 41-year-old man had right orchidectomy performed for a 4-cm tumour: pT1 pure seminoma, no vascular emboli seen. The rete testis status was not reported. The serum markers were negative pre-operatively. On follow-up MRI abdomen did not reveal any suspicious lesions, also the serum markers remained negative. What are your possible management options?
4. A 31-year-old man presented with vague abdominal pain and altered GC. CT-scan showed retroperitoneal masses suspicious of primary EGGCT since the testicles were normal. A PET-scan showed active retroperitoneal LN and biopsy revealed PLAP positive embryonic carcinoma. The tumour markers were AFP <1,000, LDH 22, β-HCG 22. The disease was staged IIa and was considered to have a good prognosis. Two PEB cycles were given with poor tolerance accompanied by weight loss and respiratory complications. Bleomycin was discontinued and the third cycle consisted of EP alone. A repeat CT revealed a persistent 1.4 cm LN in the interaortico-caval region. Markers were now negative and the patient began to gain weight although he continued to be breathless.
What is your treatment plan?
5. A 36-year-old medically fit male is married and has three children. He presented with a history of left testicular mass for 2 months. The tumour markers were beta-HCG 21, AFP 48 and LDH 329. He had a left orchiectomy which showed immature teratoma, embryonal carcinoma and yolk sac tumour. The tumour markers remained elevated and a CT-scan revealed left para-aortic lymph nodes measuring 6–7 cm. He was started on three cycles of PEB. Following the chemotherapy tumour markers normalized but CT showed a 4–5 cm persistent para-aortic nodal mass. He underwent a RPLND which revealed an immature teratoma and a small focus of positive surgical margin. What is your further management?
6. A 21-year-old unmarried medically fit patient presented with a large right hemiscrotal swelling and mild pain for 6 months. Physical examination revealed a large and hard right testicular mass. On abdominal examination a large irregular non-tender mass was palpable at the level of the umbilicus. Tumour markers were very high and did not decrease after radical inguinal orchiectomy. A CT-scan showed a 15-cm right paracaval and interaortocaval lymphnode mass extending to the right common iliac vessels. Semen analysis revealed severe oligospermia, and sperm banking was offered. He was started on four cycles of PEB but did not tolerate the treatment necessitating reduction in the dose. The patient eventually developed impairment of renal function and cisplatin was discontinued. After chemotherapy, the tumour markers were normalized and the lymph nodes shrunk to around 10 cm. RPLND was performed and revealed immature teratoma. What is your further management?
7. A 26-year-old man is diagnosed to have NSGCT stage T2N3M0 S3. Orchidectomy revealed a teratoma. He was started on four cycles of PEB. He developed shortness of breath with low oxygen saturation in room air. Chest

imaging showed wide new opacities in the lungs and the diagnosis of bleomycin-related pulmonary fibrosis was suggested. Bleomycin was withdrawn and the patient continued on EP. Tumour markers were normalized but the retroperitoneal mass was found later to increase in size after chemotherapy. What is your impression and further management?

8. A 29-year-old mentally retarded man with microcephaly was known to have a solitary left testicle after right orchiectomy was performed for undescended testis during early childhood. He presented with acute left testicular pain and swelling with no fever. Examination revealed an elevated, tender and firm left testicle. Doppler ultrasound showed a heterogeneous testis with no blood flow, suggesting a torsion. No evidence of testicular mass was seen. A transcrotal exploration was done and confirmed a testicular torsion. The testis regained a good circulation after detorsion, and a large intratesticular mass then became obvious occupying more than 50 % of the testicle. Orchiectomy was performed with high spermatic cord ligation. The histology revealed a T1 mixed germ cell. Tumour markers were normal. A CT-scan showed a left para-aortic LN measuring around 1 cm. What is your further management?
9. A 39-year-old man has a history of right testicular mass for 7 months. He is married and has two children. Tumour markers are normal and right orchiectomy revealed a classic seminoma T1. CT-scan for staging was negative. What is your further management?
10. A 32-year-old fit unmarried gentleman was found to have a small right testicular mass and normal tumour markers. CT-scan did not reveal para-aortic or caval LNs; however, 4–5 cm right common iliac lymphnodes were detected. The LN mass decreased to 3 cm after chemotherapy. What is your further management?
11. A 30-year-old man complaining of right flank pain was found to have right hydroureteronephrosis on U/S and had a right DJ stent inserted. A CT-scan performed subsequently is shown on Fig. 29.8a, b. Both testes were normal on examination. Loss of weight and fever were not apparent. What are the possible diagnoses and what is your further management?
12. A 67-year-old man has SCC of the penis with N2-3+. He undergoes a total penectomy with perineostomy and ILND. He develops post-operative infection. The perineostomy does not function well and a permanent suprapubic catheter is inserted. The patient has adjuvant chemotherapy but develops urinary sepsis. After recovery, repeat CT shows persistent pelvic nodal disease and painless metastases of the ischial bone. He develops tumour necrosis with multiple fistulae over the pubic area, the scrotum and the perineum (Fig. 29.9a, b) and his GC deteriorates. What is your management?

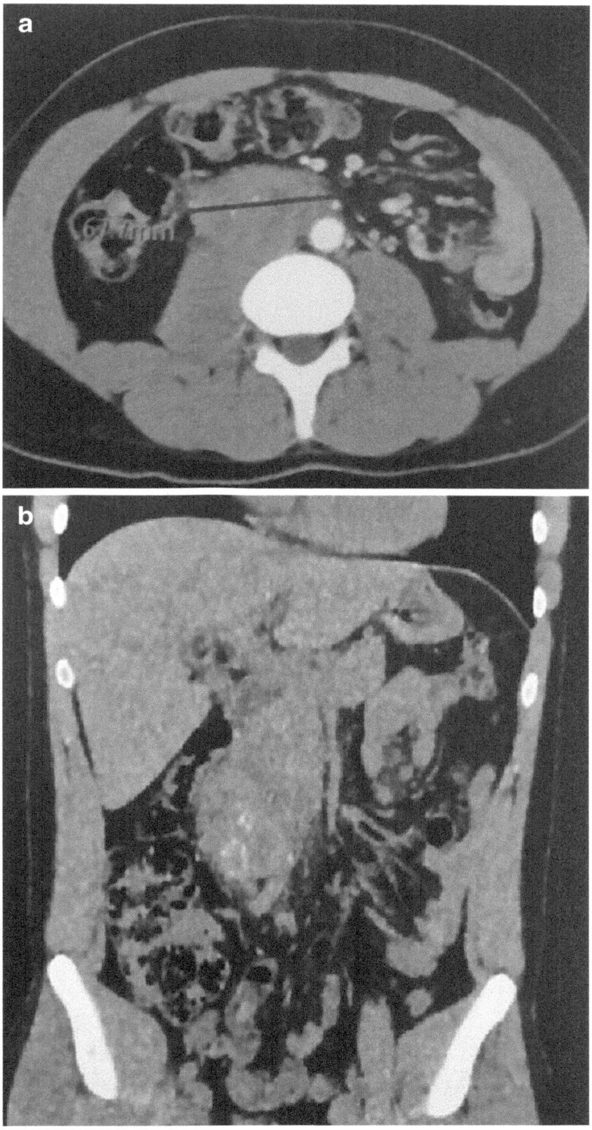

Fig. 29.8 (**a**, **b**) Retroperitoneal mass

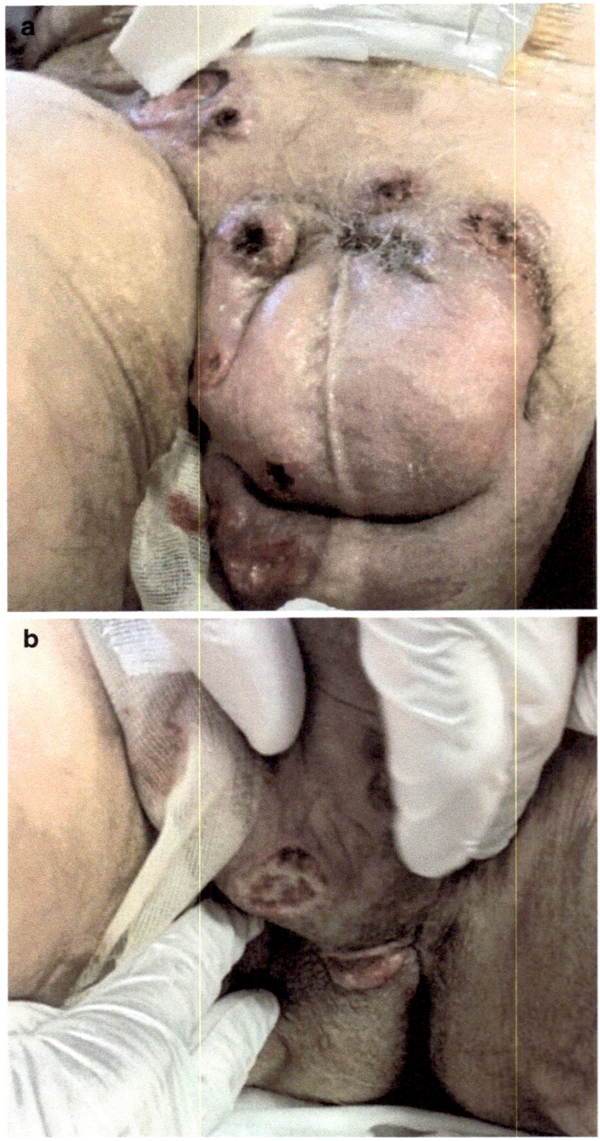

Fig. 29.9

29.6 Adrenal Tumours

1. A 65-year-old patient presented with a cough and vague abdominal pain. He has lost 5 kg but otherwise remains in a good general condition. He had a CT-scan and PET-scan shown in Fig. 29.10a–g. Discuss the diagnostic possibilities and management.

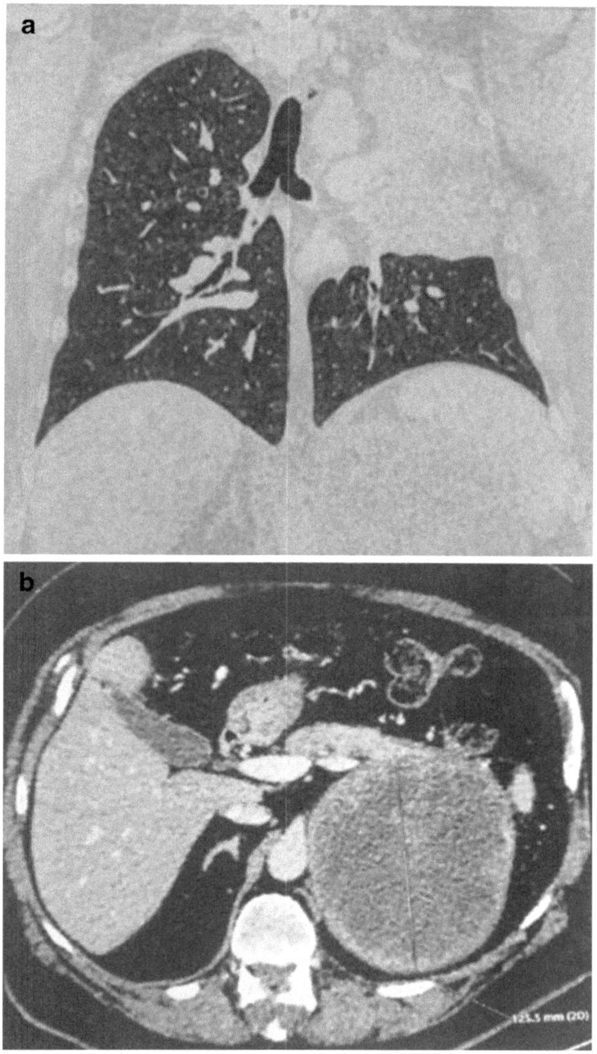

Fig. 29.10 (**a**–**g**): CT-scan (**a**–**d**), PET-scan (**e**), and combined PET-CT-scan (**f**–**g**)

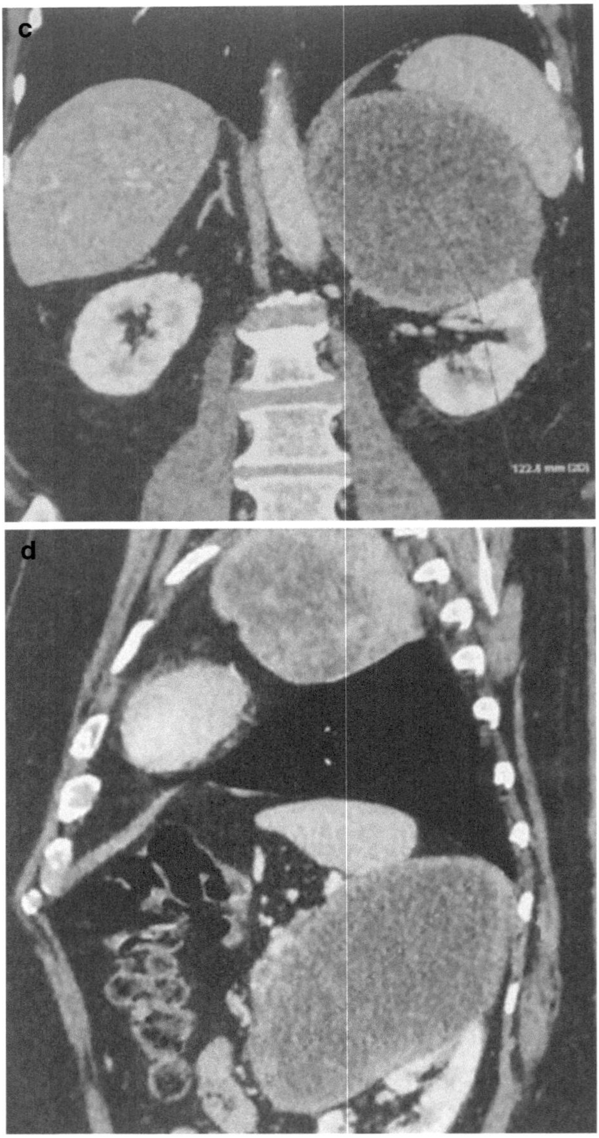

Fig. 29.10 (continued)

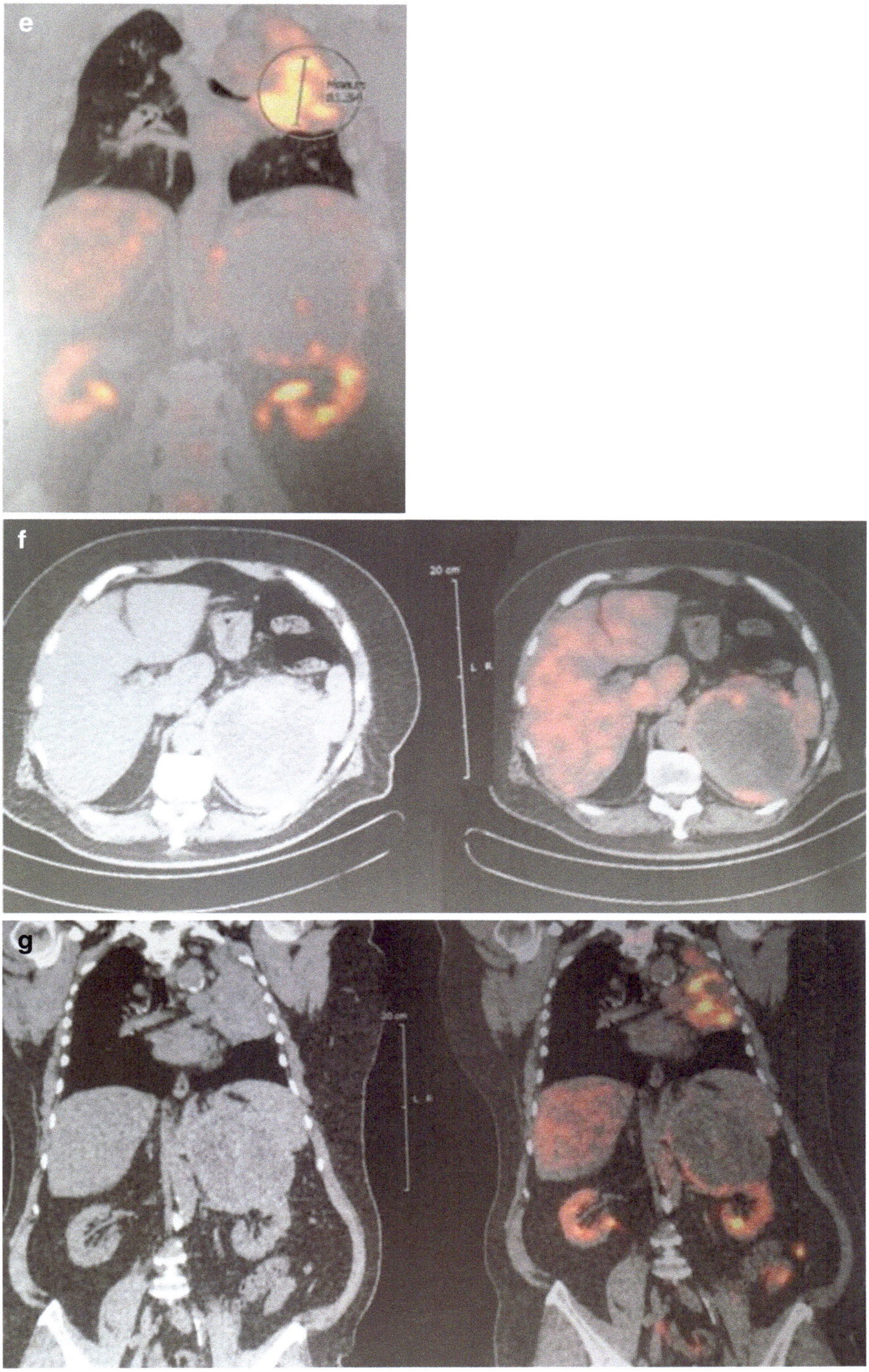

Fig. 29.10 (continued)

Chapter 30
Proposed Answers

Qais Mohamed Al-Hooti, Said Abdallah Al-Mamari, and Salim Said Al-Busaidy

30.1 Prostate Cancer

1. • Start second-line hormone therapy with abiraterone (Zytiga®).
   • Initiate treatment with zoledronic acid.
2. When the prostate is irregular on DRE, a TRUS-guided biopsy is needed regardless of the PSA value.
3. Continue surveillance with PSA estimations every 3 months.
4. Brachytherapy or intensity-modulated radiation therapy (IMRT) (radical prostatectomy is contraindicated).
5. Intermittent hormone therapy.
6. A choline-PET may be arranged. However, this has got only 50 % sensitivity in this setting. Hence, the patient should have a pelvis radiation therapy even if PET scan is negative.
7. Radiotherapy possibly with adjuvant HT.
8. Continue surveillance. Only when PSA rises to ≥0.2 ng/ml, should hormone therapy be started.
9. Combined radio-hormonotherapy (i.e. EBRT + concomitant and adjuvant HT).
10. Start immediate HT and then reassessment with MRI. May require salvage RT. A staging and debulking PLND may be needed with the targeted advantage to reduce the duration of HT as well as the extent of RT.
11. MRI does not have 100 % specificity even for high-risk group. Hence, biopsy is necessary. However, a normal MRI generally means that if any tumour is found, it will not be of a GS ≥7.
12. Combined radio-hormonotherapy.
13. Brachytherapy was performed in this case. However, other options are also suitable including RP and EBRT.

Q.M. Al-Hooti • S.A. Al-Mamari (✉) • S.S. Al-Busaidy
Urology Department, The Royal Hospital, Muscat, Oman
e-mail: sabdal67@yahoo.com; salimalbusaidy@hotmail.com

S.A. Al-Mamari, S.S. Al-Busaidy (eds.), *Urological Cancer Management*,
DOI 10.1007/978-3-319-16301-7_30

14. • T2c. This is sufficient to categorize it in the d'Amico high-risk group despite the low PSA which is indicative of low risk and GS 7 in favour of intermediate risk.
    • Nerve-sparing radical prostatectomy and adjuvant HT are indicated.
    • PLND would be justified because of the presence of three core positives in two different sextants. However, it is not necessary because PSA is only 3 ng/ml and the histopathology demonstrates mainly grade 3 disease.
15. Second-line HT with Zytiga® (abiraterone) or Ra-223.
16. • The raised PSA is probably due to the adenoma, and the second negative biopsy missed this small tumour contained in a big prostatic gland.
    • The patient needs a redo biopsy with combined ultrasound-MRI guidance. If the biopsy is positive, a radical prostatectomy is indicated targeting two goals: the relief of his voiding difficulty and tumour-related anxiety. The surgery should be nerve-sparing, and a PLND is not required.
17. Active surveillance. If he refuses AS because of anxiety, active treatment with RP or RT can be performed. The volume of the prostate precludes the possibility of a brachytherapy or focal therapy.
18. • Negative LN on histopathology is inconclusive after radio-hormonotherapy.
    • Repeat choline-PET and plan for hormonotherapy.
19. The patient has a single 6-mm core which excludes the possibility of AS. His total tumour length is 8 mm (2+6). He requires a radical prostatectomy. Moreover if the positive core at the base was 6 mm in length, an MRI would have been indicated to rule out the possibility of a T3b lesion.
20. The bone scan image is due to the spinal surgery. There is possibility of LN involvement (the risk is estimated here to be 25 %), and there is no clear evidence that radiotherapy is effective for nodal disease. Ideally nodal disease should first be excluded by a staging PLND. If it is negative, the patient will benefit from a combination EBRT+long-term HT. Otherwise, if PLND cannot be done or if it reveals a N+, then the same treatment (combined EBRT+long-term HT) may still be done, but the patient must be informed about the increased risk of failure.
21. A rise in the PSA may be associated with a benign event like UTI or retention of urine. The patient needs a repeat TURP.
22. The patient needs a second-line HT, i.e. Zytiga®.
23. This is an intermediate risk group of d'Amico because of T2b. The patient needs a RP with unilateral NVB preservation on the left side only.
24. There is a biochemical failure as per the strict definition. This appears most probably to be local in view of the negative MRI for LNs. The bone scan was not indicated here but is an additional evidence of the local nature of the failure. Salvage radiotherapy may be indicated.
25. Ba223. Continue with Xtandi®.
26. AS, brachytherapy, EBRT and RP are all possible options. The AS would be the preferred option since this is a low-risk disease and avoids overtreatment. But for anxious patients, active treatment may be indicated.

27. He needs salvage RT. However, high dose should be avoided in view of the close proximity of the sphincter to prevent urinary incontinence. Therefore, to enhance the efficacy of lower dose (<70 Gy), a combination treatment should be given with short HT course, 2 months before and 2 months concomitantly.
28. This fluctuating PSA is most probably due to the cycling. The HGPIN in two areas only is not considered extensive and does not justify a repeat biopsy. However, the patient should have a repeat PSA after 6 months, ideally 2 weeks distant from any strenuous cycling.
29. Gas is seen inside the bladder. In this scenario the most likely cause is a rectovesical fistula caused by radiotherapy. Radiation cystitis with gas-forming bacteria colonizing the bladder wall is another possibility. Diagnosis can be confirmed by cystoscopy and cystography. If rectovesical fistula is confirmed, a colostomy will be necessary.
30. The MRI was not needed in 2013. Furthermore the bone scan is not indicated for this low-grade disease in an asymptomatic patient. Possible further treatment options are:
    - RP with B/L NVB preservation and without PLND. If he still wants to have children, sperm cryopreservation is advisable.
    - EBRT is a possible option.
    - Active surveillance is not advisable in the presence of B/L disease and in such an anxious patient.
    - Brachytherapy and cryotherapy are contraindicated because of a prostatomegaly of 90 g.

30.2 Bladder Cancer

1. Biopsy must be performed from one liver lesion and P63 immunoreactivity be studied to confirm the urothelial origin of these metastases and then chemotherapy if biopsy positive. Beware of the possibility of tumour seeding during biopsy.
2. RT brain as it is a solitary lesion and a repeat CT scan later.
3. This T2-weighted MRI shows that the tumour recurrence is compressing the rectum. RT would surely end with a rectal fistula. A second-line chemotherapy would be very toxic in view of the patient's condition. An anaesthetist reassessment may be requested to see if the patient is fit for a permanent diversion colostomy which will open the possibility for a RT. If unfit, he should be left alone with only symptomatic treatment which may include a sacral neurolysis.
4. This patient needs a radical cystectomy because of the presence of CIS lesions. RT is not effective against CIS.
5. - Adenocarcinoma
   - Chemotherapy.

6. • High grade pT1 is sufficient to categorize a high-risk group for progression even if first time seen. Moreover here the disease is multifocal.
   • BCG.
   • Radical cystectomy + orthotopic replacement.
7. This patient needs adjuvant RT. However, this should be deferred until she regains her continence.
8. Neoadjuvant chemotherapy + radical cystectomy + ileocystoplasty (orthotopic bladder substitution).
9. Adjuvant therapy is not required now. The patient needs follow-up with repeat CT chest + abdomen + pelvis after 3 months. Follow-up of the incidental PC is not required for this 85-year-old man.
10. Because of the multifocality + recurrences of high-grade lesions, the patient needs cystectomy + bladder replacement.
11. There is a disease recurrence in one of the laparoscopic trocar sites in the midline. The patient needs EBRT.
12. • cT4aN2M1.
    • The patient needs a PET scan to assess the full extent of the LN as well as the metabolic activity of the lung nodule. He is a candidate for chemotherapy.

30.3 Upper Tract TCC

1. • PET scan 3 weeks after cessation of chemotherapy.
   • Radiotherapy
2. In all cases, a check cystoscopy and urine cytology have to be done at 3 months, then repeated yearly for at least 5 years. Moreover CT-urography is necessary to better define metachronous urothelial disease. It has to be done 6 monthly for 2 years and then yearly.
3. • The resection of the tumour at the left ureteric orifice may have caused a left vesico-ureteric reflux which may explain this situation. Other possible causes are stricture and tumour recurrence.
   • PET scan to see the activity of the left para-aortic LN. If negative, a radical cystectomy + ileal orthotopic bladder replacement may be undertaken.

30.4 Renal Tumours

1. • Any enhancing lesion is Bosniak III or IV. If there are nodules of solid enhancing elements, it is a Bosniak IV. In this patient it was a Bosniak III lesion because only the contour was enhancing.
   • Partial nephrectomy
2. Surveillance
3. • Stage II: T1bN0M0
   • Radical left nephrectomy.

4. Targeted antiangiogenic therapy.
5. Continue surveillance with repeat CT scan at 3 months because of Fuhrman's grade 3. If Fuhrman's grade was ≤2, the follow-up CT scan would have been 2 yearly.
6. Urgent orthopaedic referral for an intramedullary nail + cementoplasty.
7. Surveillance alone with repeat CT abdomen performed for the follow-up of both the lymphoma and RCC.
8. Partial nephrectomy.
9. There is no priority to treat the renal carcinoma in this patient with altered GC and being followed up for another more aggressive malignancy.
10. Difficult diagnosis and management options:
    - An inflammatory renal parenchymal mass is a possibility.
    - A cancer with peri-tumoral inflammatory process cannot be excluded. However, partial nephrectomy is technically difficult here, and radical nephrectomy cannot be performed unless the tumour is confirmed. Close follow-up is necessary to avoid missing an opportunity for a curative-intent treatment, i.e. a repeat CT within 3 months. If the tumour persists or progresses, a repeat biopsy is indicated. Tumour regression is indicative of a regressing inflammatory process needing consultation with infectious disease specialist.
11. An elderly patient admitted with cardiomyopathy has a high risk of mortality within 1 year which is more of a threat to him than his renal tumour recurrence. Further surgery is most likely to precipitate cardiac complications. Follow-up with repeat CT scan after 6 months and RFA if a recurrence is detected is the appropriate management.
12. This tumour location is unfavourable for conservative surgery because it is impinging on the hilar structures. Since the left kidney is normal, a radical right nephrectomy is advisable.
13. There is a 1.9 cm enhancing exophytic left renal tumour (from 28 to 58 HU). This lesion is located in the mid-pole. Normal right kidney. An ablative therapy is indicated either with cryotherapy or radiofrequency. If facilities are not available, a partial left nephrectomy can be offered. However, active surveillance is not an option for this young patient unless she refuses active treatment.
14. Radiotherapy for spine and targeted therapy with sunitinib.
15. This is a 4-cm exophytic tumour with a central stellate scar. A diagnosis of oncocytoma is most likely, but a RCC with a necrotic centre remains a possibility. The best treatment is a partial nephrectomy (Fig. 30.1). HPR confirmed the mass was an oncocytoma.

30.5 Male Genital Cancers

1. Surveillance.
2. Surveillance with a repeat TDM after 3 months.
3. Surveillance alone or single-agent chemotherapy (carboplatin) is a possible option. A risk stratification cannot be performed accurately since the rete testis

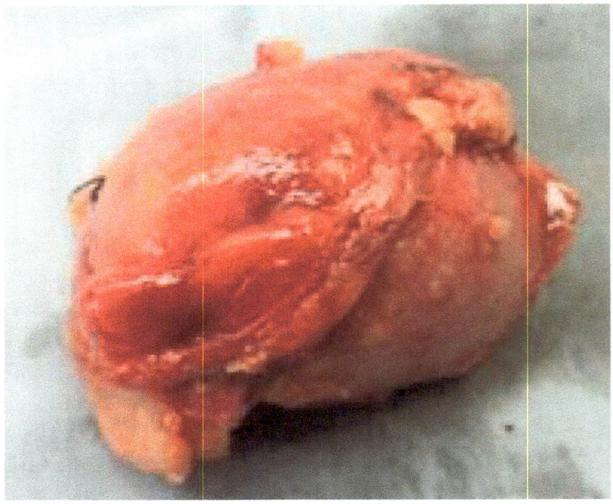

Fig. 30.1 Specimen of an open nephron-sparing surgery-wedge resection: This was proven to be an oncocytoma after histopathological study

status was not reported and the 4-cm size of the tumour is borderline. Reassessment of the pathological specimen is indicated. If the rete testis is not involved, then the patient may safely be considered low risk, and surveillance alone will be sufficient. If the rete testis is positive, he will be intermediate grade and may require chemotherapy. However even then, surveillance may still be justified to avoid the side effects of carboplatin. But the patient should be compliant and agree to regular follow-up with repeated CT and serum markers. The delay of chemotherapy up to the time of recurrence (if this occurs) will not impact negatively on the prognosis.

4. In view of his altered GC, the patient needs surveillance with repeated markers and CT scanning after 3 months. If markers increase or the lesion grows, he will need RPLND. Moreover since he has dyspnoea, a laparoscopic approach should be proposed to minimize peri-operative complications and allow early ambulation.
5. This patient needs consolidation chemotherapy with 2 PEB cycles because of the incomplete resection and the presence of embryonal cell carcinoma in the primary tumour. However, caution must be taken with regard to the cumulative dose of bleomycin. This case illustrates the necessity of having only experienced surgeons performing post-chemotherapeutic RPLND for residual tumours.
6. Surveillance with repeated serum markers and CT scanning.
7. The growing teratoma syndrome is a strong possibility. The patient needs RPLND. Significant adhesions to the aorta, large veins and other surrounding retroperitoneal organs are expected as a result of the chemotherapy and tumour mass. Complications necessitating nephrectomy, colostomy, etc., are not uncommon.
8. This is a stage IIA NSGCT. RPLND seems to be a better option here in view of the unreliable compliance of this patient. It will avoid the toxic effects of chemotherapy.

9. This is a typical low-risk case. He only requires surveillance, i.e. follow-up with repeated tumour markers and abdominal CT. However, two important criteria are missing in the scenario: The size of the tumour and the status of the rete testis.
10. The patient had a robotic iliac lymph nodes excision which showed only residual fibrosis. Then he was kept under observation with repeat tumour markers and CT.
11. There is a 43×68×70 mm interaortico-caval calcified mass. GCTs, whether gonadal or extragonadal, sarcomas or lymphomas, are possible diagnoses. The patient should have U/S of the testes and serum markers for GCTs. He also requires a CT-guided biopsy of the retroperitoneal mass to elicit the diagnosis.
12. Best supportive care. If improvement of his GC is noted which is very unlikely to occur, it may be possible to resume the chemotherapy.

30.6 Adrenal Tumours

1. The CT scan and PET scan show a large left adrenal mass measuring 164 mm (largest diameter) with SUV max 5.7 as well as a 50×60 mm left lung upper lobe tumour with SUV max 9.2. There are two possibilities: either the pulmonary is the primary and the adrenal the secondary or vice versa. Biopsy had to be performed to reach a diagnosis. The patient had a lung biopsy and pleural fluid FNAC performed, but the results were inconclusive. In view of the patient fitness, it was decided to remove in toto the most accessible lesion first, i.e. the intra-abdominal tumour. Therefore, a laparotomy with en bloc removal of the adrenal tumour as well as the left kidney and spleen (Fig. 30.2) was performed. Nephrectomy was performed because of tumour involvement and the splenectomy because of intra-operative bleeding. The histopathology was consistent with a bronchopulmonary adenocarcinoma. The patient was then managed with chemotherapy and planned to undergo a left upper pulmonary lobectomy.

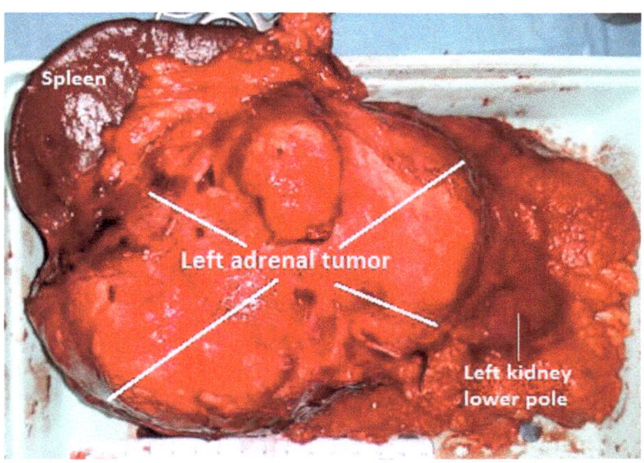

Fig. 30.2 Gross specimen of en bloc resection of a large left adrenal tumour along with spleen and left kidney (same patient of Fig. 29.10) (Courtesy of Dr J-L Hoepffner, Onco-Urologist, Saint-Augustin Clinic and Bergonié Oncological Institute, Bordeaux, France)

Index

S.A. Al-Mamari, S.S. Al-Busaidy (eds.), *Urological Cancer Management*,
DOI 10.1007/978-3-319-16301-7

MIX
Papier aus verantwortungsvollen Quellen
Paper from responsible sources
FSC® C105338

If you have any concerns about our products,
you can contact us on
ProductSafety@springernature.com

In case Publisher is established outside the EU,
the EU authorized representative is:
Springer Nature Customer Service Center GmbH
Europaplatz 3, 69115 Heidelberg, Germany

Printed by Libri Plureos GmbH
in Hamburg, Germany